A Practice of Obstetrics and Gynaecology

A Textbook for General Practice and the MRCOG

Geoffrey Chamberlain RD MD FRCS FRCOG FACOG FFFP
Emeritus Professor, Swansea

Peter Bowen-Simpkins MA MB BChir FRCOG MFFP
Consultant Obstetrician and Gynaecologist, Swansea

Third edition

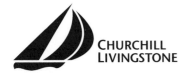

CHURCHILL
LIVINGSTONE

EDINBURGH LONDON NEW YORK PHILADELPHIA ST. LOUIS SYDNEY TORONTO 2000

CHURCHILL LIVINGSTONE
An imprint of Harcourt Publishers Limited

© Harcourt Publishers Limited 2000

 is a registered trademark of Harcourt Publishers Limited

The right of Professor Chamberlain and Mr Peter Bowen-
Simpkins to be identified as authors of this work has been
asserted by them in accordance with the Copyright, Designs
and Patents Act 1988

First Edition 1977
Second Edition 1985   11924
Third Edition 2000

ISBN 0443 051038

British Library Cataloguing in Publication Data
A catalogue record for this book is available from the British
Library

Library of Congress Cataloging in Publication Data
A catalog record for this book is available from the Library of
Congress

Note
Medical knowledge is constantly changing. As new
information becomes available, changes in treatment,
procedures, equipment and the use of drugs become
necessary. The authors and the publishers have, as far as it
is possible, taken care to ensure that the information given in
this text is accurate and up-to-date. However, readers are
strongly advised to confirm that the information, especially
with regard to drug usage, complies with the latest legislation
and standards of practice.

The
publisher's
policy is to use
**paper manufactured
from sustainable forests**

Printed in China

A Practice of Obstetrics and Gynaecology

For Churchill Livingstone

Commissioning Editor: Ellen Green
Project Manager: Ninette Premdas
Project Controller: Nancy Arnott
Designer: Erik Bigland

Contents

Preface

In 1977, Geoffrey Chamberlain and John Dewhurst (later Sir John) prepared their first edition of *A Practice of Obstetrics and Gynaecology*. It was intended for family doctors and those taking the DRCOG examination of the Royal College of Obstetricians and Gynaecologists. This was the recognized diploma for general practitioners interested in obstetrics and gynaecology in the community; many general practitioner committees required the diploma to be held by those who wished to be admitted to the obstetric list of general practice.

The role of the general practitioner changed in obstetrics and gynaecology a decade or so ago. Delivery is no longer the central point but the practitioner is responsible for much antenatal and postnatal care with a few doctors still joining in intrapartum work. In gynaecology, many changes in diagnosis and therapy have led to more being done by the family practitioner for the increasing number of women who seek his or her care in this sensitive area.

The greater recognition of the midwife as an independent practitioner in her own right and the wishes of women are but two of the factors that impact upon all practitioners in the subject. Science, too, has advanced and much that we thought useful is no longer held so, for it cannot stand the glare of evidence based medicine.

The DRCOG has yet again changed in its format while those who seek to enter general practitioner obstetrics and gynaecological practice still take this examination. While this book is not written specifically for them, it is orientated around the contents of the syllabus.

Professor Chamberlain and his co-author, Peter Bowen-Simpkins, of Singleton Hospital, Swansea, have consulted widely with their general practitioner colleagues about the contents of this book and are grateful to those who gave their advice. They present this completely rewritten third edition to a new generation of practitioners as a thoroughly up-to-date account of the subject as it relates to general practitioners and candidates for the DRCOG.

Our grateful thanks go to Ann Howell and Christine Watson for coping with the many drafts and alterations made. We are also happy to acknowledge the helpful work done by Churchill Livingstone in the production. Despite the care taken by others, any problems of clarity are the authors', and we would be happy to hear from readers about any points.

Swansea

G. C.
P. B.-S.

1

The DRCOG examination

In 1974, major changes took place to the Diploma examination of the Royal College of Obstetricians and Gynaecologists (DRCOG). Whereas the examination had previously been entirely summative, with a traditional essay paper followed by a clinical and viva examinations, the new format is now in two parts, consisting of a multiple choice question (MCQ) paper and an Objective Structured Clinical Examination (OSCE).

The changes have been made in an attempt to create a fairer examination that is more reproducible and discriminatory. It is necessary for the candidate to have been appointed to and started a recognized SHO post in obstetrics and gynaecology so that the examination can be taken anytime during or after completion of that job. It is held on a Saturday in a number of centres in the British Isles. Information about the examination can be obtained from the Examination Department at the Royal College in London (27 Sussex Place, London NW1 4RG).

Candidates will be examined within a clinical setting for the OSCE, and are advised to bring a white coat and dress formally.

The examination is aimed at assessing the knowledge of a doctor whose primary intention is to go into general practice. There is therefore less emphasis on practical aspects such as forceps delivery but more on antenatal care, family planning and primary care gynaecology. Emphasis is placed on attitudes towards women and the ability to convey or explain complex medical problems in simple terms readily understood to a layman. For instance, a candidate

Question

Decreased baseline fetal heart rate variation may be observed in all of the following situations *except*

A. fetal hypoxia
B. fetal sleep state
C. fetal gestational age in the immature fetus
D. fetal cardiac anomaly
E. fetal tachycardia greater than 180 bpm

Answers

Beware the negative question "observed in all except", i.e. which are the odd ones out that are *not* associated with loss of baseline variation

	TRUE	FALSE
A. This is the most serious and potentially treatable reason for loss of baseline variation. Lack of oxygen damps down the normal controlling and yet competing mechanisms which determine the heart rate.	●	○
B. The fetus sleeps for 20–30 minutes at a time. While this is more commonly seen in pregnancy, it can still occur in labour particularly early when contractions are less frequent.	●	○
C. By 29 weeks the fetus is showing normal baseline variability and responding to stimuli.	○	●
D. In 5–10% of reduced baseline viability with arythmics, serious abnormalities of the cardiac system are found.	●	○
E. A fetal heart beating at 180 bpm still normally shows variability of 5–10 bpm and a depression below this rate should be considered as suspicious especially since it is happening on top of baseline tachycardia, itself another signal of fetal hypoxia	●	○

Figure 1.1 A question from an MCQ paper.

might be asked to explain to a laywoman the difference between a screening and a diagnostic tests for Down's syndrome.

THE MULTIPLE CHOICE QUESTIONS (MCQ) PAPER

The MCQ paper is designed to test straightforward knowledge and not opinion.

It consists of 60 questions in a true/false format (Fig. 1.1). The paper is not truly a multiple choice examination because negative marking has been abandoned and there no longer exists a 'don't know' option. One mark is awarded for a correct answer and none for a wrong answer. At worst if you guess you will score a nought but stand the chance of gaining an extra mark. It is a good principle to remember that even when you do not really know the answer for sure, your first guess is more likely to be right than wrong. It seldom pays to mull over your answer and change it at the last moment. The majority of candidates will be able to finish the examination with plenty of time to spare. It is better to hand in your script than to go over it again and again, possibly making last minute alterations.

As the examination becomes more reliable statistically, a pass mark has been introduced. Within the questions are a proportion of markers, questions that have been used a number of times before that perform well. In addition there will be questions modified from previous papers depending upon how they performed, and a small proportion of new questions. A fixed proportion of questions that discriminate badly are removed before the final mark is arrived at. These poorly performing questions are then reviewed, and amended or removed from the bank to maintain highly discriminatory questions. In this way, the examination discriminates consistently between candidates of high ability and those of low ability.

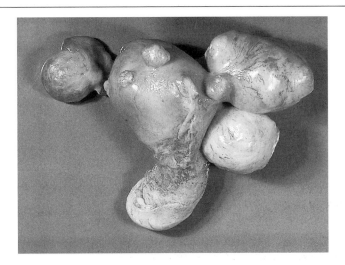

1. What is the diagnosis?

2. Give three gynaecological symptoms that may arise from this condition

3. Give three complications which may arise in pregnancy

Figure 1.2   OSCE problem-solving questions.

THE OBJECTIVE STRUCTURED CLINICAL EXAMINATION (OSCE)

This type of examination will be familiar to most young doctors, as it has been used in undergraduate examinations for some years. It consists of a circuit of stations at each of which the candidate has to perform a task. These stations may be factual, problem solving or interactive. The present arrangement for the DRCOG is that there will be 22 such stations, two being rest stations to allow the candidates a break. Six minutes is allotted for each station, at which a variety of questions will be asked.

A structured marking system has been devised which is specific to that station and allows candidates' papers to be processed effectively with a computer-operated optical marking system. Because of the very limited space, this requires a stylized answer rather than free text. Figure 1.2 is an example of an OSCE question. The advantage of this type of examination is that a variety of skills such as problem solving, clinical examination, communication, attitudes and treatment schedules can be tested objectively. Fairness is assured, because the same questions are asked using the same format for each candidate irrespective of where the examination takes place.

At interactive stations, either a task has to be completed or a communication problem has to be developed with a role player in front of the candidate (Fig. 1.3). The examiner is present, and marks the station with a structured criterion referenced assessment.

The reliability of the answers is audited, and the answers analysed statistically in order

Candidate:		Exam Number:	

			Marks	
		2	**1**	**0**
Introduce themselves	1.			
Sympathetic listener	2.			
Asked questions about the pain:				
Timing	3.			
Events triggering	4.			
Asked about menses:				
Cycle	5.			
LNMP	6.			
Explained working diagnosis	7.			
Offer to visit	8.			
Advised to go to hospital	9.			
Mention of follow-up call next day	10.			
Rapport established	11.			
Overall impression	12.			
Subtotal				

Total (Max 24)	

Figure 1.3 Assessment scheme for an OSCE interactive problem: the candidate is asked to respond in a telephone conversation to the statement 'A 28-year-old woman telephones the duty GP at 10 p.m. saying she has had 2 hours of left lower abdominal pain and vaginal spotting of blood'.

eventually to develop highly discriminatory questions. As in the MCQ paper, marker questions ensure standards are maintained and reduce variability. During the examination, real patients will not be encountered but role players will be present at the clinical stations. The role players are well briefed and rehearsed, and they have become an important integral part of the examination.

The advantage of this type of examination is that a wide variety of topics can be covered and a variety of skills tested. The examination is still evolving, and may change its emphasis in the future. Candidates should therefore write to the Royal College of Obstetricians and Gynaecologists and ask for up-to-date instructions and a syllabus of the examination.

2

Reproductive health

In many parts of the world, women do not have access to information or services that might improve their reproductive health. They are socially and economically worse off than men, and this lower status is critical. The burden of disease in general and in reproductive health in particular is greater compared with that of men (Fig. 2.1). All the pregnancy risks are theirs as well as the majority of sexually transmitted diseases. While formal medicine has a part to play, particularly in the preventative services, more important is the raising of educational standards (measured by literacy rates) and the position of women in society. A major reflection of this lies in the reproductive field.

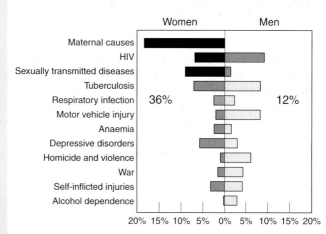

Figure 2.1 Burden of disease among women and men of 15–44 years of age in developing countries (1990). Those in the reproductive field are in black.

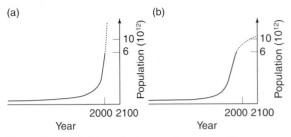

Figure 2.2a World population growth expressed by an exponential curve. **b** The contemporary valid data show the population growth falling off, reflecting the reduced population rates of many countries.

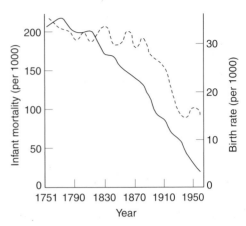

Figure 2.3 Infant mortality (——) and birth rates (– – –) in Sweden for 200 years. As infant mortality goes down, birth rates slow and level up.

WORLD FERTILITY

The population of the world is increasing. Demographers who use various theoretical formulae show by extrapolation that the population numbers could increase infinitely. This is an untenable theorem, and more pragmatic predictions include the change in total fertility rates in developing countries that occurred between 1960 and 1990. It is more likely that the world population will follow the trends in Figure 2.2, and start to level out in the middle of the next century at about 14 000 000 000 000 people.

Most of this increase is in the developing countries where the fertility rates are still high. Whilst there may be space for people, there is not enough food or fuel to cover this increase of numbers. With most people now living longer (life expectancy levels are rising), the first solution would seem to be limitation of family size. National population control policies differ according to faith, religion and the national interests of the ruling governments.

In the last 20 years, world population size has become recognized as an international problem. Slowly and at different rates, governments of the world are moving towards a balance, but care must be taken that Western countries are not seen to dictate to developing ones. Initiatives to help world population control must be perceived to give help to the entire population of any country. For example, some of the Western world's techniques of promoting contraception

in the past were too rigorous for the population at which they were aimed.

National debts to bodies like the World Bank started when the Western world (mainly the USA) was liberal in its loans of money, often with an aim to control the spread of communism. Now that the global political scene has changed, the bankers are calling in their debts, and the developing world is left with massive deficits. The interest to be repaid on these loans each year often exceeds the annual national budget of a developing country.

The association between family size and maternal mortality is not a straightforward one. Whilst the data shown in Figure 2.3 could be interpreted as a decreasing birth rate as a strong cause of decreasing mortality, it could really be that the reduced mortality persuades people to have fewer babies. Most epidemiological data could be considered in this way. Correlations derived are really more due to background such as women's education, cultural practices and basic nutrition.

The status of the women who bear the children is very different in many countries. Male domination still outweighs rational considerations. Female literacy rates relate strongly and inversely to mean family size and mortality rates of both infants and mother.

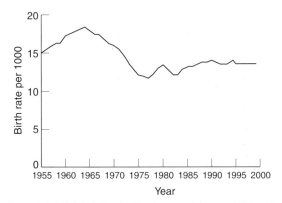

Figure 2.4   Total birth rate (England and Wales, 1955–99).

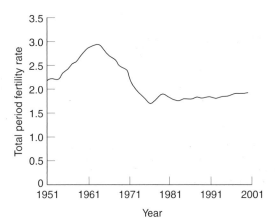

Figure 2.6   Total period fertility rate (England and Wales, 1951–99).

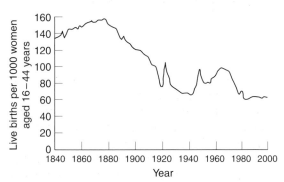

Figure 2.5   General fertility rate (England and Wales, 1840–99).

What is measured

The total birth rate can be expressed as

$$\text{total birth rate} = \frac{\text{births per year} \times 1000}{\text{midyear population}}$$

Thus, provided the number of babies born is well recorded and a census takes place in the area concerned, the total birth rate can be expressed (Fig. 2.4). This is, however, a bad denominator, for it does not relate to the process of birth. No men and few young or older women have babies, and so a more sophisticated index is the general fertility rate (Fig. 2.5):

$$\text{general fertility rate} = \frac{\text{births per year} \times 1000}{\text{women aged 15–44 years}}$$

The completed family size or the total period fertility rate can be calculated after the woman has finished her reproductive life, but this is a retrospective figure (Fig. 2.6). When the completed family size drops below 2, replacement of the population is stopped, and that society has attained zero population growth.

UK FERTILITY

The UK is a microcosm of the world, and the issues already discussed were germane here a century ago; in a lesser way they still apply, but as more limited factors. Improved literacy rates due to better women's education are still rising. The status of women in this country is superficially better, but still there are many areas of social deprivation.

The total birth rate for England and Wales is about 14 per 1000 of the population, with the general fertility rate being about 63 per 1000 women aged from 15 to 45 years. The mean family size is about 2.1 All these levels have been moderately steady for the last decade or so (Figs 2.4–2.6).

There are seasonal variations in the UK birth rate, which is highest from October to March. Whilst this might relate to social behaviour such as the timing of sexual intercourse in the year, it cannot account for the daily variation which occur consistently in the week: the lowest numbers of births on Saturday and Sunday and the highest on weekdays. This does not relate to induction of labour, and applies to spontaneous as well as to total births (Fig. 2.7). Further, the proportion of under 2500 g birth weight babies provides a mirror image of this pattern, such births having a higher rate at the weekend.

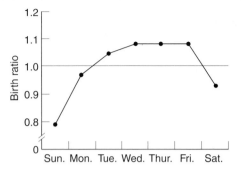

Figure 2.7 Birth ratio by day of the week. If on all days equal numbers were born, then one-seventh would occur on every day with a rate of 1.0 for each day. However, this is not so, and since fewer babies are born at the weekend, the ratios drop to 0.8 and 0.95, respectively, for those days.

RECOMMENDED READING

Miller K, Rosenfield A 1996 Population and women's reproductive health. American Review of Public Health 17: 359–382

Pitrof R 1996 The sorry state of reproductive health in women. Contemporary Review of Obstetrics and Gynaecology 8: 93–97

Obstetrics

3

Care of the woman and her fetus

Pregnancy and childbirth are natural events, but a small number of complications can occur. Women seek medical advice to try to prevent some of these problems, and it has become the norm in the Western world for pregnant women to go for antenatal care. Patterns of practice set down in the past are still followed meticulously today without much thought being given to their application. Some women often expect tests to be performed on their unborn babies, many of which are inapplicable to them. Midwives and doctors use treatments which, when subjected to scrutiny, are found to be less effective in helping mother and baby and would not pass any of the tests of evidence-based medicine, for example the giving of multivitamins during pregnancy or the induction of labour at 41 weeks of gestation to prevent postmaturity.

The objectives of obstetric care differ with different communities and different professionals providing help. Outcomes can be measured from a wide range of the final denominators: maternal mortality, stillbirth and neonatal death are at one end of the spectrum with the woman's own satisfaction and control of delivery at the other. What is good care in one area in the hands of a group of professionals would not be considered the same in another country with other doctors and midwives.

All who look after pregnant women must remember there are features in the background which may modify a woman's psychological response or physiological reaction. Her background culture, family traditions, her status and upbringing in her own childhood all are variants.

Her educational standards and ability to understand have their effect, as well as the sway of current fashions in childbirth. Add to this cluster of maternal variables those of the professionals, which include their medical education, their practice and clinical experience. In addition is the influence of expenses, and the facilities in which professionals have to work and the personnel that are there to assist them. On top of these are two more: commercial pressures from pharmaceutical and equipment companies and that overbearing Sword of Damocles the medicolegal scene – which seems to become sharper and cut wider each year.

This tangled skein needs to be unravelled to measure what is happening during care of the pregnant woman and her baby.

SOCIOECONOMIC BACKGROUND

The socioeconomic status of the woman is usually derived from a classification produced by the Registrar General from either her or her partner's occupation. It reflects the woman's past nutrition and diseases contracted when a child, her education, her parents' attitudes, the work that she and her partner do, their incomes and the position in society which they now hold. It may be a loose classification but a useful one correlating with many measures of outcome (Table 3.1)

Any socioeconomic classification using the woman's occupation may not give enough spread of jobs, and so provides poor differentiation; for this reason, the partner's occupation is used, as men have a wider range of jobs. This is not chauvinism but pragmatism. Other classifications of social status involve the income of the household, style of accommodation or years of full-time education of the mother. The correlation between the social class of the mother if measured by her father's occupation is fairly close to that of her partner.

The variation of social class in the UK is obvious, and is one of the major reasons for the differential in perinatal mortality found between the regions – the lower levels in the affluent

Table 3.1 Social class by Registrar General's classification. The proportion of women of reproductive age in each class and their perinatal mortality are indicated

Class[a]		Percentage of female reproductive population	Perinatal mortality per 1000
I.	Professional and managerial	9	7.2
II.	Supervisory	44	7.5
IIIn.	Skilled workers	12	8.3
IIIm.	Intermediate semiskilled workers	4	8.4
IV.	Unskilled workers	18	11.2
V.	Not classified	12	12.8

[a]Note that temporary occupations such as students and armed forces are not classified. The unemployed are commonly classified by their last occupation, but in many cases this was a schoolchild.

southern counties, gradually worsening with the lower class distribution in the Midlands and the more industrial North and Wales. Unemployment and undernutrition are the major features here, depriving the household of money for the provision of basic foodstuffs, heating and living standards.

A socioeconomic classification gives a useful guide to the point in the spectrum of society in which the woman lives. It is not so helpful when applied to people arriving from overseas, many of whom are employed in lower levels of skills and backgrounds than they would at home. This often happens when one moves from one country to another; the setting-up process often devalues the real socioeconomic class of the family. For example, many immigrants who came from Kenya in 1980 to escape oppression may not yet have reached a level of social class reflecting their original background.

EMOTIONAL FACTORS

Having a baby is obviously an emotional time. It is one of the four major events of a woman's lifetime – being born, finding a partner, deciding whether to have a child, and dying. She cannot remember the first, and is as yet unaware of the last, and so emphasizes her thoughts on the middle two. Childbirth and its antecedents are surrounded by a mass of folklore and tribal thoughts even among the well educated. To disentangle these would be futile, and most good doctors do not try, but will go along with any of those aspects which do not harm the mother or the unborn child.

Often the commonest emotional feature is a fear of an abnormal baby. This occurs in all women, and is not calmed until she sees the child in the cot. A mass of tests has been set up in the last 15 years to detect various types of abnormalities in the baby in pregnancy. An untoward result leads to one of three outcomes:

1. The couple may wish to remove the baby by a termination of pregnancy on the grounds of gross abnormality.

2. The couple may wish to go on with the pregnancy. The knowledge of a forthcoming abnormal child can give them more time to prepare themselves and other members of the family.

3. A small number of abnormalities are susceptible to surgical treatment very soon after birth, and therefore it is wise to have fore-knowledge of these so that the woman can deliver in a place where neonatal surgery is easily available and can be quickly called in to play.

Sometimes, surprisingly, fear of death is secondary to that of an abnormality. These days women do not often consider themselves at risk of death, but we are only two generations away from the time when it was a major risk (Box 3.1).

Box 3.1 Excerpt from the Church of England Prayer Book showing how recently the fear of death and pain of childbirth was a major aspect of a woman's life

Thanksgiving of Women after Childbirth
Commonly Called
The Churching of Women

*O, Almighty God we give Thee humble thanks for that Thou hast safely delivered this woman, Thy servant, **from the great pain and peril of childbirth**. Grant we beseech Thee that she, through Thy help, may both faithfully walk according to Thy will in this life present.*

Although in the UK maternal death is very unusual, women are still fearful of the death of their baby, a miscarriage, a stillbirth or a neonatal death.

The third deeply ingrained fear is of pain. From the Bible where God (Genesis III) laid down 'I will greatly multiply your pain in child-bearing; in pain you shall bring forth children' to *Gone With the Wind*, the image of childbirth was that it will be painful, with a knotted towel tied to the end of the bed to pull on as the only analgesic. We cannot measure pain, only its effects, and so cannot know how much pain a woman is having; only her response to what she is perceiving. Since the outcome of labour is nearly always a happy one, the retrospective perception of pain is less pronounced than it is with the sort of pain associated with an unhappy outcome such as a broken bone. Undoubtedly, fear of pain in labour is in the background of every pregnant woman, and anything the attendants can do to relieve this will be helpful by open discussion, providing suitable analgesics and showing how the woman can cope with her own skills of relaxation and control.

The result of most pregnancies and labours is a normal baby, who makes the woman and her partner happy. Happiness is the major emotion surrounding pregnancy, but the doctor must always remember that not all women come from a balanced household. In some cases the pregnant woman may be unsupported, from a difficult background or dreading the arrival of another child. These women need extra emotional support.

ETHNIC BACKGROUND

The Black and other ethnic minorities in this country make up about 10% of the women having babies, and the distribution is patchy. For example, large numbers from Pakistan and Bangladesh live in the West Midlands while West London has its Islamic population and South London its Afro-Caribbean group. The practitioner's experience of the ethnic groups will depend on where the practice is; large parts of Scotland and Wales will seldom see a coloured mother, but at St George's Hospital in South London almost 40% of the population attending the antenatal clinics are from ethnic minorities. The obstetrical problems which such groups bring range from altered genetics and inbuilt diseases, e.g. the haemoglobinopathies, to the varied faiths and cultures in the background of these women, often leading to problems such as male doctors attending women in labour. Neither of these types of problems can be removed, and action must be taken to circumvent their worst effects, preferably in calm antenatal discussion involving the members of the ethnic community, so making plans of action before problems arise.

ETHICAL CONSIDERATIONS

Ethics is a part of philosophy, and much of today's philosophical contribution in medical and obstetrical ethics is not expert enough. It is word play described as 'A departmental game in which medical issues are battered like a shuttlecock from side to side' (Gordon Dunstan at an RCOG Conference in 1994).

Ethics are mixed up with the personal ideas of both parties involved, on the one hand involving the relationship of doctors with their patients and at the other extreme the professionals with their employing authorities. On top of this is the need for medical research. Amongst this moral minefield, the doctor is an agent with individual freedom who is responsible for the carrying out of medical procedures. It is only by discussion with other doctors, with women who are having and have had babies, with other professionals and ethical philosophers that one can construct a series of templates covering the interaction of professionals with the women, women's expectations, and medical practice. It is a most difficult area, and one in which one's own conscience and ideas intrude quite rightly to the forefront, but they should not necessarily be there alone. Every now and again some urgent ethical matter hits the headlines, such as the performance of caesarean section against the woman's wishes in order to save the fetus. These events should not affect the everyday running of general practice but it needs careful and continuing surveillance.

COMMUNICATION

Communication is about passing information two ways, from the professional to the woman and her partner, about what they may expect in pregnancy and labour, and from the woman to the professionals about her requests for consideration and her questions. Communication may be:

Indirect   Books, newspapers and magazine articles
          Broadcasting
          Specially prepared leaflets for the antenatal clinic
Direct   Antenatal instruction classes (parentcraft)
          Personally in the surgery and at the couch side

Communication is improved as one descends this list.

Communication in prepregnancy

Prepregnancy instruction is often given in articles, journals, and in talks at schools and clubs, but is best when done individually with the couple concerned. They know the problems that worry them, and between their questions the professional can weave the rest of the prepregnancy advice that is needed. Time must be allowed for the interview, for the woman will often start with one query, but she and her partner will bring in other subjects during the course of the consultation.

Antenatal communication

Since it is likely that the couple may see the professional teams several times during their antenatal visits, the direct approach can be spaced through the visits. Booklets about pregnancy abound, but practitioners should ensure that the reading they recommend for women describes practices that are available locally and does not spend too much time on those which are not available. Women now want to know more, and informed choice is important. A series of leaflets is available from the Midwives Information and Resource Service (MIRS), giving both sides of most arguments, and are held to be impartial. More details may be obtained from the MIRS itself (telephone: 01179 251791).

Antenatal instruction classes are run at most maternity units, by the midwives and physiotherapists who will usually be in attendance during pregnancy and labour. Partners of the women are encouraged to attend, and most units hold some classes in early evenings to allow this. They usually include a tour of the hospital delivery suite and postnatal wards.

This is important, for it is the first time some women have ever seen inside a hospital. Many of their fears may be diminished by this brief visit, knowing they are going to be out of the hospital in a short time.

Direct communication is best when the woman knows she is going to be looked after by a small team of midwives and doctors. Rapport can be built up during the antenatal visits; usually professionals find the questions which had not been asked in earlier consultations start pouring in during the last trimester.

Some find a birth plan to be helpful. In this the woman lists all the things she wants and does not want during labour. The plan catalyses discussion, and should always be considered seriously by midwives and doctors preferably in the antenatal clinic.

Communication in labour

Ninety-eight per cent of women have their babies in a hospital or general practitioner unit where they go when labour begins. Most are accompanied by their partner, who knows the woman far better than do the professionals, and it is very helpful to have him there for communication during labour. The woman has usually been to antenatal clinic where she was able to meet her attendants, and to the antenatal classes where she learnt something of what is to happen. Members of the team who will look after the woman during labour should ensure that she knows who they are, and preferably their grading in the hierarchy. A pleasant,

informal nature is usually best, but professionals must judge this for some women prefer to be slightly distant from their advisors. As an example, it must not be assumed that all women like to be addressed by their first name. This should be asked about, and it is wise to write down the answer on the record so that others need not ask the same question later.

If the contraction rate allows, another quick tour around the relevant parts of the delivery suite on her arrival is helpful to the woman so that she can visualize important places such as the lavatory and the bathroom as well as her birthroom. By this time the professionals should know what position the mother to be wants to take up in labour and her pain relief wishes. If she has made one, it is worth going through the birth plan again. During the second stage of labour, communication becomes more intense and briefer. Some women like having very simple instructions given, such as 'Hold your breath, close your mouth and push', others consider these to be too regimented, and the good midwife or doctor will have learnt which style a woman prefers, and will act accordingly.

When the baby is delivered, remember that the woman and her child are centre stage and all the attendants are peripheral to this. It is the woman's baby, so see that all attention is on her and her child even if the professional is worried about delivering the placenta. Assuming all has gone normally, as it nearly always does, see that the woman has the child as soon as possible after delivery, usually immediately after separation of the placenta and when the child has started to breathe. The baby should be wrapped up in a warm sheet unless the mother wishes skin-to-skin contact, when they should both be covered by a warmed blanket.

Communication in the puerperium

Women after birth are very vulnerable. They like to talk about their babies to knowledgeable professionals, and will ask many questions; midwives in the hospital must have time to talk with the woman. In particular, enquiries about breast feeding need answering along a consistent and mutually agreed line from all midwives in any given ward so that the mother is not confused by different midwives' opinions.

Women stay in hospital for shorter times these days, so it is important that communication takes place between the hospital professionals, the community midwives and the general practitioner. An ideal situation is when the community midwife comes into the hospital for delivery, for she then carries on looking after the woman in her home up to the 10th day. She tells the general practitioner the next convenient day so that visits can be arranged accordingly. It is important that the hospital lets the practitioner know as soon as practical by a short note, which may be a proforma predesigned by the obstetric unit in consultation with general practitioners and the maternity liaison committee. If anything seriously untoward happened (death or congenital abnormality), it is essential that the general practitioner is telephoned and that one of the hospital team talks directly to the general practitioner before the woman goes home.

Gradually care will pass from the midwife to the health visitor, but the general practitioner stays as the constant. He should ensure that the woman attends for a postnatal visit at about 6 weeks, and then starts to make arrangements for the programme of immunization for the baby.

Communication in the case of death

Until recently, many professionals were poor at coping with a stillbirth or intrauterine death. They did not like it and tried to turn aside. The woman was often put into a side room by herself to keep her away from the other babies.

It is essential that when a death or an abnormality has occurred midwives and doctors talk easily to the couple. They might not be able to give a full explanation of events, but at least

they can keep communication going so that the couple can ask and vent their feelings. Most grief has a phase of anger in it, when the couple wonder whether any other plans of management might have resulted in a happier outcome. The professionals must be ready for this and be able to cope with it. The couple can be greatly helped by sympathetic human responses from the doctors and midwives in the first hours after the realization of death or abnormality.

It is usual in the UK to ask for an autopsy of any baby who is stillborn or had a neonatal death. This must be done with tact and skill, sometimes pointing out that it is helpful to learn more, so that the couple know about the possible problems on the next occasion if there is to be one. The idea of helping scientific knowledge or society in general is often not one that appeals to couples at this acute stage, although they would accept it in a calmer moment. Even those who belong to faiths that do not approve of an autopsy should still be asked for permission, and given a chance to permit this investigation. If not, a discussion should be made about limited investigations such as total-body radiography or computerized tomography for abnormalities, and obtaining cardiac blood, if fresh, for chromosome and viral studies, and the taking of bacterial swabs.

A properly composed Polaroid photograph should always be taken of the infant who has died. This should not be a clinical 'mug shot' but one posed with suitable clothing. It is wise always to take two copies of this. Even though the mother may not want them at the time, they should be kept in the notes as it is quite likely that she would like to see a photograph later on. A footprint or hand print has also been found to be helpful to the parents as it gives some personality to the baby they lost, and this too should be kept as part of the records.

RECOMMENDED READING

Audit Commission 1998 First class delivery. Audit Commission, London
Bewley S, Ward R (eds) 1994 Ethics in obstetrics and gynaecology. RCOG Press, London
Stillbirth and Neonatal Death Society 1993 Death before birth. Stillbirth and Neonatal Death Society, London

4

Prepregnancy care

Prepregnancy care includes the mental and physical preparation of a couple for child bearing, carried out before pregnancy starts. It has components both of education and of investigations which should lead to a healthier baby, a happier mother and a safer birth.

Antenatal care came at the turn of the twentieth century; a part of it stresses the need for early visits, but the first of these is rarely before 12 weeks of gestation. The reasons given for seeking early antenatal visits are:

1. To get a baseline of certain maternal parameters such as blood pressure and weight, so that later changes can be set in context
2. To prevent exposure to known teratogens
3. To introduce the couple into the antenatal system early.

All these could have been better dealt with in prepregnancy, for usually even the first antenatal visit is too late, e.g. teratogens affecting fetal development act mostly between 3 and 7 weeks postconception, i.e. 5–9 weeks after the last normal menstrual period. In addition, dealing with a problem, even at an early first antenatal visit, allows the couple only two options: either the pregnancy may continue or it does not. Dealing with the same problems in the prepregnancy time allows the couple another option, the postponement of pregnancy until the problem has been electively dealt with.

Prepregnancy care can be at several levels. General education at school before pregnancy as a part of biology teaching could be very important, but usually it is at first with the general practitioner at a consultation. Some doctors keep special sessions for prepregnancy counselling, recognizing the extended time some couples need. Specific questions will start the interview, but it is important to allow the discussion to widen, allowing time for this.

FAMILY HISTORY

Some conditions recur in families, and this background should be sought. Whilst the presence of diabetes and hypertension in the older members of the family may not be closely associated with problems in the consulting couple, first-degree relations with the same conditions in youth can increase the risk of affect to the mother or her unborn child. Epilepsy and multiple pregnancies, particularly on the mother's side, may be relevant.

Box 4.1 Some inherited conditions which can be detected before pregnancy

---

- Sickle cell disease
- Thalassaemia
- Haemophilia
- Cystic fibrosis
- Huntington's chorea
- Muscular dystrophy
- Tay–Sachs disease
- Fragile X syndrome

Some diseases are inherited (Box 4.1), and it may be wise to obtain specific genetic counselling on these. Risk can then be determined, and advice given whether the fetus can be tested in early pregnancy by chorionic villus biopsy or amniocentesis.

MEDICAL HISTORY

Most women in the pregnancy age group are perfectly fit, but a few will have chronic diseases that will continue. It is important in the prepregnancy interview to assess four things:

1. How may the pregnancy affect the pre-existing disease?

2. How may the pre-existing disease affect the pregnancy?
3. How may any medication taken for the disease affect pregnancy?
4. How may pregnancy affect the pharmacokinetics of any continuing drugs taken?

If the answers to these questions are not known, one should consult further, perhaps at a hospital prepregnancy service, if available. The drug information service of the hospital pharmacy may be of considerable help.

Because pregnancy changes the endocrine and physiological condition in some diseases, this needs explaining beforehand, for it may mean modifying lifestyle and work pattern. Some of these diseases occurring in the antenatal population are shown in Box 4.2.

Box 4.2 Diseases which may already be present in young women seeking prepregnancy advice

---

- Diabetes
- Epilepsy
- Asthma
- Chronic rheumatic heart disease
- Congenital heart disease
- Blood dyscrasias
- Crohn's disease
- Ulcerative colitis

PAST PREGNANCIES

The patterns of reproduction in the past sometimes give clues about what is going to happen next time; it should be remembered, however, that many problems do not recur, and the woman should be told this. It is probable that having had a previous termination of pregnancy is quite irrelevant to the outcome of the future pregnancy, provided the procedure was without complications. Enquiries should be made specifically about the conditions mentioned in Box 4.3.

WORK PATTERNS

The majority of women in the reproductive age group are working at home or in paid work, full

Box 4.3   Obstetrical conditions that may have an effect in a subsequent pregnancy

- Miscarriage
- Pregnancy-induced hypertension
- Antepartum haemorrhage
- Preterm labour
- Prolonged labour
- Operative delivery
- Postpartum haemorrhage
- Small for gestational age baby

or part time; some are worried by this. Very few of the products used in industry will have an effect on the pregnancy for most women still work in neutral environments where there is no fetotoxic or teratogenic exposure. However, very heavy, boring or repetitive tiring work may have an effect, and this should be discussed. The hazards which might lead to problems in pregnancy are outlined in Table 4.1.

Many couples enter marriage benefiting from two incomes and expect that to continue. Pregnancy will intrude upon this financial pattern. Women in most jobs outside the home can be assured that they can go on working into late pregnancy with complete safety to themselves and their babies. Further, although not generous

by the standards of some other European countries, there are maternity grants and benefits to help the finances. These change frequently as political targets alter, and the latest Department of Social Security literature should be consulted. It is now refreshingly clearly written.

MATERNAL AGE

The majority of babies are born to women aged 20–35 years. Some 9% are older than this, and they are concerned about it, but most who become pregnant have a perfectly normal time, producing healthy babies. Many women are still concerned by half-heard rumours of increasing risks of chromosomal abnormalities, and extrapolate this to other problems (Fig. 4.1). Hence they often consult about this matter.

With greater age, certain medical problems have a slightly increased incidence, e.g. hypertension and diabetes. Further, pregnancy puts an increased stress on the body's ligaments and muscles; weaknesses such as a bad back will have had more time to appear in the older mother. The effect on work might be more than in younger women, and this will need compensating for with adjustments of work programmes. The risk of certain chromosomal abnormalities does increase with age, and should be approached with frankness (Fig. 4.1). An open discussion should take place about the

Table 4.1   Some environmental hazards to which a pregnant woman may be exposed at the workplace

Chemical hazards	Physical hazards	Biological hazards
Disinfecting agents, e.g. ethylene oxide	Radiation, e.g. X rays	Contact with high-risk groups, e.g. schoolchildren and rubella cases
Solvents, e.g. carbon tetrachloride	Vibration	Waterborne infection
Herbicides	Heat and humidity	Animal contacts, e.g. lambing
Insecticides	Dust	Infections in food preparation, e.g. listeriosis
Metals, e.g. lead and mercury	Repetitive lifting of heavy loads	Health workers in contact with infections

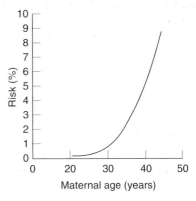

Figure 4.1   Proportions of babies with Down's syndrome by maternal age. While the risk increases after 35 years of age (and steeply after 40 years), the proportion of women having babies diminishes.

testing for congenital abnormalities, ensuring that the woman understands which abnormalities may be detected by various types of test, e.g. chorionic villus sampling assesses chromosomal problems only, whilst ultrasound is better for structural malformations, most of which are not age affected.

LIFE-STYLE

As well as work patterns, other activities may need some assessment. Some women take moderately heavy exercise in their sporting and leisure activities, and this should be assessed. Most activities are unaffected, but in competitive and contact sports the pregnant woman may give a disappointing performance as she may not be at her best. There are reports of women winning Olympic medals whilst pregnant, but these do not always record how pregnant the women were in relation to their athletic activity – some conceptions may have actually started in the Olympic Village. Some specific sports are contraindicated in pregnancy, e.g. water skiing (danger of water douche) and skiing at over 2500 m (diminished oxygen).

The problem of obesity is usually one of over-eating and eating the wrong foods. At a prepregnancy clinic the doctor can try to influence events, and sometimes the forthcoming pregnancy is stimulus enough to change the woman's eating style. Equally those who eat too little may have a problem in pregnancy and produce babies with resultant low birth weight.

About 30% of women in the pregnancy age group smoke cigarettes. In the UK most of these are fairly light smokers, with only 5% of them consuming more than 20 cigarettes a day. Without doubt smoking does affect the fetus, not just in reduced growth, but also childhood impaired development and educational standards. It is probably wise for a woman to reduce her smoking in pregnancy, a subject which can be well explored in the prepregnancy period. There is increasing evidence that passive cigarette smoking may affect the fetus, and so the partner should also be considered in the consultation. Recently, an association between the partner's smoking habit and the incidence of childhood malignancies has been mooted.

Alcohol is a tissue poison, but the doctor must weigh up the woman's satisfaction and happiness from her alcohol consumption against the need to impose bars on her behaviour. Most would probably consider that a little alcohol (e.g. one glass of wine a day in a woman who is used to drinking) would probably produce no harm, but certainly binge drinking should be strongly advised against. It takes time to alter a habit, and this is where prepregnancy care allows that time to occur.

The taking of addictive drugs affects the fetus. Those using narcotics may not come for prepregnancy care, and may be fearful or distrustful of the medical profession. If such a woman is seen, then all efforts should be made together with the drug agencies, to get her off the addictive drugs before pregnancy.

FOLATE

It has been shown that giving additional folate before conception to women who have had a previous baby with a neural tube defect (e.g. spina bifida) can reduce the risk of such defects in another pregnancy. From this was extrapolated the idea, which is now evidence based, that all women can reduce the risk of central nervous system abnormality by increased folate. This can be taken in natural diet, e.g. dark-green vegetables and breakfast cereals, but it is probably easier for many to take an extra tablet once a day for the few months before pregnancy. It should be stressed that the raised levels of folate are needed when the central nervous system is being formed at 21–28 days of embryonic life (1–2 weeks after the missed period). Since conception is often an unplanned occurrence, it is wise to have started folate taking before pregnancy in order to produce effective tissue levels where needed. Those who have had a previous neural tube defect ought to have a higher dose (e.g. 5 mg daily for 2 months before and 3 months into pregnancy), but those who have had no previous problems should have 500 µg of folate daily.

ADVICE

It should be remembered that all the factors considered are in one of two groups: those factors which cannot be changed and those which can. Amongst the former are the built-in biological and social factors and the age of the mother. These have been laid down well before the woman comes for prepregnancy consultation, and all the doctor can do is to give her the odds of the various problems related to these factors and to inform the couple of what they are facing. But, in addition, there are the many factors which can be altered. To give some idea of the types of problems seen in prepregnancy consultation, the problems encountered during 1 year at a typical hospital prepregnancy clinic are listed in Table 4.2.

Prepregnancy care can be provided by all who are in contact with young people – teachers, parents, midwives, health visitors and doctors. All have a part to play, but the medical pro-fession must be properly represented in such care, and take its correct place looking after the health and mental welfare of future mothers and fathers to improve the results of their pregnancies and the health of their children. In future, prepregnancy care could reduce perinatal mortality and morbidity in the same way that antenatal care has.

Table 4.2   A breakdown of the problems encountered during 1 year at a hospital prepregnancy clinic

Problem	Percentage of consultations
Previous maternal problems	
Problems in previous pregnancy	7
Problems in previous labour	14
Current medical problems	17
Future management of pregnancy	7
Previous fetal problems	
Previous fetal or neonatal death	39
Born with abnormalities	6
Recurrent miscarriage	10

RECOMMENDED READING

Chamberlain G 1995 Prepregnancy care. In: Chamberlain G (ed) Turnbull's obstetrics. Churchill Livingstone, Edinburgh

Paul M 1992 Occupational and environmental health hazards. Williams and Wilkins, Baltimore

5

Antenatal care

Antenatal or prenatal care has evolved this century, probably starting in Edinburgh as an extension backwards from the infant welfare clinics in a wish to prevent problems in pregnancy. From these clinical beginnings evolved a series of examinations followed by investigations, many introduced without preliminary assessment and often just added to previous care without any audit of their value. Latterly, obstetricians and midwives have tried to evaluate them, often with randomized controlled trials. Multiphasic screening with prenatal diagnosis of fetal problems has been added, so expanding the content of antenatal care in the last 30 years.

The aims of antenatal care are summarized in Box 5.1.

Box 5.1 The aims of antenatal care

---

1. To care for the whole antenatal population, dealing with:
   a. Maternal symptomatic problems, e.g. antepartum haemorrhage
   b. Fetal symptomatic problems, e.g. reduced fetal movements
2. To screen the whole pregnant population to detect subgroups at higher risk for the complications of pregnancy
3. To screen for and prevent fetal abnormalities
4. To provide special management for high-risk pregnancies, e.g. those complicated by pre-eclampsia
5. To prepare the couple for childbirth
6. To prepare the couple for child rearing

These aims may be redesignated functionally as:

- *Preventative care.* The preventive nature of antenatal care depends upon doctors and midwives knowing what might happen and then using appropriate therapy, e.g. trying to prevent open central nervous system abnormalities by giving supplementary folate. Such antenatal systems aim to prevent or detect problems early. The former is by advising courses of action to reduce the risk of unwanted events; the latter by providing extra surveillance to detect the early stages of some conditions.

- *Screening.* To detect specific problems, the total population, or a special subset of those at risk, is tested when no symptoms occur, e.g. the taking of blood pressure of all women at all antenatal clinics to detect pregnancy-induced hypertension early or the use of biochemical or biophysical tests to diagnose Down's syndrome in the fetus in early pregnancy.

- *Diagnosis.* Usually, the earlier a diagnosis in any pathological process is made the more likely it is that relevant treatment will be effective. For example, the diagnosis in early pregnancy of a fetal abnormality to enable the couple to come to terms with this. It does not necessarily indicate termination of pregnancy, but allows the woman more time to prepare herself, her partner and other children in the family for the coming of a child with an abnormality.

- *Education.* All pregnant women want to do well by their unborn child, hence they are very receptive to education at this stage. Professionals can provide much material to the willing recipients at formal and informal contacts (see 'Communication' in Ch. 3). No antenatal visit should be without its educational complement.

THE PATTERNS OF ANTENATAL CARE

Figure 5.1 shows the patterns of antenatal care laid down in the 1920s; they have hardly altered since then. Obstetricians and midwives should remember that these original patterns were planned by Dr Janet Campbell for the poor, grande multiparous and malnutritioned women

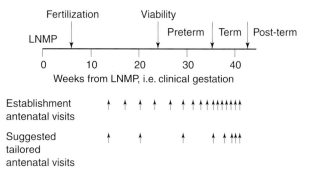

Figure 5.1 Conventional and suggested appropriate antenatal visit intervals (LNMP, last normal menstrual period).

of the East End of London. It does not mean that every middle class normal woman in the year 2000 needs this same intensive pattern, and new plans of appropriate care may be tried. However, when patterns of reduced clinic visits are introduced they can cause concern. Women have been brought up to believe that the old pattern is right, and when it is reduced there may be a feeling of undercare.

Antenatal care may be carried out in the home, in community-run clinics isolated from the general practitioners' surgery, in the general practice premises itself, or in the hospital. There has been a gradual devolution from the last to the middle two of these sites. Normal women do not need to wait the longer times that seem to be the case at many hospital clinics. In addition, at the general practice or community clinic, they can more likely get to know the midwife or small team which is going to care for them in labour.

Midwives are doing more antenatal care now, and interested general practitioners run their own clinics. Women get much satisfaction seeing somebody who has looked after them through their childhood and is going to go on looking after them and their future family. The hospital antenatal clinic should be kept for women with problems. Women are referred there by midwives and general practitioners, or are those known to have past obstetrical or medical problems and have planned for hospital care from the beginning.

The antenatal clinic has great teaching potential: medical students and student midwives should be appropriately involved as often as women permit and there is time for the senior person to do the teaching. It is undoubtedly the best place to learn about abdominal palpation and to discuss the numerous problems of normal pregnancy as well as the pathological events of abnormal pregnancies.

PLACE OF BOOKING FOR DELIVERY

At the very first visit, discussion should take place on this point. The majority of women want to deliver in hospital, perceiving it to be the safer place. A small number wish for a home-birth, and, when facilities are available, others wish for delivery in general practitioner units. The proportions are roughly 94:2:4 per 100 women at the moment.

If a woman wishes for a *hospital delivery*, then plans should be made in accordance with local custom. Some hospital antenatal clinics offer to see women for a booking visit early in pregnancy which is often combined with ultrasound scans and other tests. From then on, care is in the community until late pregnancy. Other hospitals have other patterns, and the referring doctor and midwife should know of these plans, which should have been discussed and agreed by all professionals beforehand.

General practitioner units may be on the main hospital site in a separate ward or building from the consultant beds.

If this is so, the booking facilities should be well known to the professionals. The numbers of isolated general practitioner units are reducing. It is usual to screen the women who wish to book there to reduce the number of higher-risk births taking place in the outlying unit. Assuming a woman falls into the category suitable, then she should be booked if beds are available.

The number of *home deliveries* are slightly increasing, having risen from 1% of all UK births in 1989 to 2% in 1995 (Fig. 5.2). Women who wish for a planned home delivery in the UK have the right to book one, and it is for the supervisor of midwives to ensure arrangements are made for midwife cover. The mother-to-be does not have the right to book her doctor for a home delivery, for all general practitioners do not cover domiciliary delivery, but usually in a given area one general practitioner is prepared to care for such women. Potential mothers are also screened according to laid-down criteria. A

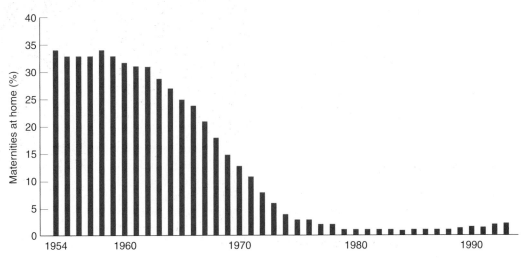

Figure 5.2   Percentage of maternities at home (England and Wales, 1954–94). (From the Office of Population Censuses and Surveys.)

booked home delivery usually has a safe outcome for mother and baby provided the criteria of booking are upheld and full care is provided by community midwives and the general practitioner obstetrician. Some 16% of women might expect to transfer to hospital care in late pregnancy or in labour. There will be a modest increase in homebirth requirements in the next decade, and practitioners should make arrangements accordingly, for the law permits women to choose this.

LEAD PROFESSIONALS

Commonly a woman goes to her general practitioner when she first thinks she is pregnant. She can now choose her lead professional, who is usually her general practitioner or a midwife. The lead professionals are the pivot of care. They are there to ensure the woman has the necessary consultations, tests and examinations at the right time, and should be available to give the woman advice during pregnancy and labour. They may well take part in her delivery at whichever site she books. They have the responsibility of advising the woman in an independent unbiased way.

If a booking is made for home or general practitioner unit delivery, antenatal care will continue in the unit or hospital setting. If she is going to be delivered in hospital, the mother-to-be will go there for some early antenatal care and be seen by the unit team of doctors and midwives. If there is a previous obstetrical problem or a medical disease warranting it, she may attend for antenatal care at the hospital throughout. These decisions are usually made at the booking visit.

DIAGNOSIS OF PREGNANCY

Most women suspect they are pregnant because their periods stop. If they have had a child before, they may have a sensation of being pregnant, which is very real in the experienced woman – the breasts tingle, pelvic organs feel heavy and urinary frequency increases. The

Table 5.1 Symptoms and signs of early pregnancy

Symptoms	Signs
Amenorrhea	Breast changes
Nausea and vomiting	Montgomery's tubercles
Breast enlargement and tingling	Skin veins
Increased urinary frequency	Areola – increased size and darker coloration
	Uterus
	Early – soft and cystic
	Later – enlarges

symptoms and signs of early pregnancy are summarized in Table 5.1.

In most cases when the doctor and the woman are both convinced of the diagnosis, there is no need for further investigation, but pregnancy tests are done very frequently now, and most practitioners' surgeries have a simple, inexpensive, test kit to check for the β subunit of human chorionic gonadotrophin (hCG) (Fig. 5.3). This is most likely to be an enzyme-linked immunosorbent assay (ELISA) test which detects hCG at very low concentrations and so gives a positive result much earlier than the older tests; a positive result is at the time of the missed period, i.e. 10–12 days postconception. The sensitivity is due to the use of two antibodies,

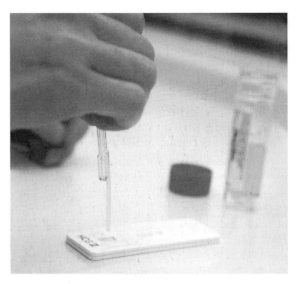

Figure 5.3 Checking a woman's urine with a simple commercial colorimetric method.

one being to both the α and β unit hCG and the other to the β unit only.

BOOKING VISIT

The first antenatal visit may be in the woman's home by the community midwife, in the practice surgery done by the general practitioner or the midwife attached to the practice, or it may be at the institution where the woman is going to deliver, performed by the hospital midwife or doctor.

Who does it and wherever it is done, the doctor or midwife should use a locally agreed antenatal proforma which is completed for every woman at the booking visit. In most health authorities, pregnant women carry their own antenatal notes, which are therefore available at all sites of antenatal care, and at any time if the woman needs emergency help. This practice has two other advantages: it leads to a lower incidence of lost notes and, since the woman can read her own records, it often encourages more questions about herself and her unborn child.

History

The booking visit commonly starts with taking a full history. This should be done in a schematic fashion; and the order is not so important as doing the same practice every time to make the records uniform.

This pregnancy

The events of this pregnancy are detailed.

The last menstrual period is noted, checking that this was a period at the expected time and also the regularity of the cycle. Any information about oral contraception taken within 2 months of the period or irregular bleeding after the last period is noted. With all these data, the speculative date of delivery can be calculated (Box 5.2). If any of these questions have doubtful answers, it is wiser not to give a precise date to the woman but instead to offer a zone of a few weeks, recommending her to await an ultrasound examination, which will add to the

---

> **Box 5.2** Dating the pregnancy
>
> 1. Determine the first day of last normal menstrual period:
>   2 December 1998
> 2. Add 9 months (actually take away 3 months and add a year):
>   2 September 1999
> 3. Add 7 days:
>   9 September 1999
>   This is the probable expected date of delivery
>
> **Do not use this method if:**
> - The cycle is not regular inside 24–35 days
> - The date of the last menstrual period is uncertain
> - The woman has used oral contraception within 2 months

---

precision of that dating. To give a precise date from imperfect information may lead to disappointment later in pregnancy.

If there is any doubt about the presence of pregnancy, abdominal ultrasound can be used to detect an amniotic sac at about 6 weeks of gestation, fetal heart movements at 7 weeks and fetal parts at 8 weeks (Figs 5.4 and 5.5). The image is greatly enhanced by using a vaginal probe, and can make these diagnoses possible a week earlier.

Medical history

Most women in the pregnancy age group are fit. The general practitioner will know of any chronic illnesses, but if the woman is new to the practice, enquiries should be made (see Ch. 4, 'Prepregnancy care').

Family history

The relevance of illness in first-degree relations (parents and siblings) is assessed (see Ch. 4). Multiple pregnancies should be asked about. There is an increased risk of dizygotic nonidentical twins if the woman's mother or one of her sisters has produced such babies, for the propensity of producing more than one oocyte during a cycle can be inherited on the female side. Obviously such occurrences on the husband's side are not relevant. However, the ability of

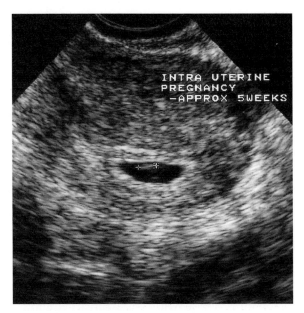

Figure 5.4 Ultrasound scan of uterus at 5 weeks of gestation showing sac.

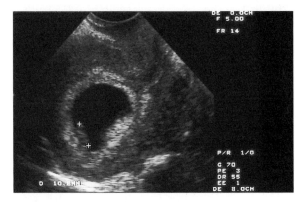

Figure 5.5 Ultrasound scan of uterus at 7 weeks of gestation showing fetal parts.

the fertilized egg to divide into two cell clusters (monozygotic twins) can be inherited from either side; this is the rarer form in humans.

Previous obstetrical history

All previous pregnancies should be listed in chronological order. Details of miscarriages should include the stage of gestation, any complications and any treatments given. Uncomplicated therapeutic abortions usually have no

> **Box 5.3** Previous obstetrical history
>
> Check all previous deliveries for:
>
> - Dates
> - Outcome (stillbirth, live born, neonatal death)
> - First names of living children (useful for future reference)
> - Birth weight and gestational stage
> - Any problems in the pregnancy
> - Place of delivery
> - Method of delivery
> - Problems with labour
> - Problems with puerperium
> - Problems with the newborn baby
> - How each child is now
>
> If there is any hint of variation from normality, previous records should be obtained from where the woman delivered previously.

effect on later pregnancies, but any related morbidity should be checked. Previous deliveries should be enquired after as detailed in Box 5.3.

Social history

It is important to know the woman's background so that she can be helped to have a suitable environment. This is obtained by a series of questions about:

- The woman's occupation
- The partner's occupation
- The age of completion of full-time education
- Details of living accommodation (owned, or rented accommodation)
- Her religion.

Some of these factors are used, but not all, in assessing the woman's socioeconomic class, for much that happens in her obstetrical career relates to that (see Ch. 4). Facilities at home and the assistance the woman will have after delivery in the home is often best discussed at this point if only to prompt the woman into thinking of these things and starting to seek help from her relatives and friends.

Tobacco, alcohol and drug use

Tobacco smoking affects the child either from the mother's own cigarettes or secondarily from her partner's smoking; this should be enquired after, and advice given about stopping or reducing the habit. Many clinics for smokers exist now to which the woman or her partner may be referred.

Alcohol also should be considered, and advice given in Chapter 4 followed.

The use of *other drugs* is much less likely, but direct questioning often brings results. If the woman is undergoing treatment for drug addiction, care of the patient should be carried out in conjunction with the doctor responsible for her addiction management. Use of opiates may lead to severe withdrawal problems for the newborn.

Examination

At the booking visit, many perform a general examination of the woman, checking for anaemia, cardiovascular and respiratory system problems, and for oedema or veins in the legs. The *breasts* may be examined, particularly if the woman is interested in subsequent breast feeding. The nipples can be checked at this time: if they are inverted, often a woman can evert them with her fingers during pregnancy to prepare them for breast feeding the child. The use of breast shields is no longer thought to be helpful.

The *height and weight* of the woman at her first booking visit are taken, the former to give warning of the difficulties that short women may have, and the latter to place the woman in her correct weight band. Most clinics do not weigh women at every antenatal visit after this, but excess weight put on during pregnancy is nearly always maternal body fat; this is very hard to remove afterwards with a new baby in the home – the woman should be warned. An overall weight gain of up to 25% of initial body weight can be expected.

The *blood pressure* is taken at the booking visit, and is used as a basal level. Readings of blood pressure will be repeated at each antenatal visit, with the woman always either sitting at the side of the desk or lying on the couch in the left lateral position having had 5 min rest. All who take the woman's blood pressure should use the same points indicating systolic and diastolic blood pressure, respectively. The former is fairly easy to obtain, but for the latter, ideally the fifth Korotkoff sound (where the beat disappears) is the correct physiological measure when adjudged against aortic catheter studies. However, many find it is very much easier to detect the change from the fourth to fifth sounds when the more staccato drum taps change to a swishing noise. Whilst this may not be strictly the diastolic blood pressure, this level acts as a surrogate with less interobserver variation than does the fading away of the blood pressure noise completely. Whichever is used it should be the same for all the observers who are going to look after the woman, and local agreements should be reached. Automatic machines can read lower than clinical observers, and are best avoided in pregnancy. Those with large forearms should have their blood pressure measured with a large cuff. Normal-sized cuffs will lead to false high readings.

Examination of the abdomen in early pregnancy usually reveals very little but a check should be made for the presence of other masses than the expected pelvic one. In a thin multiparous woman the uterus can be felt as a soft mass arising from the pelvis after 10 weeks of gestation, but in a plump woman it is only palpable much later than this. Women who have had a previous caesarean section have a uterus palpable much earlier in pregnancy.

As pregnancy goes on, palpation of the uterus and later its contents becomes more important, until the last 8 weeks, when fetal size and position in relation to the mother can be determined.

A pelvic examination used to be performed at booking in pregnancy, but this is rarely required now. The indications used to be:

- To check the woman really was pregnant
- To check the stage of gestation by delineating uterine size
- To exclude pelvic masses such as fibroids or ovarian cysts
- To check the bony pelvis shape and size.

Now in the developed world, ultrasound is used almost universally, and it can perform all

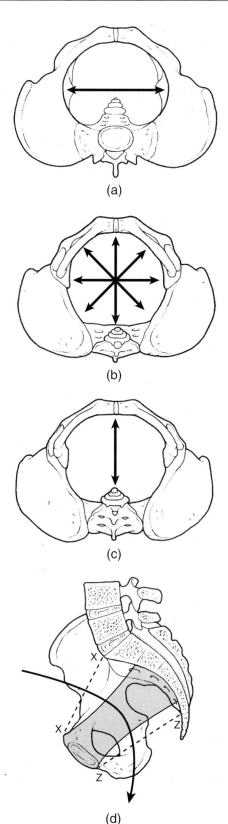

Diameter [cm]			
Antero - posterior	Oblique	Transverse	
11	12	13	Pelvic inlet
12	12	12	Midcavity
13	12	11	Pelvic outlet

Figure 5.6 Bony pelvis showing maximum diameter ←→. **a** Inlet (transverse diameter). **b** Mid-cavity (a circle, hence dimensions are all the same). **c** Outlet (anteroposterior diameter). **d** Lateral view showing zones of pelvis: x–x, inlet of pelvis 11 cm; shaded zone, mid-cavity (12 cm); z–z, outlet of pelvis (13 cm).

but the last of those functions with precision. However, vaginal examination can still be useful to check these points if ultrasound is not immediately available. Clinical checking of the bony pelvis is not usually done these days, but if it is still practised, it is best postponed until much later in the pregnancy. By 38 weeks of gestation the fetal presenting part is usually moving down the pelvis, and will give a good guide to pelvic fit. Should there be doubt about the capacity of the pelvis in late pregnancy, a vaginal assessment then will give a much better indication of maternal pelvic abnormalities, for the woman will be more relaxed about her attendants and not object to the examination so much. Further effect of progesterone relaxing the ligaments of the pelvis will be acting, so that the best assessment of the architecture of the pelvis can be made (Fig. 5.6).

A cervical smear may be carried out if vaginal examination is performed, but this is better done at the postnatal visit.

Box 5.4 Investigations that may be performed at the booking clinic (those in parentheses may not be done on all women)

Check blood for:

- Haemoglobin level
- Mean corpuscular haemoglobin level
- Platelets
- ABO and rhesus group
- Atypical blood group antibodies (Rh, ABO and Kell)
- Rubella antibodies
- Screening test for syphilis
- (Blood sugar level)
- (Haemoglobin electrophoresis)
- (Sickle cell screen)
- (Australia antigens)
- (Human immunodeficiency virus (HIV) in certain areas of the world)
- (Toxoplasmosis antibodies – in some clinics by request)
- (Leiden factor V and activated protein C resistance (APCR) – where there is a family or personal history of unprovoked thrombosis).

Check urine for:

- Protein
- Glucose
- White blood cells.

Investigations

The first screening tests of pregnancy are done at the booking clinic. Blood and urine checks are made (Box 5.4). Whilst the blood investigations first listed in Box 5.4 will be done on all women, those in parentheses may be reserved for special groups. For instance if few women of Afro-Asian or Mediterranean origin live locally, the *haemoglobinopathies* are less common, and it may be decided not to screen routinely for these.

Screening for *syphilis* is at a cross-roads at the moment. Very little syphilis is detected in the antenatal period, but the sequelae to the newborn are great, and a very effective simple treatment is available. Some still argue for the continuation of this test, but it is likely to be dropped as a routine screening test in the next decade.

Checking for *Australia antigen* is probably wise for all women, as the implications are serious for the fetus as well as for medical and midwifery staff at the delivery.

If a woman is sero-negative to *rubella* there

is little one can do about it in this pregnancy. Giving advice to avoid being in contact with german measles is very difficult for a young mother to follow in whose immediate society children abound with an infectious phase before the clinically diagnosed illness. One can, however, immunize her after this pregnancy to protect the next one and protect prophylactically higher-risk groups of young women, e.g. primary school teachers.

The testing for *HIV* is becoming more regularized, and is considered in Chapter 7.

Blood testing for *Down's syndrome* with the double or triple test may be done at 15–18 weeks of gestation. This is considered in Chapter 6.

All women should be asked if they have had *chicken pox*. If not, blood should be tested for antibodies, but as yet, immunization for varicella in pregnancy is not available in the UK.

Chest radiography is not usually performed in pregnancy unless the woman comes from a part of the world where tuberculosis is endemic or if there is a family history of the disease. If done, careful lead screening of the pelvis must be performed. The amount of radiation from a chest radiograph with a modern machine is equivalent to that which a woman will receive in a single trans-Atlantic flight.

Ultrasound investigations used to be started at about 16 weeks of gestation, but in some units now the skill of the sonographers and the excellent equipment they have allow many decisions about pregnancies to be made by an early scan done at the time of the booking clinic. The size of the fetus taken from *crown–rump measurements* will give an accurate indication of the gestational age. In expert units other checks of the fetus can be made such as nuchal translucency, but mostly in the UK ultrasound for anomalies is postponed until later in pregnancy, at 20 weeks of gestation, when it is easier to perform (see Ch. 6). However, early dating scans may be needed for the correct interpretation of serum tests for Down's screening.

Management

At the booking visit it is very important to

establish a relationship between the woman and the person who is likely to become the lead professional. They may know each other before, as do many general practitioners with the women on their lists. If, however, it is a first meeting it is the start of a very close relationship which is going to go on for many months, and trust has to be gained from the woman and her partner.

Many women like to work out what they wish to do in an ideal pregnancy and labour. If they write this down as a *birth plan*, it can be discussed during the course of the pregnancy with the midwife and doctors. Such plans should be used not as a weapon in the relationship between professionals but as a checklist to ensure that the woman's ideas are brought to the professionals' attention early and when there is time for any amendment which might be required. There are several proformata of plans available prepared by consumer groups, and these have the advantage of drawing the woman's attention to previously unconsidered aspects of the pregnancy, labour and the early days of child rearing. They are not frightening or alarming to the woman as many professionals first feared.

Make sure the woman knows where she can get more *information*. If books and leaflets are going to be recommended, ensure that they contain information which applies locally and do not consider irrelevant and unobtainable matters, e.g. there is little point in getting a woman to read about epidural analgesia if she is delivering in a hospital where it cannot be obtained.

The *social welfare benefits* of pregnancy change very rapidly, and, whilst we all try to keep up with them, it is probably better to get the woman to read them herself in the excellent literature which the Department of Social Security provides, and then ask questions after that.

Dental care is free in pregnancy (and for a year after), so ensure that the woman makes use of this.

Even as early as this, the woman may ask about *dietary advice*. One of the important things to stress is that there is no need to eat for two, for most women in developed countries have an adequate diet. Vegetarians, especially vegans, may require specialized advice, as will some Asian women who have a limited diet. Vitamin supplements are not usually needed in general, but folate is helpful in the reduction of neural tube abnormalities (see Ch. 4).

Malnutrition may be rare amongst the young in the Western world, but undernutrition of specific substances is common. An intake of 2000–2500 kcal a day is needed in the last two trimesters, while 3000 kcal a day is required while lactating.

Most calories are obtained from *carbohydrates*: mono- or disaccharides or breakdown products of more complex carbohydrate molecules. The major energy source of the fetus is glucose, and this travels across the placenta readily from the maternal blood.

Fats are taken for:

- Energy for work
- Absorption of fats and soluble vitamins
- Structural lipids.

Fats do not cross to the fetus; neolipogenesis occurs *de novo* there.

Proteins are used for:

- Structural purposes
- Energy requirements.

As amino acids they cross the placenta to the fetus. They are contained in those food items that are the most expensive to buy in the UK, and so are the most likely to be deficient in the diet. Around 60–80 g a day in pregnancy is desirable, coming from mixed animal protein from meat, fish and eggs, or vegetable protein (e.g. from lentils).

The requirements for *vitamins and minerals* increase in pregnancy. The recommended dietary allowances are probably overexpressed. Many women need iron supplementation. Some doctors prescribe iron routinely in early pregnancy, but this will often lead to constipation (or occasionally diarrhoea), and could dissuade the woman from taking iron later in pregnancy when it may be needed. It may be wise to wait for the booking visit blood test results, and then give it to those whose haemoglobin levels indicate it (e.g. less than 10 g/dl). Special attention should be paid to those who are becoming pregnant

Table 5.2 Commonly used iron preparations for pregnancy

	Dose (mg)	Equivalent dose of elemental iron (mg)
Dried ferrous sulphate	50	45
Ferrous sulphate	300	60
Ferrous gluconate	300	30
Ferrous fumarate	200	65

again soon after a previous pregnancy (within 2 years) and those who are found to have twin pregnancies. These women will certainly need iron supplementation. Remember that the haemoglobin levels fall in midpregnancy due to haemodilution, and probably the ideal of 12.5 g/dl of haemoglobin or a mean corpuscular volume of less than 84 fl are set high. A dose of about 100 mg of elemental iron per day should be aimed at, taken at the same time as food (Table 5.2).

Translating this scientific nutritional data into common-sense eating needs the skills of dieticians and dietetic journalists. There are plenty of good sources of information about eating in pregnancy which the doctor or midwife may recommend to the woman.

CONTINUING ANTENATAL CARE

At the end of the booking consultation, the lead professional will plan the subsequent visits with the woman (see Fig. 5.1). Whatever pattern these may follow, it is wise to work this out well in advance, assuming the woman is going to have a normal course. If any problems occur, extra visits can always be added, but at least the basic plan is understood by both the woman and her attendants, who will then know where, when, who and which professional team will be responsible.

Later antenatal visits

At all visits it is wise to check the blood pressure and examine the urine for protein at least and probably sugar as well.

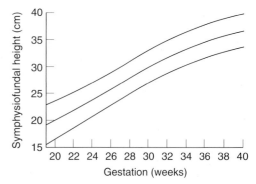

Figure 5.7 Symphysiofundal height (±2 SD) by weeks of gestation.

After 28 weeks of gestation the abdomen is checked for uterine size to ensure it is appropriate to the gestational age. This can be further checked by a flexible cloth tape measure being run from the symphysis pubis to the fundus of the uterus. This gives a fair guide to growth in pregnancy, and is probably best when it is used sequentially by the same observer, thus ensuring a longitudinal series of readings. Figure 5.7 shows that these readings rise by approximately a centimetre a week, but the range of variation of the normal widens as the pregnancy progresses, making a single reading less useful. Remember that this measures uterus, placenta and amniotic fluid as well as the fetus, a dilution of its perceived role. The uterus is most often dextro-rotated in later pregnancy, so the fundus will lie to the right of the midline.

The haemoglobin level should be rechecked at about 28 weeks of gestation in order to allow time for the correction of anaemia if detected. If the woman is rhesus-negative, a second check of antibodies should be done now. Many units screen for gestational diabetes by doing a random or fasting blood sugar test at about this time.

From 32 weeks of gestation the lie and presentation of the fetus are checked. Most babies lie longitudinally, the most economic fit of the fetal length in the irregular oval-shaped amniotic pool in the uterus. A transverse lie up to 36 weeks is not a cause for concern, but after this time it may produce problems. Such babies are undeliverable per se, and must turn to a longitudinal lie,

Fifths palpable

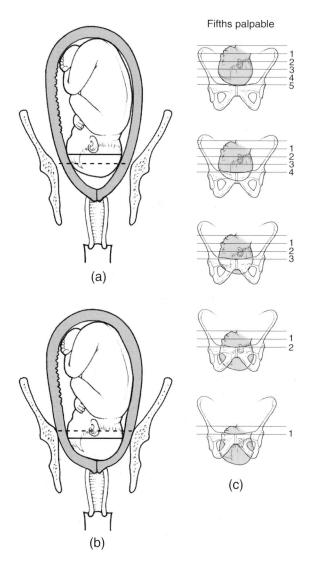

(a)

(b)

(c)

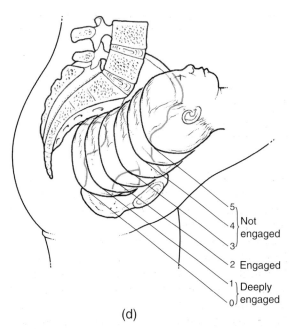

(d)

Figure 5.8 Descent of the fetal head into the pelvis.
a Head is not engaged, and maximum head diameter (–) is above brim of pelvis (– – –). **b** Head is engaged for maximum head diameter (–) is below brim of pelvis.
c Descent is measured in fifths still palpable in the abdomen. **d** Engagement is when only two-fifths or less is palpable in the abdomen.

or else be delivered by caesarean section if they stay in this position until labour starts. Breech presentations can be corrected to cephalic ones by external cephalic version. Whilst this can be done easily at about 35 weeks of gestation, the fetus will often revert, and so many wait until 38 weeks, when the gradual diminution of the amount of amniotic fluid will be against the fetus turning back. Such a version should be done without general anaesthesia, but a tocolytic may assist the technique.

From 36 weeks of gestation onwards, particularly in a primiparous woman, the fetal head will usually engage in the pelvis. This can be detected by examining through the lower abdominal wall, feeling for the maximum diameter; if it can still be felt, the head is obviously not engaged (Fig. 5.8). Descent of the head is measured in fifths. If only two-fifths of the head is palpable, it is engaged. If three-fifths or more are palpable, the head is not engaged. Since the descent of the head into the pelvis is a good measure of pelvic architecture, some obstetricians would go further. If they found the head to be not engaged in the last weeks of pregnancy, they prop the woman up on the couch on her elbows to see if the head will engage by the simple aid of gravity.

In the last weeks of pregnancy, the wellbeing of the fetus can be assessed. The *growth* of the fetus can be determined clinically or by comparing the serial ultrasound readings of previous antenatal visits with the current one. The mother can be asked about *fetal movements*. The observer can see them by looking obliquely across the abdominal surface during the examination. Some doctors and midwives will listen at each visit to the *fetal heart*. This is not necessary if movements are detected by the mother and observer, but it can be reassuring to the woman, particularly if a hand-held Doppler ultrasound machine (Sonicaid) is used so that the mother can hear the heart beat herself.

Assessment of the *amniotic fluid volume* is made to ensure there is not too much or too little. The former (polyhydramnios) is diagnosed when the uterus is ballooned out, making it difficult to palpate the fetal body or to hold the fetal head, except by dipping. Lack of fluid (oligohydramnios) allows the examiner to feel the fetal limbs too easily so that one can imagine even feeling fingers and toes through the uterine wall. Both these are clinical diagnoses and may be confirmed by ultrasound. In polyhydramnios the diameter of the largest pool of amniotic fluid is more than 8 cm; in oligohydraminos the diameter is less than 2 cm.

If the pregnancy gets to 37/38 weeks of gestation and the head is not engaged nor will engage, a gentle vaginal examination of the pelvis by experienced obstetricians can be helpful, checking the features outlined in Box 5.5.

If there is any doubt about the bimanual assessment, a standing lateral radiograph can be useful, and sometimes computerized topography of the pelvis, but fewer units are making these static measurements, preferring to rely on the dynamic test of descent of the fetal head in late pregnancy or labour.

The end of antenatal care

If a woman has been given an expected date of delivery, often confirmed by ultrasound, she becomes surprised when she passes that date. It should have been explained to her at the beginning of antenatal care, and, if not, will have to be explained now, that the date is only the *probable* expected date. She is perfectly normal if she has her baby within 2 weeks either side of that date (Fig. 5.9).

Box 5.5 Characteristics to be checked in the female bony pelvis

- Inlet:
  - Sacral promontory should be beyond the reach of the fingers of a normal examining hand. Hence an anteroposterior diameter over 11 cm
- Midcavity:
  - Good sacral curve of the fronts of the bodies of vertebrae 2, 3 and 4. If sacral vertebra 3 is protruding into the cavity, this will produce a straight sacrum with anteroposterior narrowing
  - The sacrospinous ligaments should allow two fingers on them obliquely, thus implying an opened up pelvis with good anteroposterior diameter
  - The ischial spines should not be prominent but just felt as rounded bosses of bone and ligament – a good transverse diameter
- Outlet:
  - The subpubic angle should be more than 100°
  - The width of the symphysis pubis and the pubic bones should accept two fingers to give reasonable transverse space in the outlet

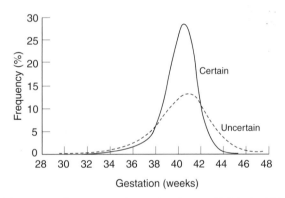

Figure 5.9 Distribution of gestational age at birth in the UK by whether the woman was sure or unsure of her last normal menstrual period. Note how both curves are skewed to the left, towards immaturity. (Reproduced with permission from the National Birthday Trust.)

The concept of postmaturity is a mathematical one. The perinatal mortality rate of babies after 42 weeks of gestation used to be much higher. Now many obstetricians would not intrude on pregnancy because of a mathematical time, but the women themselves will often try to persuade the obstetrician that sufficient time has gone by. Then the cervix should be checked, and if ripe (soft, taken up and dilated) one may well consider the use of prostaglandin gel or pessaries. In the zone of postmaturity, the indications for induction are often led by the woman rather than by the professional. If pregnancy does go past 42 certain weeks of gestation, more careful monitoring of fetal well-being should be done.

RECOMMENDED READING

Bewley S, Humphrey Ward R 1994 Ethics in obstetrics and gynaecology. RCOG Press, London

Chamberlain G 1997 ABC of antenatal care. BMJ, London

Chamberlain G, Wraight A, Cowley P 1997 Homebirths. The NBT confidential enquiry. Parthenon Press, New York

Fetal progress

EARLY DEVELOPMENT AND ORGANOGENESIS

Only a brief account of clinically applicable embryology is given here. Readers wanting more detail are advised to consult the reading recommended at the end of this chapter.

Conception

During most regular menstrual cycles, an oocyte is released from the ovary. During the previous 10 days a group of primordial oocytes (maybe 150) have been stimulated by follicle-stimulating hormone (FSH) from the pituitary. A few (maybe ten) pass to the antral (cystic) stage. In the last 3 days of this phase, one follicle becomes dominant, coming to the surface as a vesicle about 20 mm in diameter projecting into the peritoneal cavity, and is easily seen on ultrasound scanning. Cell layers give way, and the oocyte, surrounded by a cloud of supporting cells, is released under the influence of luteinizing hormone (LH). By this time the fimbrial end of the fallopian tube is embracing the relevant pole of the ovary, and so the oocyte passes straight into the lumen of the fallopian tube. There is no great transperitoneal voyage.

The follicle left in the ovary collapses, and its cells luteinize, so forming the corpus luteum. If fertilization of the oocyte occurs in that cycle, the trophoblast begins to generate human chorionic gonadotrophin (hCG) to help the fertilized ovum survive. The corpus luteum secretes progesterone for the next 8 weeks until sufficient is metabolized by the placenta to maintain the pregnancy.

Fertilization

At every act of intercourse, hundreds of millions of sperm are ejaculated into the upper end of the vagina. Within 90 seconds, the most motile pass up into the cervical mucus, where molecular barriers have been temporarily removed by higher oestrogen concentrations. They swarm in the endometrial fluid of the uterus, and some by chance reach the uterine end of the fallopian tube on the relevant side, an even smaller number travelling the length of the tube to reach the region where the oocyte will come. If the man has a normal sperm count, as many as 200 000 000 sperm are released at each act of intercourse but probably only about 400 000 will get to the region of the oocyte, the fastest taking 20 min to traverse this distance – the equivalent, body size to body size, would be a human adult running from London to Brighton in half an hour! The sperm that get there first are the most active, the fastest and, by analogy with survival of the fittest, the best.

One spermatozoon penetrates the outer layers of the oocyte, and the head is absorbed whilst the body and tail are lost. The cell membrane is converted into a barrier to other sperms by calcium-generated hostility, so preventing multiple entry. Twenty-three chromosomes from the male gamete now unite with the twenty-three of the oocyte nucleus to re-establish the normal 46 chromosomes of humans. All chromosomes are in pairs except sex chromosomes; a female will have two the same – XX – and a male will have an X and a Y chromosome. In either case it is the spermatozoon which has carried the determining chromosome. The basic phenotype is female, and development of the male embryo (XY) depends on the production of androgens leading to male gonads and genitalia. With the XX combination, oestrogen influences continue, and so female organ characteristics develop.

The fertilized ovum passes down the fallopian tube towards the uterus in a current set up in the tubal fluid by the ciliated cells of the fallopian tube working uniformly. The peristaltic action of the muscular layer of the fallopian tube is less important in this journey. In the 5 days that this takes, the ovum is receiving nutrition and oxygen from the fluid secreted by glandular cells in the lining of the fallopian tubes; similarly, catabolites and carbon dioxide are being transferred away from the ovum. Until the ovum is implanted and has a direct communication with the mother's blood many days later, survival is entirely dependent upon exchange with the contents of the fluids produced by the mucosa of the fallopian tube and the endometrium in turn. This is a much unexplored area of reproductive physiology and embryo survival.

The passage down the fallopian tube over 5 or 6 days ends, and the fertilized ovum rests on the surface of the endometrium for a day or so before implanting at 8 or 9 days after fertilization. During this transfer, development is taking place to a blastocyst (Fig. 6.1), and so a trophoblast outer layer is formed ready to digest the surface epithelium of the uterus. Inside the cystic structure an embryonic plate develops in the

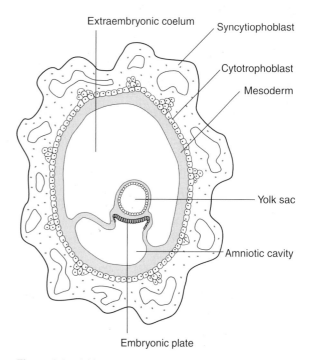

Figure 6.1 A blastocyst.

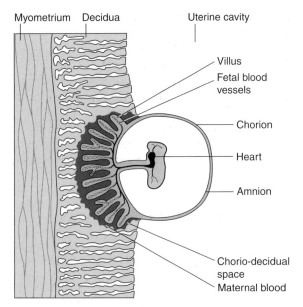

Figure 6.2 Embryo and placental formation.

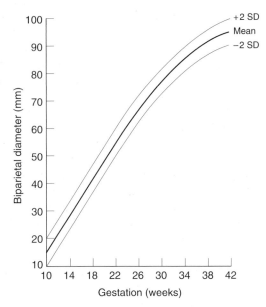

Figure 6.3 Ultrasound measurement of biparietal diameter by weeks of gestation (mean ± 2 SD).

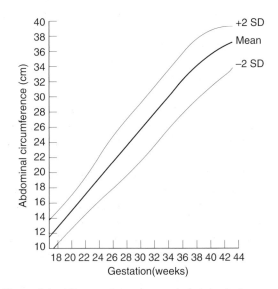

Figure 6.4 Ultrasound measurement of abdominal circumference by weeks of gestation (mean ± 2 SD).

extraembryonic coelom. The fetus develops in this plate and one portion of the trophoblast layer becomes the placenta (Fig. 6.2).

Growth

The fetus grows from one cell to about 6 000 000 in 38 weeks. This is the most rapid development in the whole life of the human body. Were growth to continue at this active phase after birth, the child would be the size of a 20-storey building by the age of 21 years. Once the fetus can be visualized, this rapid growth can be measured with ultrasound from 6 weeks. The length increases exponentially in much of the pregnancy. Fetal length from the head to the coccyx (crown–rump length) is a good measure in the first 12 weeks of pregnancy. For practical antenatal care from 16 weeks of gestation, the biparietal diameter is measured between the two parietal eminences in the head (Fig. 6.3), and this shows a narrow range of variation from the mean until about 24 weeks. From here on, increase in the abdominal circumference becomes a better guide to fetal well-being. (Fig. 6.4). Femur length is also used by some units to measure somatic growth.

Organogenesis

The *central nervous system* is formed from the sinking in of the primitive streak of ectoderm around the notocord from day 21 to 28 of embryonic life. Any noxious constraint at this time could cause a defect in the covering process, leading to a spina bifida. The cephalic end enlarges rapidly, first appearing as a hollow cyst in the tissue. The cortex increases in thickness and the central lumen diminishes to become a pair of lateral ventricles, the third and fourth ventricles communicating with the spinal cord central canal.

The *gut* forms as a tube in communication with the yolk sac by narrowing of the intestinal duct (vitellointestinal duct), which stretches the length of the body. The midgut pulls away from the back wall of the embryo on a mesentery. At the upper end a liver bud appears at about 24 days; gut rotation takes place at about 40 days to give the well-known curves of the alimentary tract. Dilatation at the upper end produces the stomach, and on the lower end the colon. The facial areas come in as a pit from the stomatodeum pressing in to join the gut tube in the pharynx. Lateral buds then lead to the gums and lips; deficiency of fusions allow cleft lip or palate to follow. At the caudal end, a pit of surface skin, the proctodeum, presses in to join the hind gut. From the area in front of this develop the lower vagina and bladder of the embryo.

The *cardiovascular system* is formed from a pair of endothelial tubes which form in the meso-thelium of the embryo very early; a thickened area towards the cephalic end becomes the primitive heart, and a peristaltic beat starts by day 21. The pair of tubes links up the blood islands outside and inside the embryo. Fast growth on the tube which is fixed at both ends produces some fairly acute bends, so making the structure of the atria and ventricles. The cephalic end of the tubes follows the pattern of the six brachial arches in the cervical region, and branches go on to the head, supplying the brain. These are greatly modified in early embryonic life to produce the complex arterial plan of the upper thorax and neck.

At the end of intrauterine life, the vascular system incorporates several bypasses which divert blood from the lungs (not a source of oxygenation in the uterus) while enhancing the placental circulation, which does provide oxygen

and nutrition, and preferring the cephalic end of the embryo. After birth when the umbilical vessels between the fetus and placenta are blocked, these bypasses close rapidly (Fig. 6.5).

The *limbs* develop as buds just before invasion of the body wall by the mesodermal cell layer. They push out from the body rapidly from about 31 days, taking with them their share of muscle and nerves; cartilage followed by bone develops in this area. Hand and foot plates

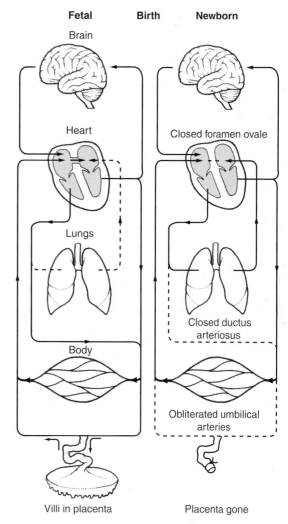

Figure 6.5   The fetal and neonatal circulations compared. Note closure of bypasses at birth. (Reproduced with permission from Chamberlain G 1996 Lecture notes in obstetrics. Blackwell, Oxford.)

appear as flattened discs at their ends at about 36 days, the arms just before the legs. Rotation of the limb buds follows different directions so that the arm rotates outwards whereas the leg rotates inwards, so allowing the preaxial border of the hand to be lateral while that of the foot is medial.

This very brief account of the embryology and organogenesis is given to provide understanding of future changes in the newborn's development. The readers are advised to consult the recommended reading for details.

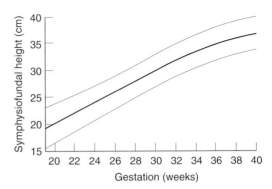

Figure 6.6 Symphysiofundal height by weeks of gestation. Note wide range of variation (±2 SD).

ASSESSMENT OF THE FETUS

Not only do obstetricians have the mother to look after but also, within her abdomen, they care for the fetus. Direct observation, except by palpation, is difficult, and indirect monitoring or other investigative methods are needed.

Clinical methods

Fetal growth

The growth of the uterus can be measured clinically and recorded as an impression using equivalent weeks of gestation as the unit. The fetus can be felt clearly in most non-obese women after 26 weeks of gestation, and the length from the head to the breech can be estimated clinically. Other aids to fetal health are the amount of amniotic fluid and the total size of the uterus. These are not as good as actually feeling the length of the fetus. Slightly more precision is achieved using a series of symphysiofundal measurements taken with a tape measure (Fig. 6.6). This method is at its best when performed by the same doctor or midwife. From 20 weeks into the pregnancy the fundal height in centimetres is roughly equivalent to the gestational age in weeks, but there is an increasing variation around the mean.

Fetal movements

Here the mother is asked to record when she feels the fetus moving in the last weeks of pregnancy. This can be made into a semiquantitative test by the use of a kick chart, showing how long it takes for her to feel ten movements or groups of movements. Most women starting at 9 a.m. will have recorded ten movements by the middle of the morning. If the day stretches on, and by 6 o'clock in the evening she has not felt ten movements, she is asked to report to her antenatal centre, where a cardiotocograph will be performed to check further on the fetus. This is not usually of importance until 28 weeks of gestation.

The advantage of this investigation is it involves the mother. Anxiety is not generated by the observation of her own fetus. Fetal movement charting is not very predictive of stillbirths among those mothers at low risk.

Biochemical tests

These depend mostly upon estimating levels in the maternal blood or urine of metabolites which arise from the fetus or the placenta. Oestriol levels used to be measured in the mother's blood or urine (Fig. 6.7), but they have a wide scatter of normal values within the normal range with a certain amount of added intralaboratory variation. Measures can also be made of placental hormones such as human placental lactogen, which is made entirely in the placenta, or placental proteins, but their use is limited to research, and probably at their best when used in assessment in early pregnancy.

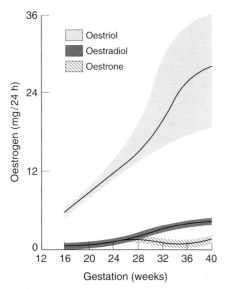

Figure 6.7 Concentrations of three oestrogens by weeks of gestation (mean ± 2 SD). The principle increase is in oestriol levels, but the range of variation is wide.

Biophysical methods

Cardiotocograph records can be made of the fetal heart rate (FHR) and simultaneous tracing of other intrauterine changes such as intermittent uterine activity, pressure changes and fetal movements (Fig. 6.8).

The FHR is recorded from Doppler ultrasound echoes for external recording through the mother's abdominal wall, or in labour when the membranes have ruptured with a direct electrode from the fetal scalp for internal recording. The important difference between these methods is that indirect Doppler measurements (external monitoring) involves a group averaging technique usually using the mean of three cardiac beats, while the direct scalp electrode picks up individual QRS complexes, and so measures individual beat-to-beat variation.

The FHR ranges between 110 and 160 beats/min, staying between 130 and 140 beats/min in most cases. A raised fetal pulse rate may be associated with maternal pyrexia, but in the absence of a maternal cause, fetal tachycardia may be a sign of fetal hypoxia. The baseline rate is not uniform, for the heart beats in response to many factors – its in-built activity, nervous stimuli of the sympathetic and parasympathetic nervous systems, the blood pH and oxygen partial

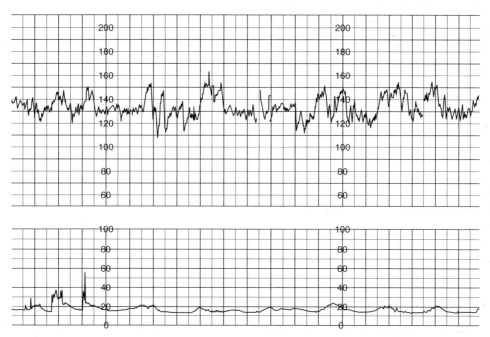

Figure 6.8 Normal antenatal CTG.

pressure in the blood, carbon dioxide partial pressure of the blood, and certain drugs such as pethidine. The rate is not absolutely steady but varies inside a range of 10–15 beats/min. When the fetus is asleep, the usual state, the reactivity of the heart is reduced, and there is a loss of baseline variability. Most fetuses sleep for up to 40 min at a time (Fig. 6.9). Occasional accelerations in heart rate for 10–15 beats/min occur: these are normal, and are often the reaction to a stimulus, e.g. a sound, a movement or a contraction (Fig. 6.10). Decelerations are not normal (Fig. 6.11), and each should be considered seriously.

An external transducer records the uterine pressures and individual fetal movements, usually of the limbs (Fig. 6.12).

Cardiotocography in practice

The external transducer is strapped on to the mother's abdomen, and the FHR and pressure changes measured for about 30 min. Monitoring of the FHR can be measured in the clinic with hand-held Doppler machines or monoauricular stethoscopes. If there is any indication that all is not well with the fetus, continuous cardiotoco-

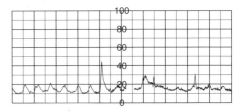
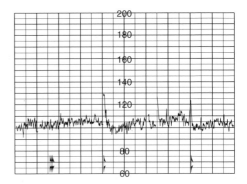

Figure 6.10 Antenatal cardiotocogram showing fetal bradycardia (105 beats/min) but good accelerations with uterine contractions.

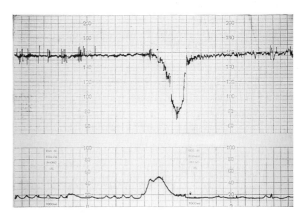

Figure 6.11 Antenatal cardiotocogram with a Braxton Hicks's contraction of the uterus showing low to baseline variability and a deep, late deceleration.

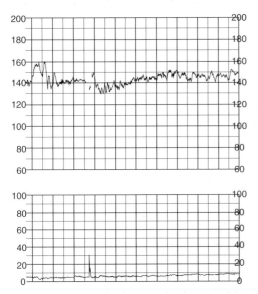

Figure 6.9 Antenatal cardiotocogram with fetus asleep.

graphic monitoring can be performed in a side room at most antenatal clinics, and the records become part of the decision making process.

Signs of abnormality are:

- Baseline tachycardia above 170 beats/min
- Baseline brachycardia below 100 beats/min
- Intermittent decelerations not associated with a uterine contraction
- Baseline variability of less than 5 beats/min.

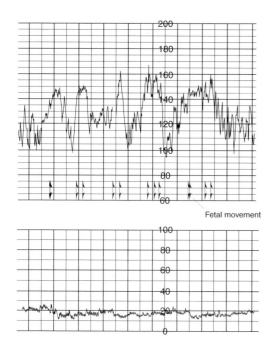

Figure 6.12 Antenatal cardiotocogram showing good accelerations with fetal movements.

The predictive value of a normal cardiotocograph is not strong, but the abnormal signs shown above should lead to greater surveillance of the woman. The signs most commonly used to indicate delivery are long and profound decelerations not associated with uterine contractions. The other signs show more gradual deterioration, which should be watched. In combination these variations may have more significance (Fig. 6.13).

Doppler wave forms

When sound is beamed at a moving target its echoes change and come back at different speeds. This is the Doppler shift, well known as the change in tone of the whistle of a train as it passes you. Ultrasound undergoes the same physical shift when it is reflected from the front of a pulse of moving blood.

The sound wave-forms can be obtained from:

1. The uteroplacental circulation. The arcuate arteries are the first branches of the maternal uterine vessels. Blood flow can be detected, and the individual characteristics of the echo projected by any given artery (its *signature*) allows an experienced ultrasonographer to locate that vessel again and again. A lack of normal invasion by trophoblast of the spiral arteries back towards the arcuate artery is associated with a high-resistance wave-form. This may be measured longitudinally, and indicate a deteriorating circulation to the placental bed which results in less oxygen to the fetus (Fig. 6.14).

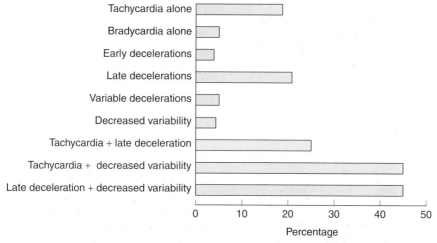

Figure 6.13 Percentage of babies born with an Apgar score below 7 at 1 min by their electrocardiogram patterns in the first stage of labour.

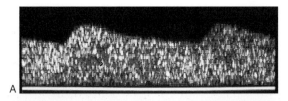

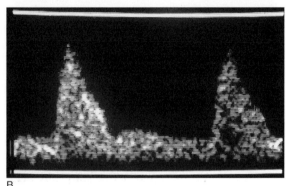

Figure 6.14 Doppler ultrasound image of an arcuate artery. **a** Normal, with good flow in systole and diastole. **b** Abnormal, with diminished flow in diastole.

2. The fetal circulation. The umbilical artery wave-forms can be measured – if there is a loss of flow in the diastolic phase, this is a serious indication of poor fetal heart action and blood flow. This is even worse should the flow be reversed at the end of diastole (Fig. 6.15).

While arcuate artery flow is the long-term guide to fetal well-being, umbilical flow is the short-term emergency guide, end-diastolic reversal being an indication for the really rapid delivery of the fetus.

Real time ultrasound

The measurement of the fetus by real time ultrasound is a useful way of telling fetal size. A longitudinal series of these measurements demonstrates fetal growth, which is a dynamic feature and cannot be measured from one reading. The first reading should be done early in the pregnancy to give a baseline. Real time ultrasound can measure:

1. *Biparietal diameter* – the distance between the two parietal eminences in the skull, a reasonable measure of brain growth. It is a reliable way to detect fetal well-being between 16 and 26 weeks of gestation.

2. *Abdominal circumference* – a measure of liver growth, a sign of fetal metabolism. This is the

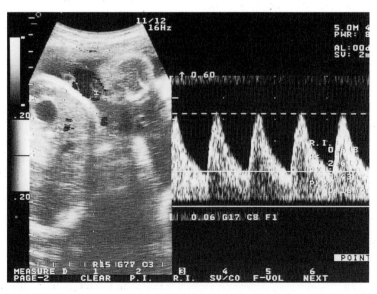

Figure 6.15 Doppler ultrasound image of the uterine artery flow pattern.

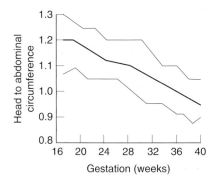

Figure 6.16 Head to abdominal circumference ratio.

best criterion for measuring fetal well-being from about 26 weeks of gestation to term.

3. *Femur length growth* – easily measured, and the sign of somatic growth, i.e. how the whole body is growing.

4. *Ratios* of various measures can be obtained, of which the best is between the abdominal and head circumferences (Fig. 6.16). Falling off of this ratio implies lack of abdominal growth, often indicating an asymmetrical small for gestational age (SGA) fetus.

Combined tests

Many countries in the West have made use of a biophysical profile, a mixture of ultrasound measures (Table 6.1).

Table 6.1 Biophysical profile

Measure	Score	
	2	0
Fetal breathing movements	For >30 s in 30 min	For <30 s in 30 min
Fetal movements	>3 body movements in 30 s	<30 body movements in 30 min
Fetal tone	1 or more flexion/ extensions of limbs in 30 min	Absence of limb movements in 30 min
Fetal reactivity	2 or more FHR accelerations of 15 beats/min in 30 min	>2 FHR accelerations in 30 min
Amniotic fluid	Largest pocket 1 cm to two perpendicular planes	Largest pocket <1 cm in two planes

By combining these facets, each with its own false-positive rate, a better predictive power is hoped for, but there is little evidence that the measurement improves fetal outcome. Whilst the full biophysical profile is not as popular in Europe as it is in the USA, parts of it such as amniotic fluid volume and cardiotocograph are used commonly as a prognosis for fetal well-being. Longitudinal readings from a series of ultrasound measures are used if a failing placental exchange system is suspected and the fetus may need early delivery.

SMALL FOR GESTATIONAL AGE

SGA is a statistical definition (which strictly should only be used when the baby has been born and weighed), when the assessment of the birth weight against the length of gestation shows the baby to be below the tenth centile (Fig. 6.17). The term is also used in the antenatal period when growth of the fetus falls below the lower second standard deviation in an ultrasound chart of either head or abdominal circumference (Table 6.2). It is probably a better concept than either:

- Immaturity – a baby who is born under 2.5 kg birth weight – or
- Intrauterine growth retardation – a concept of the lack of transfer of nutrients across the placenta to the fetus.

Impairment of fetal growth may lead to:

- *Symmetrical SGA* – the baby has both head and abdominal circumferences reduced. Its causes are shown in Table 6.2.
- *Asymmetrical SGA* is less common (40% of SGA), and is usually the result of poor perfusion of the placental bed by a diminished afferent arterial blood supply. This can lead to an increase in the rearrangement of blood flow within the fetus so that blood returning from the placental interchange surface takes the path of least resistance, diverting to the essential areas of fetal brain, coronary arteries and adrenals. This initial biological response is advantageous to the fetus for a while, but other organs become

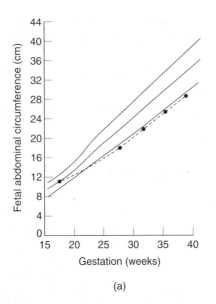
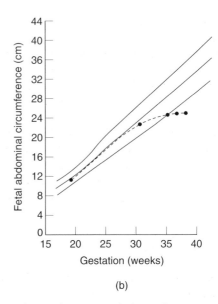

Figure 6.17 Ultrasound measurement of abdominal circumference in **a** symmetrical growth retardation and **b** asymmetrical growth retardation.

Table 6.2 Causes of SGA babies

Symmetrical SGA	Asymmetrical SGA
Genetic: small parents (mother > father)	Poor trophoblastic invasions of arcuate arteries in second
Race: White > Asian	trimester
Sex: boys > girls	Inadequate maternal response to pregnancy
Toxins	Toxins
Alcohol	Alcohol
Cigarettes	Cigarettes
Drugs	
Congenital infections	
Syphilis	
Cytomegalovirus	
Toxoplasmosis	
Maternal severe malnutrition	

underperfused if it persists, leading to the fetal bowel, kidneys and liver becoming relatively ischaemic. In severe cases this results in the neonatal complications of asymmetrical SGA such as necrotizing enterocolitis, renal failure and the reduced coagulation of the blood because of liver metabolites being deficient.

Management of SGA

Once SGA is diagnosed from ultrasound measure-ments of the head and abdominal circumference, one tries to continue the pregnancy so long as the baby is actually growing, remembering that continuing growth increments may be smaller than normal. When growth starts to fail, the method of treatment is delivery by the most appropriate route. Treatment is bed rest. So far no other management has been proven effective. Methods which have been tried but not been shown to be effective are:

- Long-term oxygen supplementation to the mother
- Abdominal decompression to increase uterine blood flow
- Protein infusions directly into the amniotic fluid for the fetus to ingest.

Some investigations may rule out specific aspects of symmetrical growth retardation. The blood can be checked for evidence of infections such as toxoplasmosis, although when diagnosed little can be done about this. It may be useful to check amniotic fluid, placental biopsy or fetal blood for chromosome abnormalities. Again nothing can be done about these, but if trisomies were to be found, the parents can be informed. The knowledge might modify a decision about caesarean section if fetal distress developed in subsequent labour.

Chronic hypoxia may be detected by measuring Doppler blood flow. Here the arcuate artery gives long-term warning while the umbilical Doppler waves provide a short-term warning system.

The postnatal period for the baby with symmetrical SGA is easier for paediatricians to manage than is the asymmetrical form. Proper sustenance and nutrition usually allows catch-up growth to occur in the first few months of life.

DETECTION OF CONGENITAL ABNORMALITIES

Abnormalities occur in about 2% of human pregnancies that are viable. Of these, about half are major, the rest being less of a problem.

The importance of the diagnosis of abnormalities in the antenatal period has increased greatly in the last 20 years: parents seek a normal healthy baby and want to know about the state of their unborn child in good time. This allows for:

- A request for termination of pregnancy if the abnormality is such that it would affect the life of the family.
- Preparations for surgical correction of the abnormality after birth. If this is the case, pregnancy and delivery should be at a unit which has neonatal surgeons and physicians who are capable of dealing with the problem.
- More time for the parents to get used to the idea of the forthcoming abnormal child and to discuss it with other children in the family.

Of these, the first is the commonest outcome for diagnosed congenital abnormalities in the UK at the moment. This is reflected in the Abortion Act of 1991, which permits termination of pregnancy on the grounds of a major abnormality well past the 24 week barrier imposed upon most terminations of pregnancy.

Most hospitals now offer an anomaly screening ultrasound scan at 18–20 weeks of gestation. The fetus is examined carefully at abdominal scan for:

- Skull and spinal deficiencies, indicating a central nervous system abnormality such as spina bifida
- Heart abnormalities (on a four-chamber view)
- Renal size.

The major groups of detectable abnormalities are considered below.

Chromosomal abnormalities

Variations of the chromosome pattern are laid down during fertilization at the fusion of the genetic material of the sperm and the egg; the commonest is trisomy 21 – Down's syndrome. Others include non-disjunction and the fusion of extra chromosomes (Fig. 6.18). The diagnosis of chromosomal abnormalities depends upon obtaining fetal cells and examining the chromosome structure with light microscopy.

The screening for such conditions may involve other biophysical or biochemical indices. The inappropriate metabolism of a baby with trisomy 21 can lead to liver function changes so that the oestriol levels in the fetal and then the mother's blood rise, as do those of hCG, but α-fetoprotein (AFP) levels are reduced. The ratio of these three to each other, taken in conjunction with the woman's age and gestational stage of pregnancy (the triple or Bart's test), can give a predictive risk of Down's syndrome. In the UK, the triple test is less frequently used now, and in 80% of cases only hCG and AFP levels are used without the oestrogen measurements.

The fetus at risk can also be labelled by indirect ultrasound surrogate measures. The width of the fat pad at the back of the neck (nuchal thickness) can be measured to within a millimetre with good ultrasound equipment. If between 10 and 12 weeks of gestation this is found to be excessive, it greatly increases the risk of trisomy 21 (Fig. 6.19). This is being used widely at the moment, for it is a non-invasive screening test and gives an answer swiftly. This risk score provides gradients, and therefore has cut-off points which are mathematical concepts of risk which need interpreting to the woman.

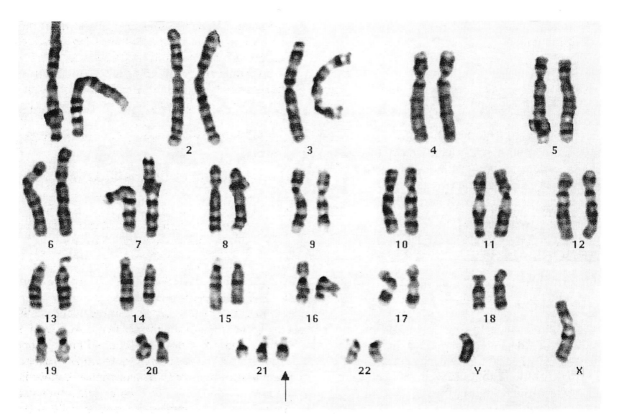

Figure 6.18 A spread of the 22 pairs of chromosomes which are in the nuclei of every cell in the body along with the sex chromosome (XX female; XY male). There is a third chromosome in the 21st pair (arrowed) – trisomy 21 – which accounts for Down's syndrome.

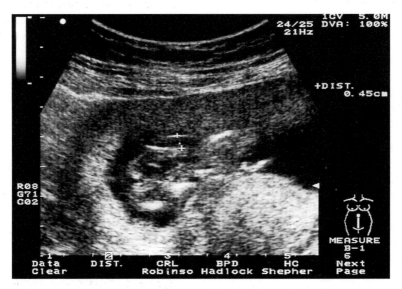

Figure 6.19 Nuchal fat pad thickness. In this case it was 4.5 mm, indicating an increased risk of chromosomal abnormality.

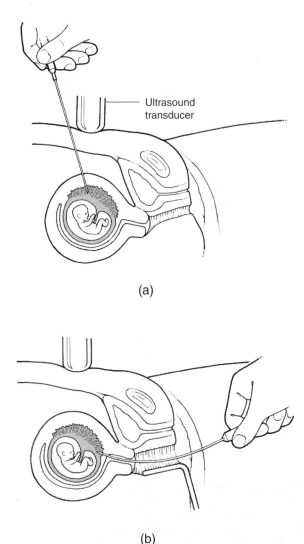

Ultrasound transducer

(a)

(b)

Figure 6.20 Chorionic villus biopsy by **a** the abdominal route and **b** the transcervical route.

With the results of the screening tests known, if the risks are considered to be appropriate, an amniocentesis may be performed to obtain amniocites and fetal cells. These are cultured, usually for about 20 days, and then a chromosome preparation is prepared. Trisomy 21 is readily seen by skilled workers in laboratories. Thus the test is diagnostic with a very low false-positive rate.

An alternative method of obtaining fetal cells is by chorionic villus biopsy. Here a needle is passed under ultrasound control either trans-cervically or through the abdominal wall, across the uterus and amniotic cavity into the edge of the placental tissue, where a sample is taken of villus tissue (Fig. 6.20). If done correctly the risk of miscarriage is about 2%, compared with that of 0.5–1% associated with an amniocentesis. Chorionic villus biopsy has the following advantages:

- It can be done at 10–11 weeks of gestation, compared with 16 weeks for amniocentesis
- It examines fibroblasts, not amniotic or fetal squamous cells, and so a result can be given inside a few days rather than 3 weeks.

For these reasons, chorionic villus biopsy is becoming more popular in the UK for the diagnosis of chromosomal abnormality.

Work is proceeding to extract fetal cells, which, having crossed the placenta, are found in minute quantities in the mother's blood. If one could harvest enough and apply DNA enhancement, these could provide chromosome material which would give an appropriate answer. Similar work is being performed on cells in the transcervical exudates from the amniotic sac; this too is still in the research phase.

The risks of Down's syndrome and other chromosomal abnormalities increase with age (Fig. 6.21). However, the distribution of pregnancies in the UK is such that, although the risks

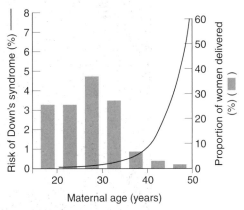

Figure 6.21 Risks of Down's syndrome by age. This increases with age, but the proportion of women having babies decreases with age.

are greater over the age of 35 years, the number of pregnancies is much fewer.

Hence, half the babies born with Down's syndrome are to women under 35 years of age. A philosophy has developed therefore of offering screening tests for Down's syndrome to mothers of all ages, although there is still a hangover of thought that tests should be offered to women of the older age group only – this is illogical and owes little to biological knowledge or an understanding of risk.

The diagnosis of Down's syndrome does not give any prognosis of the severity or the effect. Babies with Down's syndrome can be affected to all degrees; the test merely indicates the chromosome state of the babies, not their potential.

Central nervous system abnormalities

A major group of abnormalities detectable in the UK are the open central nervous system defects. Screening tests for these depend either on the detection of raised levels of AFP in the mother's circulating blood, or on ultrasound scans or both. AFP is made in the fetal liver, and provided the skin of the fetus is intact, most of it stays in the fetal circulation with only small amounts leaking across to the mother. If there is a break in the fetal skin, however, AFP leaks into the amniotic fluid, and is then absorbed over the whole surface of the amnion, so that higher maternal levels are found. Because the concentrations are not very great, it is conventional to multiply the result by 2.5 (2.5 multiples of the median) to show a normal and an abnormal zone which varies as pregnancy continues. Whilst anencephaly and open spina bifida are the two commonest causes of raised AFP in the mother's blood, gastroschesis and exomphalos also allow extra leakage. Further, certain chronic renal conditions of the fetus can cause a raised AFP amniotic fluid level.

A blood sample taken from the mother at about 11 weeks of gestation can provide the level of AFP and allow further investigations. Amniocentesis was previously used to give the level of AFP in the amniotic fluid, but now detailed ultrasound scans can detect central nervous system lesions with good accuracy. Currently the use of ultrasound at 18 weeks of gestation as a test for central nervous system and other abnormalities is being increasingly used in the UK.

Cardiovascular anomalies

The four chambers of the heart and the great vessels may be assessed at about 20–22 weeks of gestation (Fig. 6.22). This can give warning of major flow problems in the heart, and may lead to earlier warning that major cardiac surgery will be required.

A small number of babies have actually been operated upon in the uterus by balloon catheters passed into the umbilical vessels through an amnnioscope. Pregnancy has continued, allowing the baby to be born at the appropriate time without the cardiac lesion. This is still at the research stage at present.

Orthopaedic deficits

Major orthopaedic abnormalities can be detected on ultrasound. Limb length can be measured precisely; achondroplasia and other problems of limb shortening can be diagnosed.

Alimentary tract abnormalities

At the upper end of the alimentary tract, cleft palate and lip can be visualized on ultrasound, and the degree of cleft palate estimated. Blockage by duodenal atresia can be seen because of the double-bubble effect. Atresia of the rectum can be suspected, and malrotation of the intestines can be demonstrated.

Renal anomalies

The hypoechogenic anatomy of the kidneys allows renal abnormalities to be discerned in detail on ultrasound by 20 weeks of gestation. Agenesis and cystic dysplasia can be detected. Obstructive lesions of the uterovesical junction

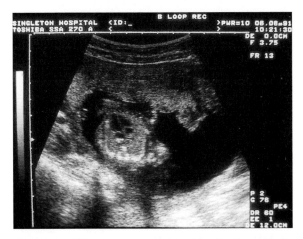

Figure 6.22 Ultrasound image of the four chambers of a normal fetal heart at 24 weeks of gestation.

(megaloureters) can be seen, and may be associated with pulmonary hypoplasia. One of the commonest abnormalities seen on ultrasound is renal pelvic dilatation following functional ureteropelvic junction derangement, preventing the initiation of ureteric peristalsis. Treatment is surgical after delivery at a hospital with paediatric urology facilities. Some obstructive lesions used to be shunted into the amniotic cavity by intrauterine placement of plastic stents, but these are being done less frequently because there are so often multiple lesions present.

All these abnormalities are mostly detected later on in pregnancy. One used to request an ultrasound scan at 14–16 weeks of gestation to obtain a baseline biparietal diameter measurement, but this is too soon for some anomalies to show; hence a second scan was done at about 20 weeks with specially trained ultrasonographers and machinery. Now some health authorities are trying to perform the booking scan and the special anomaly scan at the same time, at 18–20 weeks of gestation.

RECOMMENDED READING

Beck F, Moffart D, Davies D 1985 Human embryology. Blackwell, Oxford

Enkim M, Keirse M, Refrew M, Neilson J 1995 A guide to effective care in pregnancy and childbirth. Oxford University Press, Oxford

Moore K L 1988 The developing human, clinically orientated embryology. WB Saunders, Philadelphia

RCOG 1997 Report of the working party on ultrasound screening for congenital abnormalities. Royal College of Obstetricians and Gynaecologists, London

Abnormal pregnancy

ABNORMAL CONDITIONS OF PREGNANCY

Vaginal bleeding in early pregnancy

Loss of vaginal blood in pregnancy is a dramatic sign which will drive the woman to a doctor swiftly. The commonest diagnosed cause is a miscarriage, but a few are due to other causes. If no cause is found, such bleeding is called a *threatened miscarriage*; a diagnosis not just of exclusion but of ignorance. Doctors and patients like to feel that diagnosis has been made, but this is not so. It is only another way of describing a symptom; further, some feel that treatment must then be offered and yet there is no scientific background for the effectiveness of this.

Ectopic pregnancy

An embryo which implants outside the cavity of the uterus and goes on developing is an ectopic pregnancy. Most of these are in the fallopian tube, commonly in the outer ampullary end (Fig. 7.1).

If the ectopic pregnancy *ruptures*, there is sudden acute abdominal pain. Should the ectopic pregnancy be at the isthmial (medial) end of the tube there is less room for expansion, so the pain is very sudden and may be associated with rupture at 6–8 weeks of gestation. This is often associated with mild vaginal bleeding. On examination the woman may be shocked, with a rigid abdomen and too tender a pelvis to be assessed vaginally. The best treatment is to provide blood to resuscitate and to operate to

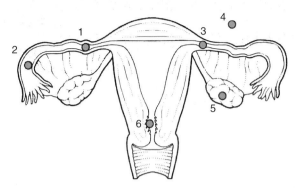

Figure 7.1 Potential sites for an ectopic pregnancy: 1, isthmial end of the oviduct; 2, ampullary end of the oviduct (1 and 2 are the most common sites); 3, cornual; 4, peritoneal; 5, ovary; 6, cervical canal.

control the bleeding area. One cannot await the full correction of the shocked state before the start of the surgery, but once the haemostasis is secured the woman gets better swiftly.

A *leaking* ectopic pregnancy may have implanted in the wider lateral ampullary end of the tube, where it can stretch more. Hence the less severe symptoms are recognized later at 8–10 weeks of gestation. A little blood may leak out of the lateral end of the tube to cause more chronic pain by irritating the pouch of Douglas. There are dull vaguely localized pains and, on examination, the uterus is tender, sometimes with an ill-defined mass behind it.

Investigations. The human chorionic gonadotrophin (hCG) levels are raised, and ultrasound shows an empty uterus sometimes with a thickened decidua. There may be fluid in the pouch of Douglas, and usually one cannot actually see the ectopic gestation sac.

Management. The management involves removal of the ectopic pregnancy tissue, and haemostasis at the site of the bleeding. This may be done via a laparoscope with an antimesenteric 2 cm longitudinal incision made in the tube to remove the ectopic pregnancy; the incision can be closed with fine sutures, but seems to close anyway. In extreme cases or with heavy blood loss, partial salpingectomy may be needed, leaving the medial end of the tube for potential future tubal surgery, often with the idea of more psychological benefit than physiological. The

embryo can be killed with laparoscopic injection of a cytotoxic drug (methotrexate) into the bulb of the ectopic pregnancy directly. Absorption of the embryonic trophoblast tissue follows. Alternatively, the injection can be given intramuscularly at a dose of 1 mg/kg. Careful monitoring with repeated β-hCG levels is necessary.

Hydatidiform mole

This is a benign tumour of the trophoblast, which if malignant becomes a chorionepithelioma.

Cause. The absence of core blood vessels in the villi allows no exchange of the oxygen and nutrients, and the embryo dies. In order to survive, the villi then become swollen and distended to provide a larger surface area. To the naked eye it may resemble a small bunch of immature grapes.

Clinical features. The woman has been feeling unwell with excessive sickness, and may have some vague lower abdominal cramping pain. She usually bleeds as the first obvious symptom; very occasionally vesicles are passed.

If detected after 14 weeks of gestation, the uterus is usually larger than expected. There is no fetal heart beat detected, and there may be bilateral ovarian luteal cysts. The blood pressure is occasionally raised.

Investigations. Ultrasound usually makes the diagnosis, with multiple cysts which look like sunlight shining through the foam on top of the washing up water (Fig. 7.2). The snowstorm effect often talked about is seen with the older B scanners. β-hCG levels rise well above those of normal pregnancy.

Management. The urgent treatment of hydatidiform mole is to minimize blood loss and evacuate pathological tissue. The woman needs to be admitted to hospital, where any excessive blood loss must be corrected. Under general anaesthetic, the uterine contents should be removed by vacuum extraction. An oxytocin infusion should be continued until the woman's uterus stays firm and there is no further bleeding.

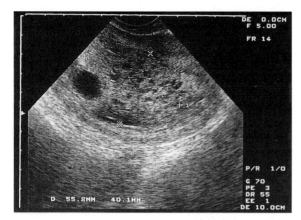

Figure 7.2 Reactive ultrasound of hydatidiform mole. Note the image is more of bubbles than the old snowstorm which was shown with B seam ultrasound.

The evacuated molar specimen should be examined histologically to exclude malignant change, and follow-up should be performed using hCG levels in urine, working in conjunction with one of the Regional Centres for Trophoblast Disease (Weston Park Hospital in Sheffield, Charing Cross Hospital in London or at Ninewells Hospital in Dundee). About 10% of women may continue to have raised hCG levels, so good follow-up is very important. If the levels of hCG reduce, the woman should still be continued with urinary hCG checks for 6 months in case of later recurrence. After this time, and if levels are normal, conception may be attempted. If hCG levels are not reduced by 6 weeks, treatment with methotrexate and actinomycin D is needed. Contraception is required during this time, oral contraceptives and IUCDs being contraindicated.

Local causes of bleeding

Anything that breaks the surface epithelium may cause bleeding in pregnancy. Sometimes *extreme infection*, particularly with candidiasis, causes spotting. A *cervical polyp* can cause scanty bleeding, and should be left alone. *Cervical ectopy* can cause spotting, and is also best left alone.

Varicose veins of the vulva can cause heavier bleeding, requiring continuous pressure to the varicose area. Surgical ligation is very difficult in pregnancy.

Carcinoma of the cervix is rare but an important cause of bleeding. If diagnosed before 16 weeks of gestation, a hysterotomy and immediate Wertheim hysterectomy should be performed, followed by irradiation. If the diagnosis is not made until after 28 weeks of gestation, the woman may wish to proceed for a few weeks longer to attain greater fetal respiratory maturity, then a caesarean Wertheim hysterectomy should be performed, followed by irradiation. By waiting, a live baby may result. This line of treatment needs very careful explanation and a full record in the notes. A frank assessment with the mother and her family is essential since, in the event of an unhappy result, the delay may be criticized later at a legal enquiry.

Vaginal bleeding in late pregnancy

Bleeding from the genital tract after the 24th week of pregnancy and before the onset of labour is defined as *antepartum haemorrhage*. Many such bleeds are not serious, but anxiety will bring the woman to the doctor very smartly.

The distribution of causes of antepartum haemorrhage are shown in Table 7.1.

Table 7.1 Maternal causes of antepartum haemorrhage

Cause	Frequency (%)
Abruption of placenta	35
Placenta praevia	30
Local causes	5
Blood dyscrasias	<1
No cause found	~30

Abruption of the placenta

Separation from the placental bed of a normal-sited placenta is an abruption. Antenatally the diagnosis is usually made clinically, but it may be retrospective, when a firm, attached clot is found adherent to the maternal surface of the placenta after delivery.

Cause. Usually the cause is not known. A small number of abruptions may be associated with:

- Overstretched uterus as in twins
- Trauma – external cephalic version.

Associated factors are:

- Proteinuric hypertension
- Multiparity (a fourth pregnancy has a fourfold risk compared with a first pregnancy)
- Previous placental abruption (increases risk twofold)
- Raised α-fetoprotein level in early pregnancy with no obvious fetal cause.

Clinical course. This depends on the extent of the abruption. Pain is usually the presenting symptom, and sometimes there is vaginal bleeding if blood from a revealed abruption trickles down between the membranes and decidua, through the cervix and vagina. Other symptoms depend on the degree of the retro-placental bleeding. The uterus is often in tonic contraction, so that fetal parts cannot be felt. In severe abruption, the fetus is dead so no fetal heart may be detected.

As well as fetal death, a severe abruption can cause the woman to go into shock due to the stretch and damage of the myometrial tissue rather than actual loss of blood from the circulation. This could lead to oliguria or anuria. In severe cases, disseminated intravascular coagulopathy (DIC) can follow.

A woman with a moderate to severe abruption is a severe emergency, and needs transport to hospital with either a flying squad or, more likely these days, with the help of paramedics trained in resuscitation. On arrival in hospital, 4–6 units of blood are cross-matched, and two large-bore intravenous cannulae inserted to allow rapid access to the vascular system. If the fetus is alive, a caesarean section may be performed to save the baby's life should gestation be far enough advanced. Ample fluid replacement is needed, for which blood is the best. An indwelling urinary catheter is commonly inserted to measure urinary output and thereby renal function.

If the fetus is dead, the woman may proceed to swift vaginal delivery. If not already in labour, the membranes should be ruptured to speed things along. Epidural analgesia is not generally used because of the possibility of coagulopathy. If this happens, the haematology unit must be involved promptly and at a senior level. Clotting tests are performed on the blood. Fresh frozen plasma is often needed in the management, and must be available to be used as advised by the consultant haematologist. Once the uterus is empty any DIC improves rapidly.

Placenta praevia

When the placenta is implanted totally or partially in the lower segment of the uterus, it is designated placenta praevia – before the fetus (Fig. 7.3). The lower segment is that thinner part of the uterus between the myometrium proper and the cervix. At term, it is a few millimetres thick, compared with a couple of centimetres in the upper segment. During later pregnancy and labour, the lower segment plays little part in uterine contractions but instead stretches passively. Any placenta implanted here peels off, and the separation is accompanied by maternal bleeding, which trickles through the cervical canal and is soon seen. Low placental implantation occurs more commonly in multiple pregnancies, and in women with a scar on the lower segment from a previous caesarean section.

Clinical course. The woman will have recurrent bright red bleeding without pain. The fetus is not usually compromised at first. The woman is usually not shocked, and examination shows a soft uterus with fetal parts easily felt, often a high head or malpresentation, and the fetal heart is easily heard – all different from the state after a placental abruption. No attempt at pelvic bimanual examination should be made, for, if the placenta is low and already separating, such manipulation can stimulate heavy bleeding. Ultrasound shows the low-lying placenta, so confirming the diagnosis. In some cases, the 20 week anomaly scan may show a low implanted placenta. This will not of necessity be a placenta praevia later, for in most cases that

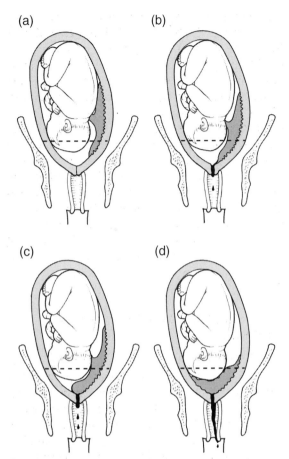

(a) (b)

(c) (d)

Figure 7.3 The four classical grades of placenta praevia: **a** grade I, placenta in lower segment but does not reach cervical os; **b** grade II, placenta reaches the cervical os but does not cover it; **c** grade III, placenta covers cervical os in pregnancy but not once it is dilating; **d** grade IV, placenta implanted centrally over cervical os. Since no clinician awaits the differentiation of grades III and IV, the words 'marginal', 'lateral' and 'central' are a better working classification. The uterine lower segment is below the dotted line.

placenta and its bed are pulled up due to differential growth of the uterus, and by the last weeks it is into the upper segment. Repeat ultrasound at 32 weeks of gestation and cautious observation without worrying the mother are needed.

If severe bleeding were to continue, a caesarean section must be done, but usually there is none, or only slight and intermittent blood loss. The woman should generally be admitted to hospital in case of repeat heavy

bleeding, and two units of blood kept cross-matched for her. When she approaches 37–38 weeks of gestation, a decision about delivery is made. Most will require an elective caesarean section performed by a senior obstetrician. Bleeding can be very heavy at operation, for an anteriorly sited placenta praevia is right under the entry incision to the uterus. Placental separation can be difficult, and as the placental bed is over the less contractile lower segment the woman may bleed heavily after placental removal. The placenta may grow into the old scar (placenta accreta) and prevent separation. Bleeding may be sufficiently heavy to warrant hysterectomy.

Sometimes if the placental encroachment into the lower segment is anterior and of a lesser degree, a carefully monitored vaginal delivery can be allowed. Usually the fetal head comes down and compresses the lowest area of the placenta against the symphysis pubis, so preventing blood loss. This does not apply to a posterior placenta praevia, for the distance from the descending fetal head to the mother's sacrum is far too great and occupied with soft tissue such as the rectum.

The prognosis for mother and baby has improved greatly in recent decades, with delayed delivery and wider use of blood transfusion for the less controlled cases.

Bleeding from fetal vessels

Occasionally the umbilical vessels run into the membranes some distance from the placenta (squash racquet placenta). On other occasions, there is an isolated cotyledon of placenta (succinturate placenta) serviced by blood vessels running in the membranes. In either of these circumstances, the unsupported vessels may by chance be over the internal os of the cervix (vasa praevia). Damage to these at membrane rupture may lead to slight vaginal bleeding. This more usually happens in labour than in the ante-partum period. Although the blood loss is not great, it is fetal blood coming from a much smaller circulation. The fetus can stand the loss less well than a similar volume of blood loss from the mother.

There may be alteration of the fetal heart rate, and Doppler ultrasound cardiotocography can indicate sudden fetal hypoxia. Any blood that is still present in the vagina can be checked for fetal haemoglobin, which is more resistant to acid reduction.

If the fetus is still alive and of sufficient gestational maturity, it is wise to deliver by caesarean section straight away rather than await another fetal bleed, which could prove fatal.

Local causes of bleeding

Whilst in early pregnancy, bleeding of unknown origin is described by the evasive phrase 'threatened miscarriage', and after 24 weeks of gestation this is labelled antepartum haemorrhage, but it may also be due to local causes. All the local causes of bleeding in early pregnancy must still be considered – infection, polyp, ectopy, varicose veins and cervical carcinoma. In addition, in later pregnancy the cause may be:

- Rupture of a *marginal sinus*. Sometimes a vein running around the edge of the placenta may rupture with a single episode of bleeding.
- *Cervical shortening*. In late pregnancy the cervix is pulled up, sometimes causing a shearing off of the membranes in the lower segment. A little bleeding follows, and this is difficult to diagnose. Often obstetricians will treat the woman as though she has placenta praevia until ultrasound localizes that organ in the upper segment.
- *Blood dyscrasias*. These are a very rare cause of vaginal bleeding at the end of pregnancy. Diagnosis rests on haematological examination of a blood film; Hodgkin's disease or leukaemia have been found. Their management depends on the causal disease, usually after delivery.

Antepartum haemorrhage of unknown origin. In retrospect, this group, comprising about a third of antepartum haemorrhages, can be assigned a diagnosis by careful examination of the placenta. There may be a ruptured marginal sinus or asymptomate abruptio placenta.

Although no diagnosis is made in pregnancy at the time of the bleed, most clinicians will treat the woman in whom they can find no cause for the bleeding very carefully. The maternal mortality rate is low but that of the fetus is higher, equal to that of abruption in some populations. The woman is admitted; and blood taken for grouping and saving of the serum. If ultrasound scanning fails to reveal a placenta praevia or evidence of abruption (as is most often the case), a gentle speculum examination is undertaken to exclude a local cause. If no cause is found, fetal growth should be monitored (for it often is retarded) and a planned delivery undertaken.

With increasing and more skilled use of ultrasound, this group of unknown causes for antepartum haemorrhages is reducing.

Pre-eclampsia and hypertensive diseases

This former term is time honoured in obstetrics but more recent classifications have produced a more logical scheme, which is shown in Box 7.1.

The older use of the triad of hypertension, proteinuria and oedema as the stigmata of pre-eclampsia (PE) is now not used, for oedema is a poor predictor, occurring in many women in pregnancy who have no pathological problems.

About 10% of the UK antenatal population will develop hypertension, about half of which will have PE. The condition occurs almost entirely in primigravidae or those having the first pregnancy with a new partner.

Box 7.1 Definitions of hypertensive disease in pregnancy

- Pregnancy-induced hypertension (PIH)
  Raised blood pressure occurring for the first time after 20 weeks gestation
- Pregnancy-associated hypertension (PAH)
  Raised blood pressure found before pregnancy or in the first 20 weeks
- Pre-eclampsia (PE)
  PIH in association with proteinuria of pregnancy

Cause

The cause of pregnancy-induced hypertension or of pre-eclampsia is not known, but Figure 7.4 gives a hypothesis. Many consider the failure of trophoblast invasion in early pregnancy is a precipitating factor, but this probably has some immunological background yet to be elucidated. In turn, a genetic cause might be responsible for triggering the whole process.

Clinical course

The rise of blood pressure is the first noted sign, and this is the raison d'être for routine antenatal care. Long afternoons in the antenatal clinic spent taking many blood pressures are worth it, for this screening test will pick up the early

stages of pregnancy-induced hypertension (PIH). As the process gets worse, symptoms may follow – a headache and visual disturbances; even more severe PIH is associated with increased reflexes (due to cerebral oedema) and epigastric pain (due to stretch of the liver capsule and to subcapsular haemorrhage).

Management

The control of PIH and PE depend upon the stage at which each is diagnosed. Early management includes extra rest either at home or, if that is impossible, in hospital (where real rest is a hard thing to achieve). The ultimate treatment is delivery, but this must await the clinician's assessment that the fetus is viable, i.e. the risks

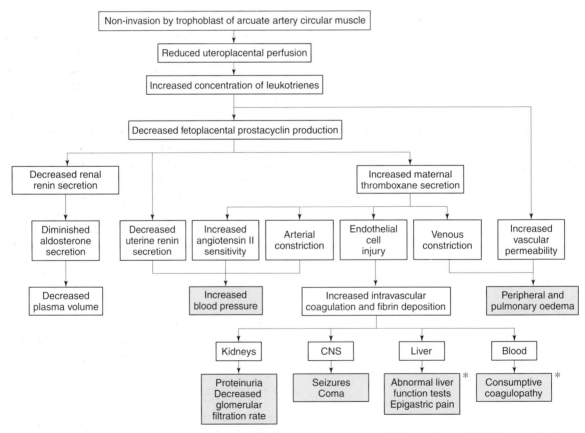

Figure 7.4 A possible aetiology of the clinical signs (tinted boxes) of PE and the HELPP syndrome (*) (CNS, central nervous system).

to the baby of being outside the uterus are less than those of continuing inside. Serial plasma urate levels are helpful in predicting deterioration, but, with their wide normal ranges, platelet counts are less so, although very low levels are prognostic.

Various pharmacological agents have been used. Aspirin and calcium supplements have been found *not to be* helpful. Acute rises in blood pressure are controlled by hydralazine, while the more chronic ones are treated with atenolol, labetalol (both β blockers) and methyldopa. The value of magnesium sulphate in the control of culminating PE is now being realized in the UK; this has been used in the rest of the world for many years but had been neglected by UK obstetricians. It is most helpful and has fewer deleterious side-effects.

Delivery of the fetus by the most expeditious route is the ultimate treatment of PIH. If the cervix is ripe and the fetus is mature and in good position, induction and a controlled labour is best. If there is difficulty in reducing the woman's blood pressure or in the presence of any other major complications, a caesarean section should be performed.

Any fetus in a mother with PIH is at increased risk. Depending upon the severity of the condition and the stage of gestation, increased monitoring should be carried out. This should include:

- Daily fetal movement charts
- Daily cardiotocography
- Weekly examination of the umbilical Doppler ultrasound pattern
- Weekly ultrasound measurements of the abdominal circumference to assess fetal growth.

A severe form of PE has been designated the HELLP syndrome. Indeed, some wish to change the term pre-eclampsia and to the pre-HELLP syndrome.

The HELLP syndrome

More recently it has been recognized that PE is characterized not just by its clinical symptoms but its biochemical and haematological ones. The combination of *Haemolysis, Elevated Liver* function and *Low Platelets* makes up the HELLP syndrome, which sometimes occurs before the clinical manifestations of fulminating PE.

Care should be taken to use normal ranges of liver function tests produced for pregnant women, as the ranges used by most laboratories include males and females of all ages, and thus the effects of age and pregnancy on the results are excluded. The basic tests to use are bilirubin with either aspartate transaminase or alanine transaminase.

The management of the HELLP syndrome is a modification of the liver dysfunction and correction of the platelet defects, combined with the treatment of fulminating PE as described previously.

Eclampsia

Fits in association with hypertension were one of the first antenatal pathological states to be recognized at the end of the last century; antenatal care started in an attempt at their prevention.

Actual fitting in pregnancy is rare in the UK, for antenatal care detects and treats many women with potential eclampsia. Still, women can fit, particularly in the early third trimester, having had a perfectly normal blood pressure measured at an antenatal clinic visit a few days before. Probably less than 0.1% of women in the UK who have moderate to severe PIH will develop eclampsia, so the incidence is about 1:2000 pregnancies.

Cause

There is cerebral oedema with a concomitant vasoconstriction leading to localized cerebral ischaemia which can trigger off signals to fit.

Clinical course

The onset of eclamptic fits is divided equally between the antenatal intrapartum and postpartum periods. The fit is similar to an epileptic fit, with tonic and clonic phases followed by a coma. The fits may be repeated frequently, and this is a seriously bad prognostic sign.

Management

The management of a woman having an eclamptic fit is to keep her alive during that fit by turning her on her side, maintaining an airway and stopping the inhalation of vomit. This is combined with stopping the fit with intravenous diazepam, often hard to give whilst the woman is fitting, but, with a little assistance, venous access can usually be found. The next aim is to prevent more fits, and in this magnesium sulphate is probably the best drug, although diazepam and phenytoin are still being used. The woman should be transferred to hospital as an emergency, with anticonvulsants such as phenytoin given during the transfer, if magnesium sulphate is not used. Arrival at hospital allows a rapid delivery of the baby by the most expeditious route. If vaginal delivery seems likely because of a ripe cervix, this should be performed; if not, a caesarean section is needed.

Often a woman may have only one or a few fits. If she is early in pregnancy and the fetus is immature, obstetricians may decide to wait a week or two. This is sitting on a powder barrel, as she may fit again. It must be realized that fetal growth is not as good as normal in such cases, so the increase in maturation of the fetus might not be all that is hoped for by this delaying tactic.

Blood group incompatibility

Rhesus incompatibility used to be a major problem, but with its startling reduction, following Anti-D prophylaxis other ABO blood group incompatibilities are becoming relatively more important, although there is no evidence of an increase in actual numbers.

Rhesus incompatibility

Rhesus genes are found in 15% of the female population in the UK. The mother may have been immunized by blood transfusions of an incorrect rhesus group, but this is rare in the Western world, although it can still take place in developing countries.

The commonest method of sensitization is for the red cells of a rhesus-positive fetus to pass across the placenta during pregnancy, or during the third stage of labour. This can occur at miscarriage, ectopia, abruption, amniocentesis or an external cephalic version. Since the commonest immunizing stimulus is at separation of the placenta, obviously antibodies will not be generated in that pregnancy, and the baby usually escapes without any effect. Subsequent pregnancies, however, allow an accelerated response in a sensitized woman, and so the fetus may well be affected. Antibodies return across the placenta to the fetus, breaking down fetal red cells, which leads to anaemia and, after birth, to hyperbilirubinaemia. This used to lead to a grossly anaemic and oedematous fetus who might die of heart failure. Other major sequelae used to be kernicterus, where the basal nuclei of the brain were deeply stained with bile products, leading to an atharoid state. Thirty years ago up to a third of the young children in the mental institutions in the UK were there because of a neurological rhesus-caused problem.

All this has changed with Anti-D IgG routine prophylaxis. At all deliveries of a rhesus positive baby to a rhesus negative mother feto-maternal haemorrhage may occur. This may also have happened at a therapeutic abortion, a spontaneous miscarriage or an ectopic pregnancy. Whatever the clinical cause, the mother is given 500 i.u. of Anti-D IgG within 72 hours (and more if the Kleihaur test indicates a larger fetal infusion). Now that Anti-D IgG is more readily available many obstetricians are changing to antenatal prophylaxis for all Rh negative women. They are given 500 i.u. at 28 weeks, the same dose at 34 weeks and again after delivery. This is a more expensive regime but is claimed to be more effective (Joint Working Group RCPE/RCOG 1998).

Management. All women should have their rhesus status checked at booking. If negative, antibody levels should be checked. The latter should be repeated in midpregnancy, and if the level is rising they should be under the care of a specialist rhesus unit. Too few of us see rhesus disease these days to allow the luxury of looking after the rhesus affected in peripheral hospitals. If the antibody levels go on rising, amniocentesis allows amniotic fluid to be examined for levels of bilirubin products by absorption curves. Levels at which action is recommended become lower as the pregnancy goes on. In most specialized centres the haemoglobin level is now checked by direct intrauterine sampling from the umbilical cord, and if below certain levels, treatment is offered. This used to be intra-peritoneal transfusion of rhesus-negative blood, for this was easily absorbed by diapodesis across the fetal peritoneal membranes. Now most people perform intrauterine exchange transfusion directly into the fetal intravascular compartment by cannulating the umbilical vein in the uterus. This may need to be repeated, and delivery can be expedited when the baby is considered mature enough.

Once born, the baby is checked for blood group, rhesus antibodies, haemoglobin, and bilirubin, and a direct Coombe's test is per-formed. The arrival of new antibodies will obviously stop at birth, but the old antibodies already transferred across the placenta and the bilirubin are still leaching out of the tissue fluids, and so the rhesus effect can continue for a limited time after delivery. This is usually dealt with by exchange transfusion to wash out the affected fetal blood, if necessary repeating the procedure.

Other blood group incompatibilities

About 20% of pregnancies have an incom-patibility between maternal and fetal ABO blood groups, but only 5% of these (i.e. 1% of all) have signs of haemolytic disease. Anti-A and anti-B antibodies do not pass across the placenta easily while there is a wider distribution of A and B factors through the tissues of the fetus, which absorb anti-A and anti-B antibodies thus protecting the fetal red cells. The diagnosis is commonly not made until after delivery, when jaundice develops in babies of mothers who are group O with a baby who is group A or B. There is no specific test of compatibility as there is in the rhesus effect. Rarely is the disease severe enough to require exchange transfusion, and phototherapy is usually sufficient.

Rarer blood groups can cause incompatibility, e.g. Kell. The diagnosis is confirmed on serological grouping of the mother's and father's blood, checking for antibodies in early preg-nancy. The treatment can be by exchange transfusion of a suitable donor blood, but top-up transfusions usually suffice.

Abnormal production of amniotic fluid

The amniotic fluid is made by the entire amnion with a contribution from the fetus. In early preg-nancy there is a transudate across the un-cornified fetal skin which ceases after 20 weeks of gestation and an increasing amount of amniotic fluid is formed from the fetal urine to increase the amniotic fluid volume. The range of normal values of amniotic fluid present varies greatly throughout the pregnancy. By term between 500 and 1300 ml is present. However, too much or too little amniotic can be produced.

Polyhydramnios

An excess of amniotic fluid can be easily detected clinically. The uterus is too round, and the fetus cannot be easily palpated. Ultrasound may confirm the excess fluid, and a semi-quantitative measure can be made by finding the largest diameter (column) of a pool of amniotic fluid. Columns above 8 cm are diagnostic (Fig. 7.5). A full fetal ultrasound examination should be performed to exclude twins or structural abnormality.

Polyhydramnios may be associated with maternal diabetes, fetal abnormality, particularly oesophageal atresia, and monozygotic twins.

Clinical course. The woman may present with pain due to the tense, stretched uterus between 30 and 36 weeks of gestation. Otherwise, poly-hydramnios is noted at antenatal clinic examination.

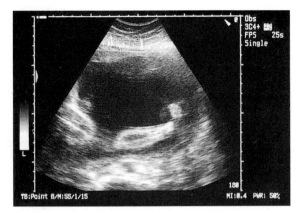

Figure 7.5   Ultrasound scan showing polyhydramnios.

Management. Bed rest works well, but diuretics are not helpful. If the excess fluid is causing symptoms, slow amniocentesis may help. Indomethacine may also be of use.

Oligohydramnios

The lack of amniotic fluid is much rarer than polyhydramnios. Oligohydramnios is associated with abnormalities of the genito-urinary tract, small for gestational age fetuses, fetal abnormality or premature rupture of the membranes.

Clinical course. The woman usually has no symptoms or signs. Oligohydramnios may be detected by the clinician who finds the uterus too full of fetus – one can feel elbows, knees and even hands, which is unusual. Ultrasound will show a lack of fluid, a column of 2 cm or less being considered diagnostic.

Cause. Oligohydramnios is often associated with renal agenesis with adhesions in the fetal skin to the amnion and intrauterine growth retardation. There is a higher rate of limb abnormalities, and congenital dislocation of the hip and talipes, possibly due to pressure.

Management. Often oligohydramnios is associated with the signs of fetal malperfusion. After renal abnormalities have been excluded, an expedited delivery may be helpful if a mature enough stage of gestation is reached.

SYSTEMIC DISEASES IN PREGNANCY

In the UK, young women who get pregnant are usually fit, but a few have long-standing illnesses which may worsen in pregnancy or might affect the progress of pregnancy. Further, the treatments given for these diseases could also have some effect on the fetus or the progress of pregnancy, and might need to be modified. For the needs of this book only a brief account of each disease condition will be given to enable the reader to relate pregnancy and the disease. It is important to know how pregnancy may affect progress of the disease and how the disease could affect pregnancy. For further details of the diseases, readers are referred to the recommended reading at the end of the chapter.

Heart disease

Cause

In the UK, just under half of heart disease seen in pregnancy is still rheumatic in origin, with a mitral valve being the most affected. Congenital defects of the septum and reverse shunts make up about 40%.

Clinical features

These will depend on the exact cardiac lesion. With left-sided disease such as mitral stenosis, damming back may cause pulmonary oedema, and right-sided congestive failure may occur.

With aortic stenosis, left-sided congestive failure could follow, but this is rare during pregnancy.

With congenital abnormalities, the right-to-left shunt is the more dangerous of the two, producing gross symptoms of breathlessness on even slight exertion.

The appropriate signs for the lesion will be found on examination.

Investigations

The woman should be checked with a chest radiograph, an electrocardiogram and an echocardiogram. In some cases, catheter studies may be required for pressure and blood gases.

Management

In pregnancy, extra loads to the heart should be avoided. Flare-ups of rheumatic fever can occur which may lead to arrhythmia; PE with its attendant hypertension means harder work to pump the blood around the body. Anaemia involves circulating more dilute blood, which is inefficient. Potentially infective procedures such as dental extraction may lead to acute bacterial endocarditis. Women should be seen by a senior cardiologist and an obstetrician throughout pregnancy. Anaesthetists and paediatricians should be involved towards the end of pregnancy to help make plans for labour.

In labour the onset of congestive failure should be prevented. Sit the woman with her head high, and go for a short second stage, which may be assisted with forceps or a vacuum extraction. Do not use syntometrine unless absolutely essential, and be ready to manage pulmonary oedema, which may occur immediately after delivery. A litre of blood can suddenly be shunted into the inferior vena cava from the uterine veins constricted by sustained uterine muscle contraction.

Asthma

Bronchospasm usually starts in youth or teenage, and may well be under treatment by the time the woman becomes pregnant. There is nothing about pregnancy that causes it to deteriorate; indeed, many women with asthma are actually better in association with the higher circulating corticosteroid levels.

Clinical course

This is the same as in non-pregnant women, with a shortage of breath, with especial difficulty in the expiratory phase. There may be signs of rhonchi in the chest. The lower lung on each side is less aerated as pregnancy goes on, and so signs are best elicited from the upper lobes.

Investigations

These women should be seen by a chest physician with knowledge of pregnancy who may order flow studies as well as gas studies. Chest radiographs of women not in an acute attack are not very helpful.

Management

Bronchial antispasmodics should be continued, and antibiotics added if required. Steroids are rarely required for the first time in pregnancy, for the cortisol level is raised naturally.

Prognosis

Pregnancy does not usually affect the bronchial condition, but the baby may be small if the control of the mother's asthma is not good.

Anaemia

Anaemia follows a reduction in the haemoglobin level in the blood, so providing a poorer circulation of oxygen to the tissues. It is often associated with malnutrition in those from developing countries.

Cause

Anaemia may be:

- *Haemorrhagic* due to blood loss
- *Haemolytic* due to increased breakdown of red cells
- *Haemopoietic*, following the poor production of red blood cells.

Most anaemias associated with pregnancy are haemopoietic due to a lack of iron or folate, usually following dietary deficiency. Lack of iron usually leads to a microcytic anaemia, while folate lack causes a megaloblastic pattern.

The normal values of various blood levels in pregnancy are given in Table 7.2.

Table 7.2 Normal haematological values in pregnancy

Blood test	Normal range
Total blood volume (ml)	4000–6000
Red cell volume (ml)	1500–1800
Red cell count (10^{12}/l)	4–5
White cell count (10^9/l)	8–18
Haemoglobin (g/dl)	10.5–13.5
Mean corpuscular volume (fl)	80–95
Mean corpuscular haemoglobin (µg)	32–36
Serum iron (µmol/l)	11–25
Serum folate (µg/l)	6–9
Serum ferritin (µg/l)	10–200

Box 7.2 Iron- and folate-rich foods

- Animal sources:
  - red meat (iron from the haemoglobin and myoglobin)
  - white meat (iron from the myoglobin)
  - fish (iron from the myoglobin)
- Plant sources:
  - breakfast cereals (rich in folate)
  - lentils and beans (moderate amount of iron but rich in folate)
  - dark-green leaf vegetables (rich in folate)

Clinical features

Severe anaemia can be associated with tiredness, but this is a common symptom in pregnancy for other reasons. The woman may look pale, particularly the conjunctiva of the eyes and the palms of her hands.

Investigations

A haemoglobin level and a blood film examination usually give the answer. In *iron deficiency anaemia*, the haemoglobin level is reduced below 10 g/dl, and the mean corpuscular haemoglobin level is also reduced. The serum iron and serum ferritin levels are low if the anaemia has been present long enough. Blood cells may be hypochromatic.

In *megaloblastic anaemia*, the blood cells may appear normal, although often there is some poikilocytosis and occasionally nuclear cells. White cells may show hypersegmentation of the nuclei. The haemoglobin level can be greatly reduced, but the mean corpuscular volume and corpuscular haemoglobin levels are not lowered and may be increased. Serum folate levels will be reduced, as may be the serum iron level. Occasionally a marrow sample from the iliac crest is required to show megaloblasts, for one cannot rely upon macrocytes being present in the peripheral blood.

Management

Ensure that the woman is taking sufficient iron- and folate-rich foods (Box 7.2).

Ensure that the woman is taking prophylactic iron tablets. If she cannot swallow tablets, use a liquid preparation. If all forms of oral iron are precluded, give it parenterally:

- Iron sorbitol (Jectofer) given intravenously or intramuscularly on alternate days
- Iron dextran (Imferon) given intramuscularly on alternate days after a test dose of 50 mg.

If a woman is in the last weeks of pregnancy and has a haemoglobin level below 7 g/dl, she should have a blood transfusion before labour, for her bone marrow would need 4–5 weeks to correct an anaemia of this degree.

Folic acid anaemia should be prevented by folate supplements and treated with folic acid 5–10 mg daily orally. If the anaemia is severe, then blood transfusion may be required.

Progress

If neglected, anaemia becomes worse, and if the woman then has a heavy blood loss at delivery, she will be at higher risk of death. Additionally, an anaemic woman embarking on baby care after delivery is chronically fatigued and at risk of intercurrent illness.

Prognosis

The prognosis is usually very good with appropriate treatment.

Thalassaemia

Cause

Thalassaemia is due to defective formation of haemoglobin side-chains. It may be

- *Homozygous* – thalassaemia major – which is usually fatal in youth, and the woman seldom reaches sexual maturity.
- *Heterozygous* – thalassaemia minor – in which the β chain form is more serious.

Symptoms

If very severe, there may be pain in the bones or in the abdomen. Women presenting with this disease used to come predominantly from Mediterranean countries, but with the widespread changes of population they can now be from any part of the world. The anaemia is usually mild.

Investigations

Electrophoresis will detect the abnormal haemoglobins.

Management

Iron levels are kept high to prevent a severe anaemia, but there are usually adequate iron stores. Haemolytic crises and stresses should be covered. Delivery between crises is aimed at.

Progress

Thalassaemia often worsens. The reader is directed to the recommended reading list for haematology intricacies.

Prognosis

The prognosis is poor in the long run but good in pregnancy.

Haemoglobinopathies

Cause

Defective genes affect the side-chains of the haemoglobin molecule in the haemoglobinopathies. The red cell envelope is also defective, allowing easier and earlier breakdown of cells, so releasing haemoglobin into the serum. There are many abnormal haemoglobins, the commonest being found in the Middle East, Africa, and southern Europe. Sickle cell disease is one of the more common.

Clinical features

There may be an infarct causing sudden pain in the chest or abdomen but there are usually few signs.

Investigations

The haemoglobin level is low; the blood film may show target cells with polychromatophilia. A haemoglobin electrophoresis will make the diagnosis.

Management

Hypoxia and dehydration should be prevented, and folate given prophylactically at a dose of 1–2 mg/day.

If the haemoglobin level drops sharply, packed red cells with a fast acting diuretic are provided simultaneously. If a red cell breakdown crisis occurs, heparinize and consider exchange transfusion.

Epilepsy

Cause

The cause of epilepsy is unknown but may be due to local foci in the brain cortex.

Clinical course

Often an epileptic woman on treatment will have consulted her family doctor at a pre-pregnancy appointment in order to discuss the future, and she will have been well warned of what may ensue. A few women have more fits in pregnancy, some have less, but most stay about the same. The antiepileptic drugs can in themselves be a potential hazard, for most are teratogenic. In addition, epileptic women have an inherent increased risk of having babies with malformations, particularly neural tube defects. Should the partner of a woman be an epileptic man, the risk is further increased. To stop all antiepileptic drugs leaves the woman with a greater chance of fitting, and possibly hypoxia associated with the fits could damage the fetus.

Investigations

An electroencephalogram might be even more confusing during pregnancy than in the non-pregnant state.

Management

The dose of established antiepileptic drugs must be considered, and the lowest possible dose of a single antiepileptic drug used. Phenytoin has a slightly lower association with neural tube defects than valproate or carbamazepine. The new antiepileptic drugs lamotrigine and gabapentin work in animals, but their use in humans in pregnancy is yet to be established. The fetus should have ultrasound screening for spina bifida, and extra folate should always be given, for the antiepileptic drugs reduce its absorption. Vitamin K should be given to the baby after delivery.

Prognosis

The progress of the mother's disease is not usually affected by pregnancy. The baby may have abnormalities and has an increased risk of epilepsy, which is higher if both parents are epileptic.

Diabetes mellitus

Cause

Diabetes is a metabolic disease resulting in the underproduction of insulin in the pancreas. Disturbances in the metabolism of carbohydrate,

fat and protein occur, and there can be a sustained rise in the blood glucose level, associated with damage to organs such as the heart, kidney and eye. Diabetes may be:

- Pre-existing
- Gestational – discovered for the first time in pregnancy and disappearing after the baby is born.

Clinical course

An established diabetic woman on balanced management should have no symptoms. An increase in thirst may arise for the first time in pregnancy. Examination usually reveals no abnormalities of the mother, but an established diabetic woman may show an increased growth of the baby and the volume of amniotic fluid as gestation proceeds.

A known diabetic woman should have been to a prepregnancy clinic, where a rigid regime of insulin/glucose balance is instituted, to maintain the blood sugar between 5.6 and 6.7 mmol/l. An Hb A level should be checked after at least 2 months on the above regime, and should be lower than the norm at the local laboratory.

Many antenatal clinics perform routine antenatal screening of blood glucose levels at booking and later in pregnancy.

Once a diabetic woman becomes pregnant she should be seen at a diabetic antenatal clinic by her physician and senior obstetrician together. Normal glycaemia is aimed at; the woman monitors herself with blood sugar sticks at home, and the use of a specialist diabetic unit nurse is helpful in continuing antenatal clinics and overall specialist supervision from very early pregnancy. Insulin requirements usually rise, but fall rapidly after delivery. A watch for urinary tract infection is maintained, and fetal growth is reviewed with ultrasound every few weeks, checking the pattern of growth and the volume of amniotic fluid. In the last trimester, weekly clinic visits are advisable.

Women with nephropathy or retinopathies deteriorate more rapidly, and some may recommend a termination of pregnancy for a woman with such pathology, depending upon its severity.

Complications

Well-controlled women do not of necessity deteriorate, and careful consultation with those expert in this condition in pregnancy should be sought early on to avoid false and worrying advice or treatment being given.

There is an increased incidence of first- and second-trimester miscarriages. In some populations the congenital abnormality rate is raised threefold above the background level. There is an increased risk of hypertension.

Delivery is not usually allowed to go past 40 weeks of gestation, but there is no specific need to intervene at 38 weeks; caesarean section should only be needed on obstetrical grounds, but is done more frequently in diabetic women because of:

- Suspected disproportion
- Failed induction
- Abnormal lie
- Fetal distress in labour.

Labour is covered by intravenous glucose, with intravenous insulin infusions given separately, monitored with the woman's blood sugar levels checked using blood sugar sticks every hour. Those babies with macrosomia have an increased risk of sudden intrauterine death during the last weeks of pregnancy, and the overall perinatal mortality rate can be as much as twice that of the rest of the population unless meticulous control has been maintained.

Associated with the increased risk of macrosomia is birth trauma, including shoulder dystocia and asphyxia. After birth the baby may be hypoglycaemic and hypercalcaemic. Both the respiratory distress syndrome and hypothermia are increased risks. The breakdown of excess red cells in a baby with a diabetic mother may lead to hyperbilirubinaemia in the infant.

Gestational diabetes is diagnosed when abnormal glucose tolerance patterns are discovered for the first time in pregnancy. The immediate risks to the mother are only slightly increased,

Box 7.3   Indications for glucose tolerance tests on suspicion of abnormal glucose metabolism

- Maternal weight over 100 kg
- Previous baby with a birth weight over 4.5 kg
- Diabetes in a first-degree relative
- Glycosuria once before 20 weeks of gestation or twice after 20 weeks
- Previous unexplained stillbirth or neonatal death
- Polyhydramnios
- Random glucose >6.5 mg%
- Ultrasound showing a grossly large baby (over the 90th centile on growth chart)

but for the fetus they are similar to those of established diabetic problems. Indications for glucose tolerance tests are shown in Box 7.3. A number of these women do develop full diabetes later, in the years after pregnancy.

The patterns for abnormal glucose tolerance test are shown in Figure 7.6.

INFECTIONS IN PREGNANCY

Normal young women are no more susceptible to systemic infections in pregnancy than are the non-pregnant. There is superadded maternal and paternal anxiety in case the fetus is affected,

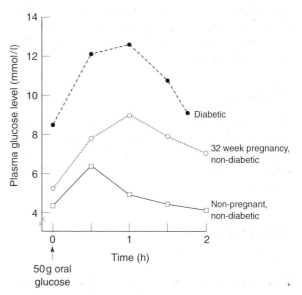

Figure 7.6   Standard tests of glucose tolerance showing full 50 g load with $\frac{1}{2}$ h readings.

as some organisms can cross the placenta and could damage the unborn child even though the maternal infection is mild. In very early pregnancy, non-specific effects of severe infection might cause a miscarriage, and later on, both systemic and local infections may be associated with preterm labour.

In this section, emphasis is placed on the obstetrical aspects of these conditions, and more general facts should be sought from books on infectious diseases and genitourinary medicine.

Systemic diseases

Rubella is a virus infection, usually of little import which most people acquire in their childhood or teens. However, if it occurs in pregnancy the virus can cross the placenta and affect the fetus. It is often a subclinical disease with an incubation period of 12–24 days from contact to the onset of the rash. Hence women may well harbour the virus while being unaware of it. Since the beginning of active immunization of young girls in school, rubella is much less common as a disease during the pregnancy age group.

Fetal infection is most probable, and damage is likely when the virus is present in the first 12 weeks of gestation, leading to cardiac, eye and ear abnormalities. After this time the fetal effect is less likely, though it may be associated with deafness and mental retardation. After 17 weeks of gestation, infection is most unlikely to be linked with abnormality.

The management of the rubella-affected baby is often termination of pregnancy if the parents wish. However, in order to be more certain that the fetus is affected in a mother with rubella, specific rubella IgM in fetal blood can be assessed by fetal blood obtained by cordocentesis after 17 weeks of gestation (Table 7.3).

All women at booking should be tested for rubella antibodies. If these are present, this knowledge can remove the woman's worries during pregnancy, for reinfection is unusual. In the UK about 5% of women only are susceptible. They should all be advised of this, although it is often too late to prevent contact with those with

Table 7.3 Transmission of rubella virus from mother to fetus

Gestation (weeks)	Fetal infection (%)	Fetuses affected (%)	Abnormality
<8	90	Up to 100	Cardiac Eye Ear Neurological
9–12	80	65–85	Cardiac Eye Ear Neurological
13–16	40	35	Deafness Mental retardation
≥17	50	Rare (<1%)	Deafness Mental retardation

rubella by the time the test is done. Women should be advised to have rubella immunization when the pregnancy is over.

Malaria is caused by a protozoan transmitted by female anophelese mosquitoes. It is endemic in most tropical and subtropical areas, and over 100 million cases occur every year. It is the most common infectious disease in the world, and, although not seen in this country among the indigenous population, malaria can arrive here via travellers or those who have been brought up overseas. Although we have known the cause for over 100 years, the incidence of malaria is not declining in the world.

During pregnancy an acute attack may cause a miscarriage or preterm labour due to maternal pyrexia. There is an increased risk of parasitaemia in pregnancy, leading to anaemia and placental infection, where the large surface area of villi allows infected red cells and parasites to attach themselves. The parasites pass across to the fetus, and this may lead to retardation of exchange and so to reduced fetal growth, and hypoxia in labour. In addition to the mechanical blockage the parasites rapidly proliferate and use up oxygen.

Travellers to malarial areas should request geographically specific advice, for the parasites vary in different parts of the world. Malarial reference laboratories can be consulted in

London, Liverpool, Oxford, Birmingham and Glasgow. Generally, maloprin and inefloquinine should be avoided in early pregnancy. Extra folate may be needed.

Congenital malaria is more likely to occur in infants and non-immune women, and may present as fever later in infancy associated with anaemia and hyperbilirubinaemia and jaundice.

Tuberculosis is spread by the anaerobic bacillus *Mycobacteria*. Whilst the disease has become relatively uncommon in the young in the Western world, in Africa and South-East Asia it has a higher prevalence, possibly due to an increasing association with human immuno-deficiency virus (HIV) infection. Chest radiography was mandatory at booking in the antenatal clinics 40 years ago. Now it is used only for those coming from countries with a high rate of tuberculosis or when there is a family history. In a properly controlled radiology department the irradiation to a fetus from a maternal chest radiograph is minimal – equivalent to that received on flying the Atlantic.

Systemic tuberculosis may be associated with infertility, and, once pregnant, the miscarriage rate is increased. There is no effect on congenital abnormalities, but the condition itself may worsen without proper care. Antituberculosis drugs which have been started may be continued despite the earlier thoughts of teratogenesis. Streptomycin is rarely used now in pregnancy, and probably the best drugs are isoniazid and ethambutol.

Transplacental transmission to the fetus may occur, with the greatest risk around the time of labour. Tubercle can be transmitted in the milk of the mother and by direct contact with the newborn baby after delivery. If the mother has been treated successfully and there are no tubercle bacilli in the sputum, the baby may be nursed by the mother. BCG immunization of infants is still recommended.

Less common are women with active bacillae in the sputum or with haematogenous disease. It is probable that separating the mother and infant is less useful than thought previously, but the child should be checked by culture for the organism *Mycobacterium tuberculosis*, and treatment with isoniazid and rifampicin given for 6–12 months.

Cytomegalovirus (CMV) is transmitted by a virus similar to herpes virus but rather larger. The woman is usually asymptomatic, and the infection is commonly acquired in parts of the world where standards of hygiene are not good. Pregnant women may acquire infection from contact with young children.

The virus can cross the placenta to the fetus, and is present in maternal urine and saliva. Extrauterine infection may occur during delivery.

In-utero CMV may be associated with growth retardation, ascites or hydrocephalus. After birth there may be enlargement of liver and spleen with a petechial rash. Jaundice occurs later. Microcephaly is reported, and another common sequela is deafness.

In pregnancy, examination of the maternal blood may show IgM antibodies, but repeated titres are needed to see whether the infection is a recent one or if the antibodies are a result of previous infections. At present we do not screen for CMV, but if a woman is suspected of being at high risk then direct incubation of culture combined with sensitive tests for IgM would be helpful. CMV vaccine does exist, but the use of live vaccines in pregnancy is problematic. Acyclovir may reduce viral shedding, but there is no evidence of any benefit to the fetus.

Toxoplasmosis is a protozoan infection which can be transmitted to humans through either undercooked meat or faecal or urine contact, particularly of the cat. It is less common in the UK than in France and Germany, where raw meat is consumed in greater proportions. The occurrence rate is said to be 10% for every 10 years of life.

It is a mild, often asymptomatic disease, although sometimes there is localized enlargement of the lymph glands in the neck. Transmission to the fetus occurs readily, producing choroidoretinitis, hydrocephaly and intracranial calcification, the last being associated with convulsions and mental retardation, perhaps not occurring until the child is 10 years old or more.

During antenatal care, routine screening is not performed in this country as it is not considered to be cost-effective. IgG antibody may be detected, and results interpreted against the time since infection. The status can be checked by repeating the IgG levels 2 or 3 weeks later, when increasingly raised levels would indicate recent infection. This infection can be confirmed by fetal blood sampling and testing for IgM.

Treatment is with spiramycin, although some women may elect a termination of pregnancy if there is firm evidence of fetal involvement. General precautions are to wash all fresh vegetables, wash hands after handling raw meat and to wear gloves when handling cat litter. There is no need to get rid of the cat.

Listeria is a Gram-positive bacillus found widely in wild and domestic animals. It is unusual in humans, excepting at the extremes of maternal age in pregnancy. It is associated with a high rate of miscarriage and stillbirths and is probably transmitted by ingestion of milk, cheese and uncooked vegetables contaminated by the droppings of infected animals.

The maternal illness is a mild, non-specific flu-like illness; abortion rates are high in animals, and on small studies seem to be so in humans if the infection is early enough. Later in pregnancy it is associated with stillbirth in a high number. Those born alive are likely to have respiratory distress due to congenital pneumonia, and convulsions; a spotty rash and conjunctivitis may occur, coming on within 3 days of birth.

Infant listeria is diagnosed usually after birth with a cerebrospinal fluid culture. It is sensitive to many antibiotics, and a combination of gentamicin and ampicillin is commonly used.

Infection by *HIV* is a worldwide disease of young people, including those who are pregnant. The virus acts by attacking the T4 helper lymphocytes which control many of the immune functions, and is spread by direct tissue contact, i.e. semen through a break in the epithelial protection of the cervix or a split in the anal mucosa, by the use of contaminated needles for intravenous drug injection or by contaminated blood transfusion. In the Western world the latter two are the common means of infection, but in the world generally, homo- and heterosexual intercourse is the major cause of transmission.

Tests for HIV are readily available and have a high specificity and sensitivity.

In the few months of pregnancy, the clinical condition may not deteriorate very much in the mother but transplacental transmission occurs in about 40%. The role of local infection during passage of the baby through the birth canal is less certain. However, if it exists then bypass by caesarean section may be justified. Certainly cleaning the vagina with chlorhexidine at delivery reduces vertical transmission rates. Milk is another source of infection, and it is probably wiser if the mother does not breast feed her baby. While this may be a satisfactory answer in Western countries, in the developing world this must be weighed up against the relative safety of breast feeding against infant infection and its usefulness as a method of contraception.

Screening for HIV is a controversial subject. In some areas of the UK, such as south London, the disease is present in 3/1000 pregnant women, whilst in the county of Surrey there is a very low incidence. Because of the implications of a diagnosis of HIV, counselling must be a major part of any screening programme, but the added knowledge that detection and treatment helps their unborn child usually outweighs the mother's anxiety. This is very labour-intensive, and now prescreening discussion is replacing counselling. From society's point of view, it is probably worthwhile to screen in areas of high risk (London, Dundee and Edinburgh) but not in low-risk areas. Some advocate routine screening if prevalence levels are above 2/1000 in the pregnant population. This should either be done with the woman's specific consent or by means of an opting out policy in which all women are tested unless they request not to be.

The diagnosis of HIV in pregnancy has led to an active intervention treatment with acyclovir and lamirudine. This seems to be helping the fetus, for vertical transmission rates are reduced, but much more work is required before it is proven. Trials are proceeding of other combinations of drugs, including protease inhibitors and non-nucleoside reverse transcriptor inhibitors. The active treatment during pregnancy reduces the fetal risk of infection from 25 to 5%.

The knowledge that a woman is HIV-positive has an effect upon the health care staff. They are naturally worried, and tend to take precautions which may seem excessive to the woman and other observers. Perhaps such precautions against infection transmission should be taken for every woman.

The most effective treatment at the moment is prevention. In the developed world, high-risk groups have responded with varying degrees of success to the use of condoms and clean needles. Lack of money and education has not allowed this to happen in the developing world, where:

there is a widespread and growing sense of inadequacy, confusion on how best to proceed, failure to link AIDS with other health issues, increasing bureaucratisation, and lack of commitment to caring for people with HIV and AIDS.

(Tarantolad L 1994 Health and disease in developing countries. Macmillan Press, London)

The increasing number of HIV strains becoming resistant to antiviral therapies and the galloping increase of tuberculosis may limit pharmacological treatment. For the moment we are therefore thrust back to prevention.

Local infections

Human papilloma virus (HPV) *infection* is caused by a group of DNA viruses. It is spread by direct contact in adults, almost always sexually transmitted.

Genital HPV manifests itself as a series of flourishing warts in the fourchette and perianal region, often associated with chronic candidiasis. It may advance up the vagina to the cervix, and show up on colposcopy as aceto-white zones. The warts increase during pregnancy, and present two problems. The enlarged warts can intrude physically on delivery or, because they are so vascular, may cause heavy bleeding. Podophyllin is not used in pregnancy because of the risk of absorption and toxicity to the fetus.

Cutting diathermy can be tried, but this will lead to much blood loss. Cryotherapy is less bloody, but probably laser surgery is the best way to deal with large lesions. None of these are cures but merely reduce the bulk and risk of potential haemorrhage at a vaginal delivery.

Transmission to the infant can occur at delivery, and may manifest itself with laryngeal papillomata later. Rarely, intrauterine infection may follow ascending organisms, as transplacental transmission is unlikely. The management of the fetus and the mother is often delivery by caesarean section to avoid the potentially hazardous bleeding areas.

Herpes simplex virus (HSV) is a DNA virus, of which there are several phenotypes. The virus enters through breaks in the epithelium in the cervix and possibly lower genital tract, causing ulceration and vesicles. In the lower genital tract they can be very painful. The fetus can be infected either transplacentally from infection of the endometrium or on passage through an infected cervix and lower genital tract. HVS is also excreted in breastmilk, where the levels are high. The infant may show affect by cutaneous herpes or by encephalitis.

Women in pregnancy with lesions of herpes should have these checked by culture of the fluid from the intact vesicles or cells scraped from the ulcerated areas. If positive, then the classical advice has been to perform a caesarean section in order to avoid infant infection during vaginal delivery. However, because of the poor pick-up of the virus, for many women are asymptomatic and have no signs in late pregnancy, currently caesarean section is restricted to those with active lesions when labour commences. During pregnancy, treatment is with vidaravine and acyclovir.

Chlamydia infections are caused by bacteria which can only multiply within cells. It is spread via sexual contact, and diagnosis is limited by the difficulty in culturing the organism.

Commonly chlamydia attacks the fallopian tubes, leading to reduced fertility, and does not present at the antenatal clinic. The woman may have a chronic vaginal discharge which may smell of fish, particularly when the discharge is rendered alkaline, as happens when semen is deposited in the vagina after intercourse. In pregnancy its spread may be enhanced by the increased blood supply. Its effect on the length of the pregnancy and preterm labour is difficult to assess, as this is complicated by other socio-economic factors. The fetus may be infected during delivery, causing conjunctivitis, pneumonia and rectal infection.

Treatment is best with tetracycline or erythromycin.

Gonorrhoea is spread by a Gram-negative diplococcus transmitted by direct contact. It is a common disease in the UK, and is prevalent in developing and underdeveloped countries. It is usually asymptomatic, although local pain and joint pain may follow chronic illness. Trans-placental infection of the fetus is most unusual, and most infant cases follow passage through an infected and untreated vagina. Gonococcal ophthalmia was a common cause of blindness, but is now rare following better eye hygiene after delivery.

The original treatment with sulphonamides has become less effective with the rise in resistant strains. Currently a large dose of one of the third-generation penicillins is helpful; if not, many of the other antibiotics will kill the organism, e.g. tetracycline.

Syphilis is probably the commonest infectious condition tested for in the antenatal clinic and yet it has a very low prevalence in the Western world. However, effective treatment can be given during the antenatal period to the fetus, and the results of congenital syphilis are so severe that it is considered wise at the moment to continue screening, although this may change in the next few years in the UK. The disease is caused by a treponeme, and is usually sexually transmitted; it passes across the placenta readily and affects the fetus.

In antenatal clinic screening, the Wassermann complement fixation test has mostly been replaced by the Venereal Disease Research Laboratory (VDRL) test. If this is positive, it is usually followed by a test for specific treponemal antibody. Because of the comparative cheapness of the tests compared with the expense to society of caring for a child with congenital syphilis, it is still cost-effective to perform routine antenatal testing. Indeed, there is a move from genitourinary physicians to press for a second test to be done in the third trimester, particularly for those at higher risk of sexual transmission, for a late infection during pregnancy would still allow congenital syphilis to occur in the newborn baby. This is under discussion at the moment.

The affect of the baby is usually late, for there are few symptoms early on. Birth weight reduction, mental retardation, microcephaly and chorioretinitis are reported. Other effects include peg-shaped teeth, eighth-nerve deafness, mental retardation, epilepsy and syphilitic osteitis.

The treatment is with penicillin in large doses during pregnancy and afterwards for the baby.

Bacterial vaginosis (also known as anaerobic vaginosis) is a common infection in women, characterized by a frothy offensive discharge. It has been implicated in midtrimester loss and premature rupture of the membranes. The infecting organisms are predominantly *Gardnerella*, *Ureaplasma* and *Mobiluncus*, all sensitive to metronidazole and clindamycin. Diagnosis is made by the presence of *clue cells* in an air-dried vaginal wall smear that is Gram stained. Treatment is with metronidazole or clindamycin.

Urinary tract infection

Stasis in the upper urinary tract and mild obstruction to the bladder provide potential media for growth of bacteria.

Asymptomatic bacilluria. About 5% of pregnant women are found to have more than 10^5 bacteria per millilitre in the urine. If present, it is wise to treat it, for this could proceed to acute pyelonephritis. If the infection occurs in pregnancy, it would be wise to check the urinary tract for structural abnormalities when the pregnancy is over, when intravenous urography and ultrasound show a 20% pick-up rate. The infecting organisms are usually *Escherichia coli*, and are sensitive to rotating courses of 2 weeks each of amoxycillin, trimethoprim and nitrofurantoin.

Symptomatic infections. The symptoms depend upon the level of infection:

- Dysuria – urethritis
- Increased frequency – trigonitis
- Backache – pyelonephritis.

The woman may be febrile, feeling unwell and with tenderness over the affected area. A mid-stream specimen of urine should be examined for white cells and organisms for sensitivity. The treatment is bed rest with ample fluid intake, using a broad-spectrum antibiotic at first, which can change when the sensitivities of the organisms are revealed. A 7 day course should be given at least, and the urine should be recultured a few days after the end of this course.

RECOMMENDED READING

Brocklehurst P, French R 1998 The association between HIV infection and perinatal outcome. British Journal of Obstetrics and Gynaecology 105: 836–848

Chamberlain G 1997 ABC of antenatal care, 3rd edn. BMJ, London

Department of Health 1996 Report on confidential enquiries into maternal deaths in UK 1991–1993. HMSO, London

de Swiet M 1996 Medical diseases of pregnancy 3rd edn. Churchill Livingstone, London

Gilbert G 1991 Infectious disease in pregnancy and the newborn infant (No. 2 of a series). Hawood, Chur, Switzerland

Howard RJ, Tuck SM, Pearson TC 1995 Pregnancy in sickle cell disease in the UK. British Journal of Obstetrics and Gynaecology 102: 947–951

Jardine Brown C, Dawson A, Dodds R *et al* 1996 Report of the Pregnancy and Neonatal Care Group. Diabetic Medicine 13: S43–S53

Joint Working Group RCPE/RCOG 1998 Consensus conference on Anti-D prophylaxis. British Journal of Obstetrics and Gynaecology 105: S1–2

Smith J, Cowan FM, Munday P 1998 The management of herpes simplex infection in pregnancy. British Journal of Obstetrics and Gynaecology 105: 255–259

Teoh T, Redman C 1996 Management of pre-existing disorders in pregnancy; hypertension. Prescriber's Journal 36: 28–36

Normal labour

During labour the fetus, placenta and membranes are expelled from the uterus through the birth canal. This event usually occurs after a normal pregnancy, between 38 and 42 weeks of gestation, most commonly at about 40 weeks. By this time the uterus is almost filling the abdominal cavity, and the fundal height is 36–40 cm from the symphysis pubis.

In the third trimester the lower part of the uterus becomes the lower uterine segment, and is much thinner than the upper segment. At caesarean section it is easily recognized because the peritoneum is only loosely attached. If the fetal head is fully flexed on the chest, and the occiput is lying anterior, then a circular aspect of the head is presenting – the biparietal diameter (10 cm) and the suboccipital bregmatic diameter (10 cm) engaging in the pelvic brim. When this has actually passed through the pelvic brim, the head is said to be engaged (Fig. 8.1). In a primigravid this usually takes place around the 38th week of pregnancy, although in a multigravid it may not occur until labour ensues. With the head fully flexed in the occipitoanterior position, that part of the head which is lowest is known as the vertex, and lies midway between the anterior and posterior fontanelles. The head now separates the uterine cavity into two compartments. When the membranes are intact, a small amount of fluid is trapped between the membranes and the fetal head – the fore-waters. The much larger hind-waters lie above.

During labour the process of thinning of the lower segment continues, so that the cervix itself is pulled up and effaced in a dilating and

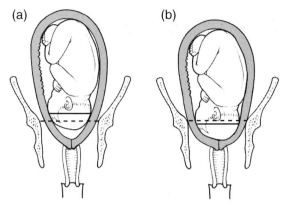

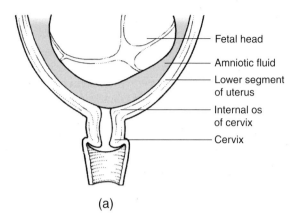

Fetal head

Amniotic fluid

Lower segment
of uterus

Internal os
of cervix

Cervix

(a)

Figure 8.1   Engagement of the fetal head. **a** The head is not engaged as its maximum diameter (——) is above the inlet of the mother's pelvis (– – –). **b** The head is engaged with its maximum diameter below the inlet.

thinning process. Once it has been pulled up, then cervical dilatation occurs (Fig. 8.2).

This sequence of events is seen most clearly in primigravid patients, for in multigravid patients effacement and dilatation may occur simultaneously, often in late pregnancy. The onset of labour is not precisely timed; it is typified by the presence of regular painful contractions occurring at least once every 5 min and the presence of a show – a plug of blood and mucus indicating that the cervix is beginning to dilate. Sometimes the membranes have ruptured prior to the show, and in the presence of regular contractions this is also considered to be labour. Otherwise, in the absence of these two signs, there must be evidence of progress which means progressive dilatation of the cervix and descent of the presenting part.

Labour is divided into three stages, with very different durations:

* The first stage – from the onset to full dilatation
* The second stage – from full dilatation to the delivery of the baby
* The third stage – from the delivery of the baby to the expulsion of the placenta and membranes.

MANAGEMENT OF LABOUR

Labour should be a normal physiological

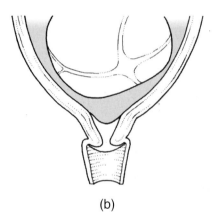

(b)

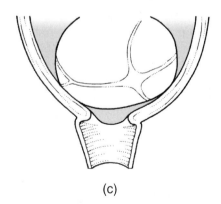

(c)

Figure 8.2   Effacement and dilatation of the cervix. **a** Non-effaced – before labour. **b** Partly taken up – late pregnancy or early labour. **c** Dilated 2–3 cm – early labour.

process in which no harm comes to either the baby or the mother; this happens in about 80% of labours. However, problems can arise, and for this reason a skilled team should be available to assist the mother. Every woman must have a midwife in attendance who, where necessary, may summon medical assistance. The midwife's functions are to achieve the delivery of a normal, healthy child at the same time ensuring that the mother is comfortable and that she will remember it as a happy, satisfying event. The midwife must be able to anticipate conditions which may lead to problems with the mother or baby and to summon medical aid when appropriate.

Since the Second World War there has been a rapid steady progression of women seeking delivery within a hospital, so that by the 1970s few women had home confinements. This remained so until recently: the number of women who wish to have their babies at home is now increasing (approximately 2% of deliveries are now at home). A compromise between these two situations is when mothers are brought into hospital with their midwife, delivered by that midwife and go home again within 6 h. The Domino scheme (DOMiciliary IN and Out) aims at providing the best of both worlds with the attention of a known midwife and the safety of a hospital environment for the delivery but the ability of the patient to return to her home and family as soon as possible.

It is desirable for women who elect to have their babies in hospital to know the midwife who is going to look after her in labour, and that midwife should stay with her if at all possible through to delivery. The woman's partner is encouraged to stay with her throughout, and he should be involved with the mother in decision making. Any birth plans discussed in the antenatal clinic should be brought into hospital and consulted.

In the majority of well-equipped delivery suites, medical staff consist of a senior house officer and registrar who are immediately available, together with a consultant obstetrician on call. There should also be available an anaesthetist and a paediatrician of appropriate seniority. In the majority of cases they will have no part

in the management or delivery of the woman but must be in the hospital.

On most sites, the obstetric unit is an integral part of the general hospital; ideally the delivery suite should have its own operating theatre. Similarly, a special care baby unit should be close by. The mother should be accommodated in the same room throughout labour. In some units, where space is short, a number of women may be accommodated in a first-stage room and only moved to the delivery suite for the second stage of labour.

The modern birth room should be a comfortable, airy room which is carpeted and curtained and where medical equipment should be as inconspicuous as possible. There should be comfortable seating for the mother and her partner as well as the delivery bed. However, the room must be large enough to contain a number of medical staff in the case of any operative intervention, and there must be adequate storage space for resuscitation equipment. Similarly there must be properly planned lighting for operative delivery, suturing or resuscitation if required.

EQUIPMENT

In the modern well-equipped unit there should be a cardiotocograph machine available in each birth room. All midwifery and medical staff should be trained and refreshed at intervals in the correct interpretation of cardiotocogram (CTG). In addition, there should be an oxytocin infusion pump for each room, anaesthetic equipment and resuscitation equipment for the newborn infant common for several rooms but within the labour unit. An essential requirement is a facility for the assessment of fetal pH and acid–base status, and at least one member of the obstetric team on duty must be able to perform these measurements.

NORMAL LABOUR
The first stage of labour

The first stage of labour is characterized by

regular strong contractions lasting often for a minute or more and occurring every 3–5 min. The contractions force the presenting part against the internal cervical os, leading to its effacement and then dilatation. The fore-waters probably have little part to play in this dilatation, for there seems to be little difference between the speed of dilatation whether they are intact or not.

The first stage of labour is divided into two phases: the latent phase and the active phase. The latent phase is fairly prolonged, and on average lasts for about 7 h in nulliparous patients. Dilatation of the cervix may be to 4 cm. The active phase is much more rapid, and is associated with more rapid cervical dilatation, usually 1–2 cm per hour. For practical purposes the mean dilatation rate for the whole of labour in a nulliparous patient is 1 cm per hour (Fig. 8.3).

The second stage of labour

The second stage of labour starts when the cervix is fully dilated to 10 cm. This stage of labour concerns the expulsion of the fetus, and often is diagnosed when the presenting part is visible at the introitus. It is at this point that the mother has the desire to bear down, for the fetal head is now pressing on the rectum and pelvic floor, producing a desire to push. This is particularly acute during a contraction.

The position the mother adopts is largely left to her. It is commonest in the UK for women to deliver in the propped-up, half-sitting position with a large rubber wedge to support them (Fig. 8.4). This is probably the most comfortable for the mother, and gravity may assist in the expulsion of the baby. Some find squatting or resting on the hands and knees a natural position to give birth. A very small proportion make use of a deep-water bath for comfort, and where it is available, a birth chair can be used.

As the mother pushes down, the vulva becomes progressively dilated by the head of the baby. A pad should be placed over the anus to protect the baby from faecal soiling, and the advancing head is controlled by the midwife's left hand. The aim is to allow release of the head as smoothly as possible and with minimal perineal damage. However, if there is undue stretching or early signs of skin splitting of the perineum, an episiotomy may be necessary. It is important that the head should be flexed until the occiput appears beneath the mother's symphysis pubis. After this the chin is freed, and the head is allowed to rotate through 90° as the shoulders negotiate the pelvis moving to the anteroposterior diameter. A check should be made that there are no loops of umbilical cord around the baby's neck (nuchal entanglement), and with the next contraction the anterior shoulder should be delivered. This may be assisted by gentle lateral extension of the fetal head in a backwards direction.

After the anterior shoulder is delivered, the baby is directed forwards towards the mother's abdomen, thus allowing the posterior shoulder to pass down the posterior vaginal wall. Once this is delivered, the trunk and legs follow rapidly. An oxytocic such as a mixture of ergometrine and oxytocin (Syntometrine) is usually given intramuscularly to promote contraction of the uterus and to minimize bleeding. The umbilical cord should be divided between clamps, and the infant is given to the mother, wrapped in a warm blanket, as soon as possible after its nasopharynx has been cleared and respiration is established.

The third stage of labour

The mother has an injection of Syntometrin at the time of the delivery of the anterior shoulder to minimize the risk of postpartum haemorrhage and encourage contraction of the uterus. The first sign of placental expulsion is that there is lengthening of the cord with an accompanying small loss of blood. It is usually then to support the uterus by placing a hand immediately above the symphysis pubis, so keeping the uterus in an extrapelvic position. The cord is grasped, and steady traction is applied. The placenta, which has separated when the baby was born, slips out of the uterus into the vagina. The cord can then be released, and delivery of the entire placenta can gently be encouraged with maternal effort.

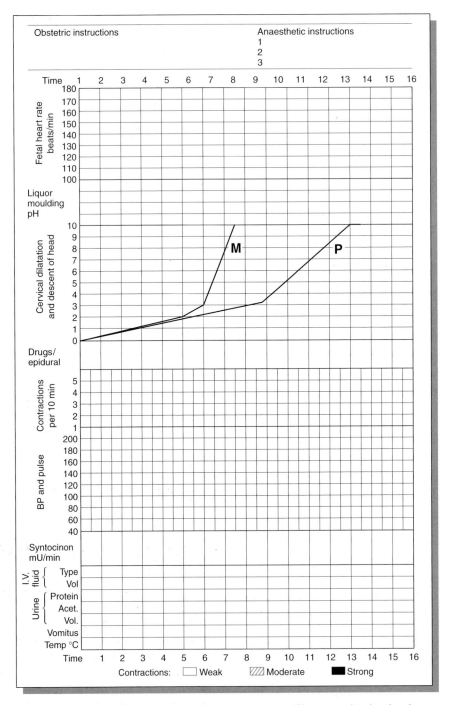

Figure 8.3 Partogram of multiparous (M) and primaparous (P) women showing the slower latent and the faster active phases of labour.

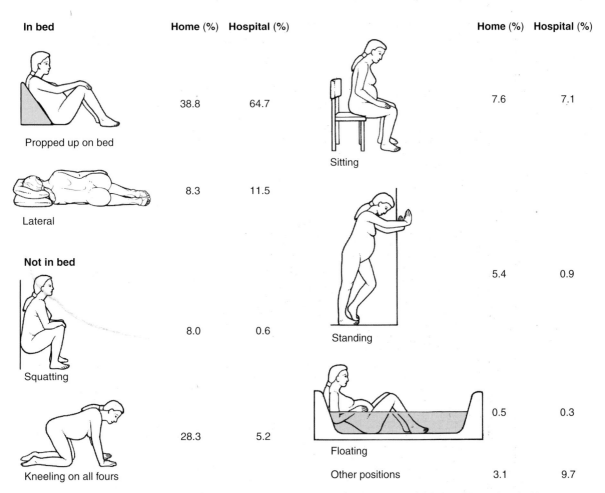

In bed	Home (%)	Hospital (%)		Home (%)	Hospital (%)
Propped up on bed	38.8	64.7	Sitting	7.6	7.1
Lateral	8.3	11.5			
Not in bed			Standing	5.4	0.9
Squatting	8.0	0.6			
			Floating	0.5	0.3
Kneeling on all fours	28.3	5.2	Other positions	3.1	9.7

Figure 8.4 Positions reported by midwives for women delivering in the booked place of delivery. (Reproduced with permission from Chamberlain G, Wraight A, Crowley P 1997 Home births. Report of the NBT survey of 1994. Parthenon Press, London.)

Care must be taken that the membranes follow. Following this, both placenta and membranes are inspected carefully for completeness.

If the placenta is retained for more than 15 min or blood loss is considered to be excessive, then further action is taken. Firstly, a contraction is encouraged by rubbing the fundus of the uterus, the bladder should be catheterized and blood should be taken for cross-matching. If bleeding continues, despite a firmly contracted uterus, it is suggestive of trauma of the reproductive tract. If the placenta remains within the uterus, then arrangements must be made for a manual removal (see Ch. 9).

ASSESSING THE FETUS DURING LABOUR

This is colloquially known as 'monitoring', and it encompasses a number of measures to assess fetal welfare during labour.

Fetal hypoxia or asphyxia can be as a result of chronic malperfusion of the placental bed in late pregnancy exacerbated by the cut-off accompanying each uterine contraction in labour. It may also follow a rapid loss of oxygen to the baby from cord compression, particularly if the cord is wrapped around the baby's neck. If the fetus becomes hypoxic, it is distressed, and there are three clinical signs of this:

- Changes in the baby's heart rate particularly tachycardia over 160 beats/min
- The passage of meconium into the liquor
- Excessive fetal movements.

Abnormalities of the fetal heart rate can be detected by auscultation. However, such observations are seldom made during a contraction, and yet it is precisely at this time that changes in the heart rate are most important. To overcome this problem the availability of electronic fetal heart monitoring or cardiotocography is now almost universal in the labour wards of the UK.

If the membranes are intact the cardiograph signal is obtained with an ultrasound head attached to the mother's abdomen. When the membranes have ruptured, an electrode can be applied directly to the fetal scalp, generally ensuring a better signal. In both cases tocography is carried out by strapping a displacement pressure transducer to the maternal abdomen. This produces a pair of signals which are printed out as a continuous tracing of both

the fetal heart and of uterine contractions – a cardiotocogram or CTG (Fig. 8.5).

CTG baseline changes

The normal fetal heart rate lies between 120 and 160 beats/min. Although this rate appears steady by auscultation, there is in fact slight variation due to vagal and sympathetic activity on the heart (Fig. 8.6). This is recorded as the baseline variability. In a healthy trace this is about 8 beats/min (range 5–10 beats/min). A loss of baseline variability to less than 5 beats/min is an indication of some impaired response of the baby. This can be seen during fetal sleep, and also as the result of depressing drugs, but should not continue if the baby is stimulated by uterine contractions, abdominal palpation or even loud noises. A tachycardia of more than 160 beats/min may be associated with hypoxia. When it is above 180 beats/min it is considered to be severe, but between 160 and 180 beats/min and not complicated by any other alterations in the fetal heart rate, it is probably of little import.

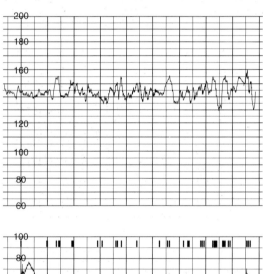

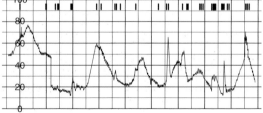

Figure 8.5 Normal CTG in labour at 3 cm of cervical dilatation.

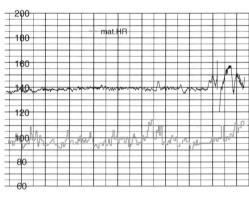

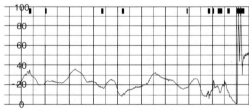

Figure 8.6 CTG in early labour with loss of baseline variability in one of two twins. The fetus appeared to wake at the end of this 10 min trace.

When combined with other changes it takes on greater significance.

Bradycardia between 100 and 120 beats/min is of no significance when accompanied by good baseline variability. However, when below 100 beats/min it is considered to be severe, and again may be associated with severe acidosis.

Variable changes in the CTG

These may be accelerations or decelerations.

Accelerations usually occur as a result of fetal movement, uterine contraction or external stimuli. They are normally associated with good baseline variability and a normal heart rate, and are said to be reactive. They are evidence of a baby in good condition.

Decelerations are of more importance:

• *Early decelerations* are synchronous with the contractions (Fig. 8.7), are V shaped and the fall rarely exceeds 30 beats/min. It is considered to be due to head compression and vagal stimulation. It can also occur due to cord compression.

• *Late decelerations* (type II dips) are usually U shaped. These decelerations usually commence 20–30 s after the start of a contraction

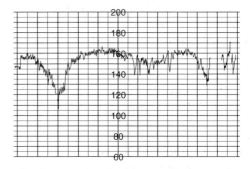

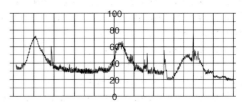

Figure 8.8 CTG in labour showing late decelerations from baseline of 160 beats/min to 90 beats/min. The start of the deceleration occurs over 30 s from the start of the uterine contraction, and the fetal heart rate is slow to recover.

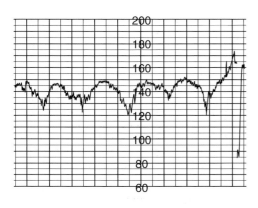

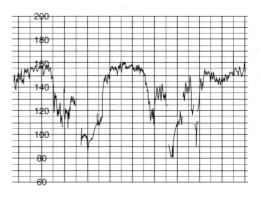

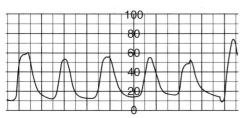

Figure 8.7 CTG in labour with early decelerations. Although they are deep, they are within 30 s of the uterine contraction and return to the baseline quickly.

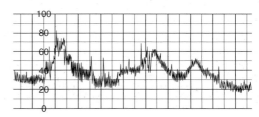

Figure 8.9 CTG in labour with variable decelerations. They vary in their relationship with uterine contractions.

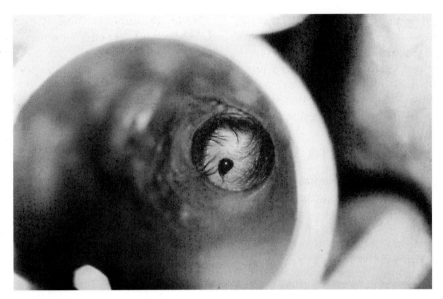

Figure 8.10   The fetal scalp has been pricked and a bead of fetal blood is produced for sampling.

(Fig. 8.8). They are much shallower than early dips, and may be evidence of placental insufficiency. When associated with a tachycardia or loss of variability, they are then considered to be a sign of severe asphyxia.

• *Variable decelerations*, often unrelated to the contraction, are of varying depth and shape (Fig. 8.9). A variety of such dips are described, and are often due to acute cord compression. Their severity is dependent upon the concomitant changes in the baseline and the variability.

Interpretation of CTGs is notoriously difficult, and many babies are born in excellent condition after traces which appear to indicate prolonged asphyxia. On the other hand, babies born in poor condition may sometimes only show a short-term abnormality in the CTG. Further, severe CTG changes may be a manifestation of previous damage to the fetus in the antenatal period and not reflect acute episodes in labour.

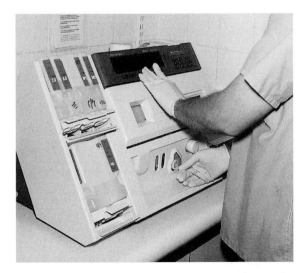

Figure 8.11   Analysis of the pH of blood gases of a sample.

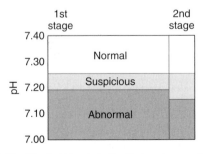

Figure 8.12   Fetal pH levels in the first and second stages of labour indicate hypoxia if below 7.20 in the first stage of labour or below 7.15 in the second stage. These low levels indicate a speedy delivery.

It is for this reason that it is essential that fetal blood sampling is available as a necessary adjunct to cardiotocography.

Obtaining a fetal blood sample is relatively simple (Fig. 8.10). An amnioscope is passed through the cervix, exposing the fetal head. This is dried with a swab, and then sprayed with ethyl chloride to encourage reactive hyperaemia. A small amount of silicone gel is smeared on, to get blood droplet formation, and the scalp is lanced with a guarded blade to a depth of about 2 mm. The blood sample is collected in a heparinized capillary tube, and the end sealed immediately with plasticine. The blood is then taken for pH and base deficit estimation, which can be assessed in many machines (Fig. 8.11).

The normal fetal pH during labour lies between 7.30 and 7.45, and borderline levels are between 7.25 and 7.20. Levels below 7.20 are considered to be acidotic, and confirm fetal hypoxia. When the levels are below 7.20, immediate delivery should be planned, although in stage II of labour the lower accepted limit may be decreased to 7.15 in normality (Fig. 8.12).

RECOMMENDED READING

Chamberlain G 1999 ABC of labour. BMJ, London

Problems in labour

INDUCTION OF LABOUR

Induction of labour involves the initiation of labour with the intent to end the pregnancy. Although the procedure is usually technically simple, it is not without its hazards, and a decision to induce labour should not be taken lightly.

The indications for induction are numerous, but the guiding principle must be, except in the case of intrauterine death, that the obstetrician considers the extrauterine milieu safer for the fetus than staying in the intrauterine environment. Induction rates vary considerably from one unit to another, and average about 20% of all pregnancies depending upon how the above indication is interpreted and by whom. The following represents a broad group of fetal and maternal indications for induction.

Indications for induction

Fetal

Intrauterine growth retardation has multiple causes, of which pre-eclampsia and hypertension are the most common in the UK. Postmaturity, maternal age, maternal diabetes, smoking, social class and nutrition of the mother all have a bearing on this. The condition is one of progressive fetal malnutrition and hypoxia leading to a slowing of the growth rate and, in the extreme, to intrauterine demise. Present day assessment of fetal condition by serial ultrasonography, biophysical profile of the fetus, fetal activity as judged by a kick chart, symphysis-to-fundus height measurements and, where necessary, antenatal cardiotocography, all play an important part in monitoring fetal intra-uterine welfare.

If and when these indicate compromise, judicious intervention may save the life of the baby. The timing of induction in relation to the maturity of the infant is of paramount importance. When preterm delivery is considered before 34 weeks of gestation, it may be more usual to perform an elective caesarean section rather than subject the infant to the stresses of labour, which could still fail to end in a vaginal delivery.

Where a previous large baby has been born and the present pregnancy ultrasound investigations indicate that the baby is again a large size, induction at term may be considered to avoid shoulder dystocia, provided the cervix is ripe (see Table 9.1).

In the presence of an abruption of the placenta in later pregnancy with its attendant risk of disseminated intravascular coagulopathy, if the fetus has not died then induction of labour is preferred to caesarean section in the majority of cases. Labour is usually rapid.

Rhesus iso-immunization and other causes of haemolytic disease of the newborn may lead to early delivery of the baby, depending upon the antibody titre. Gross congenital abnormalities incompatible with life may lead to very early induction of labour but are usually diagnosed before 24 weeks of gestation, when a termination of pregnancy is performed. Intrauterine death is a strong indication for induction of labour, mostly for psychological reasons but also because of the theoretical risk of disseminated intravascular coagulation affecting the mother.

Maternal

Maternal diseases such as hypertension, diabetes and renal disease are not usually grounds in themselves for induction of labour, but the conditions may lead to a worsening of the intrauterine environment such that induction is best for fetal survival. Very occasionally induction may be needed where the mother has a terminal malignant condition.

A far more common indication these days for induction is maternal wishes – social and domestic. There are many occasions when a woman may request to have her baby delivered at a particular time that is important to her. If the cervix is ripe and providing that the theoretical risks of induction and the problems associated with its failure are explained carefully to her, then many clinicians would agree.

Assessing suitability for induction

Prior to attempting induction, it is important to establish that the procedure is likely to succeed and not lead to problems greater than if the baby was allowed to remain *in utero*. In the past a major problem was miscalculation in the gestational age leading to premature delivery. Following the almost universal introduction of ultrasound dating in early pregnancy, this gives a much more accurate estimate of the date of delivery, so this is now a lesser problem.

It is common practice to assess the cervix prior to induction to determine the likelihood of establishing labour. A point-scoring system (Bishop score) which takes into account the dilatation, effacement, consistency and position of the cervix and the station of the presenting part is usually carried out (Table 9.1). Where scores are greater than 7, induction is likely to succeed but when less than 5, induction is less likely to succeed, and consideration given to either abdominal delivery or to delaying the induction if that is safe.

Table 9.1 Bishop's score to assess the condition of the cervix. A score above 7 indicates ripeness for induction

Cervix	0	1	2
Dilatation (cm)	0	1–2	3–4
Consistency	Firm	Medium	Soft
Length (cm)	>2	1–2	<1
Position	Posterior	Mid	Anterior
Station of head above ischial spines (cm)	3	2	1

Methods

Prostaglandin

The use of prostaglandin E$_2$ gel given intravaginally is now the most commonly used mode of induction in the UK. The gel (1 or 2 mg) is deposited into the upper vagina, and if labour has not ensued within 6 h the application is repeated. The method has the advantage that labour takes time to ensue and mimics the onset of natural labour closely. It is therefore more acceptable to the mother. The use of prostaglandins also has the benefit of ripening the cervix (improving the Bishop score), and therefore has advantages over more traditional methods when there is an unfavourable cervix. Vaginal prostaglandin tablets have been used in the past, but these have largely gone out of favour; other routes of delivery of prostaglandins are no longer used for this indication because of side-effects.

Artificial rupture of the membranes (ARM)

Rupture of the fore-waters – amniotomy – is a most efficient way of inducing labour if the cervix is favourable and the os dilated to 3 cm or more. Amniotomy is performed using a sharp, pointed instrument, some of which have been especially designed for the purpose (Fig. 9.1). Once the membranes have been ruptured, a

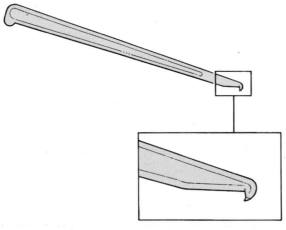

Figure 9.1 An amnihook for low rupture of the membranes.

quantity of liquor is allowed to escape. Hindwater rupture can be carried out using a specially designed metal catheter with a sinusoidal curve, but this is now rarely done in the UK because of the dangers of injury to the placenta or the baby.

Although amniotomy alone will lead to delivery within 24 h of at least 60% of babies, it is usual to combine this with an intravenous infusion of oxytocin. Synthetic oxytocin (Syntocinon) in 5% dextrose is infused into the patient at variable rates. Each labour ward will have its own protocol for the infusion of Syntocinon, and this should be adhered to within that unit.

Utilizing amniotomy and simultaneous oxytocic infusion, induction-to-delivery intervals of approximately 8 h can be expected in primiparous women, and 5 h in nulliparous women. The woman needs to be carefully observed during labour, especially to avoid hyperstimulation and its effects on the fetus.

Complications of induction

These are most uncommon when using prostaglandin gels, although disturbance of the gastrointestinal system has been reported. The major complication is failure, when caesarean section may need to be contemplated.

With amniotomy there is a risk of infection should the interval between rupture of the membranes and delivery exceed 24 h. Broad-spectrum antibiotic therapy should be considered in these circumstances. Very unusual complications following amniotomy such as umbilical cord prolapse or rupture of a large vessel traversing the membranes (vasa previa) may be encountered.

The greatest problem encountered in large units is the psychological impact on women when delivery does not ensue rapidly following a prostaglandin induction. This can, to a large extent, be obviated by careful counselling prior to the introduction of the gel.

PROLONGED LABOUR

The successful progress of labour is classically

defined as being dependent upon three factors. The powers (uterine contractions), the passages (the birth-canal) and the passenger (the fetus). Each of these plays an important part in the normal progress of labour. Where abnormalities of labour exist, there are dangers primarily to the fetus but also to the mother. Metabolic changes occurring in the mother as a result of dehydration and a low blood sugar level can lead to a direct effect on uterine powers. She may become mentally and physically distressed. Uterine infection becomes a greater possibility with the passage of time and, very occasionally, there may be a risk of uterine rupture.

Fetal distress with the attendant risks of cerebral damage due to fetal hypoxia are a major problem. It is therefore important to establish a normal pattern of labour, and this can be illustrated pictorially on a partogram, a chart that shows both cervical dilatation and descent of the presenting part against time (see Fig. 8.3). It has become customary to establish an action line on such a partogram, illustrating an ideal progress of labour. Should the line representing cervical dilatation cross this line and exceed 4 h without progress being made, it is then normal practice to accelerate or augment labour in an attempt to avoid maternal or fetal distress (Fig. 9.2).

To assess progress in labour it is necessary first to establish that labour has begun, using the criteria of the presence of regular uterine contractions and the demonstration of either progressive cervical dilatation or descent of the presenting part. In effect this means that a vaginal examination of the cervix needs to be carried out at least every 4 h and sometimes more often. Should there be significant delay in labour, appropriate action must be taken.

Management

Once delay has been established, the first action is to rupture the fore-waters if this has not occurred spontaneously. This will often lead to a descent in the presenting part. It also offers an opportunity to study the amniotic fluid for meconium staining, and, if cervical dilatation is more than 2 cm, for the application of a fetal scalp electrode for improved cardiotocographic monitoring of the fetus.

Oxytocic infusion

Oxytocin is used if there has been prolonged rupture of membranes or if there is no progress 2 h after the artificial rupture of the membranes. An increasing rate of oxytocin infusion is

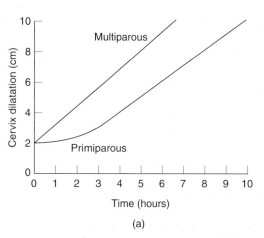

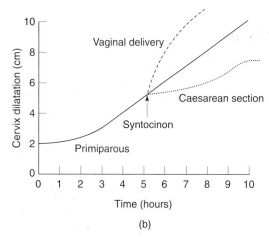

Figure 9.2 Dilatation of the cervix. **a** Normal progress. **b** Syntocinon at 5 h leads to either rapid dilatation (vaginal delivery), or failure of dilatation (caesarean section).

necessary, and a suitable labour ward protocol should be established. In general such measures prevent prolonged labour, the abnormal moulding of the fetal head and fetal distress. However, where there is no further progress, despite these measures, caesarean section should be undertaken. Where there is evidence of dystocia, careful fetal monitoring with cardiotocography and the appropriate fetal blood sampling is mandatory.

Causes

The powers

Poor uterine action may be the result of overdistension of the uterus, as occurs in a multiple pregnancy or where there is obstructive labour. If amniotomy and oxytocic infusion fail to restore normal uterine contractions, then caesarean section should be undertaken.

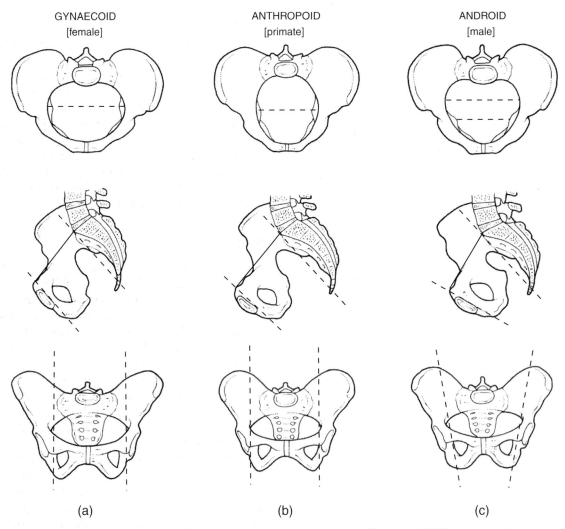

Figure 9.3 Major types of pelvic bony architecture found in the human female. **a** Gynaecoid (50%): rounded with good sacral curve. **b** Anthropoid (25%): brim is an ellipse with a smaller transverse diameter. **c** Android (20%): brim is triangular with the transverse diameter shifted backwards; the pelvis funnels as the fetus descends.

The passages

The shape of the maternal pelvis is an important factor in the way in which the fetus traverses the birth canal. Anthropoid and android pelvises are associated with a narrowed subpubic arch, prominent ischial spines and a narrowed inlet (Fig. 9.3). They are more commonly associated with a persistent occiput posterior position or transverse position of the fetal head. The labours are often long and associated with marked back-ache; little help in judging the progress of labour comes from pelvimetry, clinical examination, radiography or cardiotocography. There is usually a combination of a narrowed pelvis and a malpresentation of the fetal head that leads to cephalopelvic disproportion and obstructed labour, and a controlled trial of labour is the best way of answering the question.

The passenger

The fetus usually presents by the head, which is fully flexed on to the fetal chest, and the occiput is anterior. Delay may be due to poor flexion, a malpresentation or just too large a baby. A clue to the latter is non-engagement of the head in the presence of good contractions. The management is a caesarean section timed before either the mother or fetus is disturbed. Malpresentations are considered later in this chapter.

PRETERM LABOUR

Preterm is defined as labour that commences more than 21 days before term, so it is prior to 37 weeks of gestation. It occurs spontaneously in about 5% of all pregnancies, but elective preterm delivery, because of obstetric complications, will lead to a further 3%.

Aetiology

Epidemiological factors such as low social class, small stature, extremes of reproductive age and increased smoking are all associated with an increased incidence of preterm labour. Possible causes are shown in Table 9.2.

Table 9.2 Factors associated with preterm labour

Obstetric	Mechanical	Premature rupture of membranes
Antepartum haemorrhage	Cervical incompetence	Polyhydramnios
Polyhydramnios	Previous cervical tears	Cervical incompetence
Multiple pregnancy	Uterine congenital deformities	Multiple pregnancy
Uterine abnormalities, e.g. fibroids		Chorioamnionitis
Fetal abnormalities		
Severe hypertension		
Maternal infection		

Management

Prophylactic measures to prevent preterm labour are generally unsuccessful. It is important to ensure a good diet and to reduce smoking as much as possible. There is no evidence that rest in bed in hospital has any effect on the incidence of preterm delivery, but when it has happened before with disastrous results, it may be of considerable psychological benefit to the woman to be in hospital. Where there is proven cervical incompetence, then cervical circlage, early in the second trimester, is often helpful.

Presentation

Women will present either with regular painful contractions, a bloody show or, in a third of cases, with premature rupture of membranes, all the signs of onset of a normal labour but too early. The woman should be admitted to hospital and assessed. An initial abdominal examination should elicit how often the contractions are coming, and a speculum examination of the cervix can be carried out to ascertain whether the membranes are ruptured from the leak of amniotic fluid through the cervix. If the membranes are intact, a digital vaginal examination can then be performed to assess the effacement and dilatation of the cervix.

If the gestational age of the pregnancy is before 34 weeks, it is good practice to administer betamethasone 24 mg given in divided doses over a period of 48 h, to reduce the incidence of respiratory distress syndrome by increasing surfactant. Although it is common to repeat

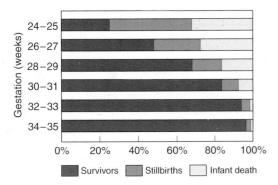

Figure 9.4 Survival to 1 year old by gestational age at birth (1993–95).

these injections on a weekly basis if the patient remains undelivered, there is no good evidence that this practice is of any benefit.

Wherever possible an attempt should be made to delay delivery to allow administration of steroids, and this can be achieved by the use of tocolytic agents, such as ritodrine, a β-sympathomimetic drug, which has been used extensively in the UK. Unfortunately its use is associated with tachycardia, vasodilation and hypertension. It is given by intravenous infusion at a rate of 50 µg/min, increased over the subsequent 24–48 h. Its use is contraindicated where there is hypertension controlled by β-blockers or a previous antepartum haemorrhage. In addition, those whose asthma is controlled by sympathomimetics should avoid ritodrine.

The major problem with preterm labour is the prematurity of the infant and the consequences of that. The respiratory distress syndrome has, in the past, been the main cause of infant mortality, but this is being tackled by the judicious use of steroids as detailed above. In a well-equipped modern special care baby unit, particularly where there are facilities for intensive care, two-thirds of babies born after 28 weeks of gestation survive without neurological damage (Fig. 9.4).

Management in subsequent pregnancies

Where premature labour has occurred in a previous pregnancy a cause should be sought. Factors associated with preterm labour are listed in Table 9.2, but many of these are individual to a specific pregnancy. However, uterine abnormalities such as fibroids can be removed prior to a subsequent pregnancy, and this may be advisable.

Cases of cervical incompetence classically present with the onset of relatively painless labour and rapid dilatation of the cervix, with rupture of the membranes being a later event. Between pregnancies it is difficult to demonstrate, but the passage of a dilator greater than size 6 Hegar suggests an element of incompetence of the internal os. Hysterography can demonstrate dilatation of the internal os. In these circumstances the insertion of a cervical suture at or around the 13th week of pregnancy may be of benefit. Although this may be helpful in an individual case, a randomized multicentre controlled trial in the UK failed to show any major benefit of cervical circlage.

In cases where a suture has been inserted, the woman should be warned that if she develops uterine contractions or bleeding at any time during the pregnancy she must report immediately to the hospital. The suture may have to be removed if there is evidence of cervical effacement and dilatation. Under normal circumstances the suture will need to be removed at approximately 37 weeks of gestation.

Chorioamnionitis is an important cause of premature labour and rupture of membranes. It may be associated with an anaerobic bacterial vaginosis, the common organisms being *Gardnerella* and *Mobiluncus*.

MALPRESENTATIONS AND MALPOSITIONS

Transverse and oblique lies

These lies occur when the long axis of the fetus is not parallel to that of the mother: the head or breech of the baby in one or other of the iliac fossae or the baby might be lying entirely transversely across the uterus (Fig. 9.5).

Aetiology

- Prematurity: it is not uncommon to find an

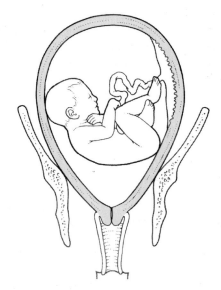

Figure 9.5   Transverse lie.

oblique lie up to 30 weeks of gestation in primigravid patients and 34 weeks in multigravid patients.
- Multiple pregnancy.
- Fetal abnormalities.
- Placenta praevia.
- Polyhydramnios.
- Abnormalities of the uterus.
- Extrauterine pelvic masses such as ovarian cysts.
- Severely contracted pelvis.

Management

Inevitably the first line of management is to discover the cause; ultrasound will be valuable in excluding a low-lying placenta or multiple pregnancy. External version is usually very easy but often pointless, as shortly after the fetus will return to its abnormal lie. It is usual practice to admit patients to hospital after 37 weeks of gestation if the lie is still unstable because of the risk of cord prolapse if the membranes rupture.

In multigravid patients where there are no obvious abnormalities then a longitudinal lie is often obtained once labour starts. However, if this fails to occur then caesarean section should be carried out.

Cord prolapse

The umbilical cord can lie beside the presenting part – occult prolapse – or below it – frank prolapse. If the membranes are not ruptured and the cord lies below the presenting part, this is a cord presentation. The overall incidence of prolapse of the umbilical cord is approximately 1/200 deliveries. The aetiological factors associated with it are very much the same as for transverse and oblique lies.

Diagnosis

Prolapse of the cord will only occur with rupture of the membranes, and occasionally the cord may pass out through the introitus. Presentation of the cord with the membranes intact can be watched carefully, for often with further descent of the fetal head the cord will slip to one side. With prolapse through the cervix, loops of cord may be felt or even seen if the descent extrudes through the vagina to the vulva. Check if the cord is still pulsating, so showing the fetus to be alive.

Management

The main factors in avoiding fetal distress are to prevent the cord from cooling or drying, so causing spasm, and to check that the presenting part is not compressing the cord. Immediate action needs to be taken. Place the woman in the knee/chest or exaggerated Sims position so that gravity allows the presenting part to move away from the pelvis. A sterile gloved hand is placed in the vagina to further push up the presenting part away from the cord. An alternative to this is to fill the bladder with a large quantity of saline. If the cord has prolapsed out of the vagina, this should be replaced into the vagina. The woman should then be taken as rapidly as possible to the operating theatre and caesarean section performed. It will be necessary for someone to keep the presenting part off the cord by transvaginal digital pressure until the baby is delivered from above.

Breech presentation

A breech presentation is when the buttocks or lower extremities of the baby present at the pelvis. The incidence is about 2–3% of all deliveries, but is dependent upon the stage of pregnancy when the woman goes into labour. At 28 weeks of gestation, about 25% of babies will be presenting by the breech, but most undergo spontaneous version by 34 weeks as the ratio of fluid to fetus reduces.

Aetiology

Causes include multiple pregnancy, placenta praevia and fetal malformations such as hydrocephaly.

The maternal factors are usually uterine, and are associated with malformations of the uterus – a bicornuate uterus or unicornuate uterus – or tumours of the uterus such as fibroids.

Types of breech presentation

- Frank breech: the legs are extended at the knee and flexed at the hip. This presentation represents the majority of cases.
- Complete or flexed breech: this presentation is next in frequency; in these circumstances the legs are flexed at the knee and hip.
- Footling breech: one or other of the feet is present at the cervical os.

Diagnosis

Most typically the head will be felt immediately below the right costal margin, and the mother may often complain of pain or tenderness in this area. On palpation the head can easily be located in this position, and the round soft mass of the breech is felt in the pelvis. The fetal heart is usually heard maximally at a much higher level. Nowadays if doubt exists about the presentation, rapid ultrasound examination can confirm the presentation.

Persistence beyond 36 weeks of gestation

If the breech presentation persists beyond 36 weeks of gestation a decision has to be made antenatally as to how to deliver the baby. A number of options are open to the mother.

Caesarean section. In primigravid patients there is an increasing tendency in the UK to offer an elective caesarean section. When one considers that among women with a breech presentation allowed to labour spontaneously 55% end up with a caesarean section, many opt for an elective procedure anyway. The main theoretical problem of vaginal delivery is that the pelvis is untried and there is always the risk that the largest part of the fetus, the head, which is last to be delivered, may be too large to traverse the birth canal without injury after passage of the rest of the baby. X-ray pelvimetry has been performed to assess the suitability of a vaginal delivery but this has largely gone out of favour, as has its successor, computerized tomography scanning. Sometimes these techniques are combined with an ultrasound measurement of the fetal head also, but the comparison of measurements obtained from two entirely different biophysical methods is imprecise.

External cephalic version. This used to be carried out between 32 and 34 weeks of gestation, but the overall incidence of breech presentation at term was not decreased by this procedure, for many underwent spontaneous version back to breech. At present, many units will offer external cephalic version at or around 38 weeks of gestation. This is often carried out with tocylitics to relax the uterine muscle, and has a higher success rate.

Mechanisms of vaginal breech delivery

The extended breech is by far the most common presentation in the primigravid woman. The baby's bottom is smaller than the fetal head, and therefore engagement usually takes place. Engagement is said to have occurred when the bistrochanteric diameter passes through the inlet of the pelvis. The breech usually presents with the sacrum anterior. The sacrum rotates so that the hip lies immediately below the symphysis pubis, and as the body descends there is lateral flexion of the body of the baby as it negotiates the curve of the birth canal. When the breech reaches the perineum the sacrum will be in the lateral position and the bistrochanteric diameter will lie in the anteroposterior diameter. Once the pelvic girdle is delivered there is restitution through 45° so that the sacrum lies in the right anterior position. Once the leg and trunk are free, the shoulders pass down the birth canal in the anteroposterior position. The head has to pass through the pelvis rapidly. Engagement best takes place with the suboccipitobregmatic diameter passing through, but there may be deflexion of the head. The back of the baby's neck will then rest under the symphysis, and the head is delivered over the perineum, usually under the control of a pair of forceps.

Management during labour

Breech deliveries are nearly always assisted, and it is necessary for an experienced obstetrician and midwife to be present together with a paediatrician and anaesthetist. Ideally the woman will have an epidural block. She is placed in the lithotomy position and is encouraged to push with contractions to expel the buttocks. An episiotomy is often performed at this point. Once the baby is born to the level of the umbilicus, a loop of cord is pulled down. From this point on, the cord may well be compressed and the baby will receive little or no oxygen, and it is therefore advisable for delivery to be completed within 5 min.

Once the knees are visible, or easily palpable, the lower limbs are flexed, and the legs delivered. The body rotates to become sacro-anterior. The baby is then allowed to hang down, and the effect of gravity will pull the baby down through the birth canal. A warm towel is placed around the baby's pelvis, and gentle traction may be applied, at the same time rotating the baby so that the anterior shoulder passes beneath the symphysis. It may be necessary at this point to disengage the arm and pull it down. Then the baby is rotated through 180° so that the posterior shoulder becomes anterior, and this too is delivered beneath the symphysis pubis, and the arm pulled down.

The baby is allowed to hang down, encouraging flexion of the fetal head, until the hairline becomes visible. This usually takes 15–30 s. Forceps are applied to the baby's head, and the baby's feet are swung upwards, encouraging the baby's face to pass over the perineum. The speed at which the head is delivered is controlled by the forceps. Once the mouth and nose appear at the introitus, mucus is extracted, and the baby is able to breathe. The remainder of the head is then allowed to gently escape from the pelvis.

An alternative method of delivery of the head (the Mauriceau–Smellie–Veit technique) is sometimes used. The baby is placed astride the obstetrician's arm, and flexion of the baby's head is maintained by placing the middle finger into the baby's mouth. The ring and index fingers are placed on the baby's cheeks on either side. The other hand is held gently over the occiput, encouraging the flexion, and the head is then delivered by drawing the baby downwards and then swinging upwards over the mother's abdomen.

Breech extraction. This is rarely performed nowadays. Extraction is indicated if there is slow progress in the second stage of labour accompanied by fetal distress, and should only be done if there is good anaesthesia (usually epidural). With an extended breech, the obstetrician's finger is placed in the groin of the baby, who is gently pulled down until the legs can be freed by flexion at the poplitial fossa. If there is a footling breech, the foot is grasped and pulled down, applying traction on the body of the baby. These methods should only be used in an emergency, and it is more usual to resort to caesarean section in such emergency situations, provided facilities are available.

The occipitoposterior position

This is the commonest malposition, and may occur in as many as 10% of women at the onset of labour. The head is often somewhat deflexed and has to rotate through 180° from the normal. As a result there is larger presenting diameter to the pelvis, and a relative cephalopelvic dispro-portion may exist. In the majority of cases, rotation of the head takes place spontaneously during labour, but occipitoposterior positions may lead to delay in the first and second stages of labour, with the necessity for instrumental delivery.

The occipitoposterior position is more likely to occur in a woman with an anthropoid pelvis, that is, one in which the pelvis is deep and the subpubic arch is relatively narrow. The diag-nosis can often be made by palpation of the abdomen. The fetal limbs can be felt anteriorly, with the back posterior and difficult to define. Both the occiput and synciput can be palpated because the head is relatively deflexed. On vaginal examination in labour the anterior fontanelle is often felt more easily than the posterior – the anterior fontanelle is diamond shaped and has four sutures running from it whereas the posterior fontanelle is triangular and has only three sutures. As labour progresses and a caput forms, it becomes progressively harder to distinguish between the anterior and posterior fontanelles, and it is this that often leads to mistakes. In these circumstances and provided that the cervix is sufficiently dilated, an ear on the side of the head can be identified, to aid diagnosis.

Mechanism. The outcome of labour is deter-mined by the shape of the pelvis and also the strength of the uterine activity.

Anterior or long rotation occurs in 60–70% of women; the head rotates through 135° to the anterior position, and then the mechanism is exactly as for a normal occipitoanterior position but it is achieved a little later in labour.

Posterior or short rotation is most likely to occur with an anthropoid pelvis, and occurs in about 20% of women. In these circumstances, rotation is only through 45°, and labour, descent of the fetal head and engagement occur as for an anterior position, but when the head reaches the pelvic floor the occiput rotates backwards to posterior. When the head reaches the perineum, maximum flexion is obtained, and the brow and the face are applied to the symphysis pubis, as opposed to the back of the neck in the occipito-anterior position. When the head crowns, the face is then delivered by extension. This is often accompanied by perineal tearing, and delivery must be aided by an episiotomy.

Deep transverse arrest. In about 10% of cases, rotation is arrested in the transverse position, often at the level of the spines. This is usually because of an unfavourable pelvic shape and deflexion of the head. Once in this position, flexion of the head occurs in a lateral posterior direction (asynclitism), and no further advance is possible. Delivery then has to be by rotation to the occipitoanterior or direct posterior position so that the long axis of the fetal head is in the long axis of the pelvic outlet. If this cannot occur, delivery has to be by caesarean section.

Management. For second-stage delay, instru-mental delivery may be necessary, depending upon the abnormality.

Posterior position (face to pubis)

This is best managed by a large episiotomy and either forceps or vacuum extraction.

Transverse arrest. The head needs to be slightly disimpacted, and then:

- manually rotated to the occiput anterior position followed by forceps delivery
- rotated using Kjelland's straight forceps or
- using the Ventouse vacuum extractor, the head is subject to a linear pull and so rotates when reaching the pelvic floor.

These methods should be used by only experienced personnel. The Kjelland's forceps, in particular, is a dangerous instrument which can lead to severe maternal injury (to the bladder and rectum) and occasionally fetal injury.

Brow and face presentations

These are the results of varying degrees of deflexion of the head. With moderate deflexion a brow presentation will occur. Because the presenting diameter is the largest (the mento-occipital), a baby with a normal sized head

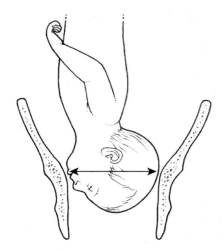

Figure 9.6   Brow presentation with the mentovertex diameter as the largest part of the presenting head (↔). This is usually 14 cm, making an average-sized baby undeliverable vaginally in this presentation.

cannot pass through a normal pelvis, and caesarean section is mandatory (Fig. 9.6).

Face presentations represent extreme extension of the baby's head. Provided that the chin is anterior, then vaginal delivery is possible.

Diagnosis. On vaginal examination, the diagnosis of a brow presentation can be made once the cervix is reasonably well dilated. The ridge of the nose can often be felt, as can the orbital ridges. In addition, the large anterior fontanelle will be palpable. It may be possible to convert the brow into a face presentation provided that the chin is anterior, but, more often than not, this is difficult in a term baby.

On vaginal examination for a baby with a face presentation, the findings may be confusing. The fetal mouth may be confused with an anus, and a breech presentation diagnosed. The most useful landmarks are the nose and the orbital ridges.

MULTIPLE PREGNANCY

The incidence of multiple pregnancy in the UK has increased considerably since the introduction of assisted conception. The incidence is approximately 1:100 as a natural occurrence, but represents up to 25% of all conceptions by assisted conception. Triplets naturally occur at a rate of 1/6000.

Most twins born are binovular (75%), that is, they are dizygotic or originate from two separate eggs. There are racial differences in incidence, with West Africans and Caribbean populations having a higher occurrence of multiple ovulation. In addition, the older a woman becomes the more likely it is for her to have binovular twins. It is more common amongst multiparous patients. Perhaps most alarming is that the incidence of repeated binovular twins is increased tenfold. Binovular twins obviously can only have a hereditary factor on the female side while uniovular twins may have a factor on the male or female side.

With binovular twins there are two placentae, amnions and chorions, and although at delivery one large placenta may be delivered, careful inspection will show that there are two separate organs grown together (Fig. 9.7). No interrelationship between blood vessels has been shown. Uniovular twins, on the other hand, show a wide variety of placentation depending upon the stage when embryo division occurs. In the majority of cases there are separate amnions but a single chorion with vascular connections. This can lead to imbalance, with fetofetal transfusion making one twin polycythaemic and big and the other anaemic and small.

Problems of multiple pregnancy

As a generalization, all complications which occur in the antenatal period are likely in a more exaggerated form in a multiple pregnancy. The mother is more likely to develop both iron and folate deficiency anaemia. Pre-eclampsia is considerably more common. Hyperemesis gravidarum may occur earlier and last longer. Pressure symptoms such as oedema, varicose veins and haemorrhoids are considerably more common. Inevitably, stretch marks are more likely to occur because of the overdistension of the abdomen, and gastrointestinal disturbances such as constipation and heartburn occur frequently.

In the first trimester there is an increased rate of miscarriage. Because of the introduction of

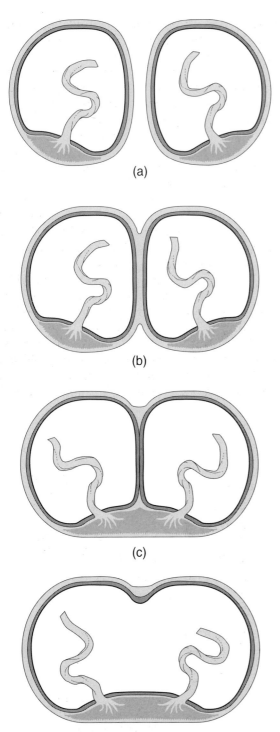

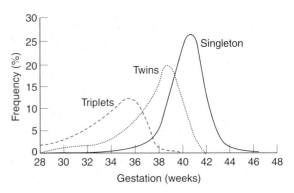

Figure 9.8 Distribution of weeks of gestation at delivery of singletons, twins and triplets in the UK.

early pregnancy units it has now become apparent that a number of cases of threatened miscarriage represent the demise of one fetus of a twin pregnancy. In most instances the pregnancy continues successfully. The average length of a twin pregnancy is 37 weeks, although 10% of them will deliver before 34 weeks of gestation. The average length of a triplet pregnancy is 34 weeks (Fig. 9.8).

Other common problems that can occur antenatally are:

- antepartum haemorrhage, because of the very large size of the placenta which may encroach upon the lower segment, leading to placenta praevia
- premature separation of the placenta following the delivery of the first baby, which is a major problem to the second twin, although abruption does not seem to be more common
- polyhydramnios, which is specifically associated with uniovular twin pregnancies and particularly where there are vascular interconnections between the two.

Diagnosis

In the past, about 3% of twin pregnancies were not diagnosed until after the delivery of the first baby. However, with the wide use of ultrasound this is now an uncommon event in the UK. The first indication of a multiple pregnancy will be

Figure 9.7 Placentas from a twin pregnancy. **a** Completely separate, hence binovular twins. **b** The fetuses are separated by two chorionic and amniotic membranes – probably binovular twins. **c** The fetuses are only separated by amnion – probably uniovular twins. **d** Only one sac – definitely uniovular twins.

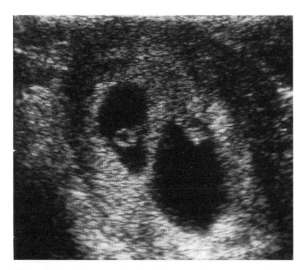

Figure 9.9 Ultrasound scan of a twin pregnancy at 9 weeks of gestation. The sacs can be clearly seen.

either exaggerated signs of pregnancy such as hyperemesis or a uterine size larger than dates. This, of course, can be due to mistaken dates or even the uterus held high in the abdomen by a previous caesarean section scar. Other simple problems such as a full bladder or rectum may lead to the impression of a uterus larger than dates. In all cases it is likely that an ultrasound scan will be carried out to estimate the number of fetuses present and their gestational age (Fig. 9.9). Later in pregnancy, when parts of the fetus can be palpated, a clinical diagnosis of multiple pregnancy is made by the presence of at least three poles (e.g. two heads and a breech). The detection of two fetal hearts using Doppler ultrasound is very unreliable unless two distinct different rates are detectable. Radiographic examination of pregnancy is very rarely undertaken nowadays because of the wide availability of ultrasound.

Antenatal care

The diagnosis of multiple pregnancies is made early, often shortly after the booking visit, because of the size of the uterus and confirmed by ultrasound. It is not necessary to see the patient more often than usual until 28 weeks of

pregnancy, but the patient should be encouraged to take iron supplements and folic acid at the increased dose of 5 mg/day.

It is common practice from 28 weeks of gestation to see the patient usually every 2 weeks, and ultrasound examinations for fetal growth rate to be performed at 28, 32 and 36 weeks. Up to 28 weeks of gestation the growth rate on ultrasound scanning is the same as that for a singleton pregnancy, but after this time, growth rates tend to fall off (Fig. 9.10).

There is no consensus of opinion about admission for rest in an attempt to prevent premature labour, but the best available evidence at present suggests that it is unnecessary unless the woman feels that she needs it.

A particular problem that occurs for older women with a multiple pregnancy is screening for Down's syndrome, and it is therefore necessary to screen using ultrasound soft tissue markers. Diagnostic tests such as chorionic villi sampling and amniocentesis have problems: with the presence of twin sacs one must be certain from which fetus fluid or tissue comes. A

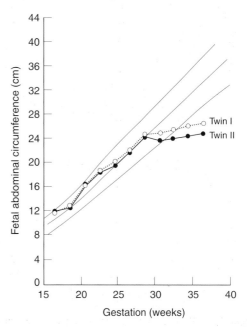

Figure 9.10 Ultrasound measures of biparietal diameters of both twins. Until about 26–28 weeks of gestation, growth rates are as singletons; thereafter they fall off.

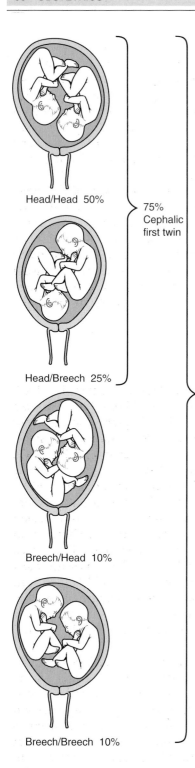

Head/Head 50%

Head/Breech 25%

} 75% Cephalic first twin

Breech/Head 10%

Breech/Breech 10%

} 95% Longitudinal lie first twin

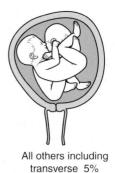

All others including transverse 5%

Figure 9.11 Presentation of twins at onset of mature labour (≤ 36 weeks of gestation).

screening test using blood values is not discriminatory.

Labour

The commonest presentation for multiple pregnancies is head and head, and most of the other presentations still have longitudinal lies (Fig. 9.11). Other presentations can occur, but the leading fetus is usually lying longitudinally, presenting by one pole or other. Labour usually follows a normal course, and the latent phase may be shorter than usual. For the delivery of two babies, an increased number of neonatal personnel will be needed in the delivery room, and it is important to explain to the woman and her partner beforehand that there will be more people than usual present. It is usual for an experienced obstetrician with an assistant to be present, an anaesthetist and usually two paediatricians. In addition there will be several midwives. Epidural analgesia is preferred, and makes manipulation at delivery of the second twin easier.

Delivery

In the majority of cases the first fetus will present by the head, and delivery is conducted in the normal manner. Similarly, a breech presentation is managed in the conventional way. Once the baby is born the cord is securely clamped and divided. As soon as this has occurred, the uterus is palpated to ensure that the second twin is in a longitudinal lie. If it is not, external version is performed. The forewaters are then ruptured, and it may be best to do this with a uterine contraction, although it is not necessary. It is good practice to have an intravenous infusion running at the time so that oxytocics can be given to encourage uterine contractions if they do not return spontaneously.

The second twin is managed as for the first, depending upon the presentation. On the rare occasion of a persistent transverse or oblique lie, either caesarean section will need to be undertaken or, in the presence of a very experienced obstetrician, internal podalic version to a breech followed by breech extraction can be carried out. It must be stressed that this manoeuvre should only be carried out by somebody with considerable experience.

Third stage of labour

Following delivery of the second twin, it is important that oxytocics are given because the uterus, which is overdistended, may become atonic, leading to a large postpartum haemorrhage. It is usually wise to give intravenous syntocinon as well as an intramuscular dose.

Triplets

Because of the variable presentations of triplets it is now common to deliver them by caesarean section, although vaginal delivery is sometimes achieved, especially if the patient goes into premature labour, which is rapid. In all cases of premature labour, prior to 34 weeks of gestation, injections of dexamethasone should be given to improve fetal lung maturity. If the full 48 h needed ideally does not follow before delivery, even a few hours worth is helpful to the fetus.

ABNORMALITIES OF THE PUERPERIUM

Primary postpartum haemorrhage

This is defined as a blood loss exceeding half a litre occurring within 24 hours of delivery, usually in the first hours.

Causes

- An *atonic uterus* accounts for the vast majority of haemorrhages. A *retained placenta* is a further common cause. Factors that make these complications more likely to occur are increasing parity and multiple pregnancy, an antepartum haemorrhage, prolonged labour, and operative delivery. Coagulation disorders may present at this time.

- *Trauma* can occur in any part of the lower genital tract, and each must be examined carefully in turn, starting with the perineum and vagina, where tears or an episiotomy which has extended may lead to rapid and severe blood loss. The cervix can be torn, especially following forceps delivery. Similarly, lacerations may extend up into the uterus, sometimes involving the uterine vessels.

Management

Once it is realized that a woman is bleeding heavily, and it is likely that the loss will exceed 500 ml, it is important to carry out one or two immediate manoeuvres. Intravenous ergometrine 0.25 mg should be given, and the uterus should be massaged vigorously to ensure that it its contracting. The bladder must be catheterized because a full bladder can be associated with uterine atony. Blood should be taken for cross-matching, and intravenous fluids commenced. The usual observations of pulse and blood pressure must be made, and one midwife should be allocated to this task along with keeping a written and timed record of all that happens to the woman and especially all the drugs and transfusions she is given.

If the placenta has not been delivered, efforts must be made to ensure that it is. Following the treatment with ergometrine, controlled cord traction should ensure delivery of the placenta if it is trapped in the cervix. If the cord snaps, a gentle vaginal examination may reveal part of the placenta extruded through the cervix into the vagina; it can be hooked with the middle finger and removed.

Manual removal of the placenta

This should be carried out either under regional block or general anaesthesia because the procedure is uncomfortable, possibly increasing the shock of the woman. She must be placed into the lithotomy position, and the fingers of one hand inserted into the vagina. The uterus is pushed down into the pelvis. The fingers should be then passed through the cervix, dilating it if it has partially closed, and the edge of the placenta found. The placenta should then be separated and pulled down in the cupped hand. It is obviously important to inspect the placenta and membranes carefully immediately afterwards to make sure that they are complete. It is common practice to give antibiotics to cover the procedure because of the likely introduction of bacteria from the vagina.

On very rare occasions the placenta may become morbidly adherent to the uterus, often at the site of a previous caesarean section scar. If the patient wishes to conserve her reproductive capacity, then the adherent placenta can be left *in situ* provided that there is not continued bleeding. It will probably become necrotic over a period of weeks and be expelled. If not, or in the event of continuing haemorrhage, then hysterectomy is necessary.

Injuries to the birth canal

Tears of the perineum, vulva and labia are common, but the superficial ones heal rapidly. Wider ones may require suturing if there is continued bleeding (Fig. 9.12). Vulval haematomas can occur insidiously over a period of 24 h. Because of the loose nature of the tissues, a large amount of blood can be retained within the area, and drainage will be required.

Extension of episiotomies can sometimes occur, particularly with a delivery of a baby in the occipitoposterior position. These tears may involve the anal sphincter, and it is essential that a careful rectal examination is performed following the completion of the third stage of labour and before suturing commences. Repair of the sphincter should be performed by an experienced obstetrician.

Cervical injuries

These are relatively rare and occur as a result of forceps deliveries, particularly rotational forceps delivery. It is usual for them to be sutured under general anaesthesia although regional analgesia may be sufficient. Very large retractors are required, and a competent assistant is necessary. The best retractors commonly found in the

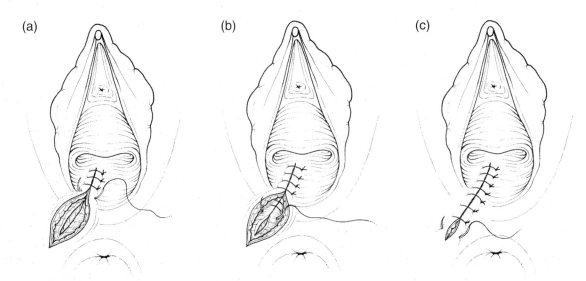

Figure 9.12 Repair of an episiotomy: (a) vagina, (b) perineal muscle, (c) skin.

delivery room are a pair of obstetric forceps used as simple spoons with the concave side turned outwards and moved to follow the operator. The apex of the tear must be identified, and the tear can then be sutured with interrupted sutures.

Uterine rupture

This is, fortunately, extremely rare and follows either injudicious use of oxytocics, operative intervention or obstructed labour. It is much more common in developing countries, where prolonged obstructed labour is common and obstetric facilities not easily available. Fistulae between the bladder and the uterus are not uncommon in these circumstances. Surgical treatment is indicated promptly and, on occasions where there is bleeding into the broad ligament, ligation of the uterine artery may be necessary. Occasionally a hysterectomy is needed for haemostasis.

Secondary postpartum haemorrhage

This can occur any time from 24 h after completion of the third stage of labour up to 6 weeks postpartum. It is usually the result of retained products of conception, and leads to a brisk loss. Ultrasound examination is commonly requested, but is an unnecessary investigation. If the bleeding is heavy, then one should proceed to an examination under anaesthesia and exploration of the uterine cavity. If it is relatively mild, antibiotic therapy should be given because there is usually an associated endometritis. The most common cause is retained decidual tissue, retained membranes or retained clot.

OPERATIVE DELIVERY
Forceps delivery

Obstetric forceps have been in use for over 350 years. The name associated with their popularization was Chamberlen, and later Chapman and Smellie refined the design of forceps in the UK. Since then, many eponymous forceps have

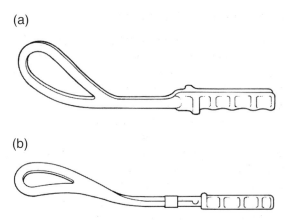

(a)

(b)

Figure 9.13 **a** Simpson's forceps with pelvic curve. **b** a Kjelland's straight forceps.

been invented although the essence of their components remain much the same. They consist of blades, a shank, a lock and handles. The blades are curved so that they might fit around the baby's head, the cephalic curve, and, except for the case of rotational forceps, they also have a pelvic curve to adapt to the shape of the mother's birth canal (Fig. 9.13). The shank and lock allow the two blades to be fitted together and held in position. With rotational forceps (Kjelland's) the lock allows the blades to slide up and down on each other. The size of the handle varies. Midcavity forceps have a fairly substantial handle, but low forceps (Wrigley's) have virtually no handle.

Indications

Forceps deliveries are conducted to control the delivery of the baby in cases of a prolonged second stage of labour or where fetal distress exists. Occasionally they are used prophylactically for the delivery of a premature baby or for protection of the after-coming head in a breech delivery.

Forceps deliveries are either midcavity or low cavity. Midcavity presentations are when the head is in the pelvis but the vertex has not reached the pelvic floor. Low cavity is below this, and the high cavity position is where the head is above the pelvic brim. There is no longer an indication for a high forceps delivery in the UK; caesarean section is always preferred.

For a forceps delivery to be undertaken, certain prerequisites must be met:

- The cervix must be fully dilated
- The head must be engaged
- The pelvis must be adequate
- The head must be in a suitable position (such as occiput–anterior)
- Anaesthesia is needed – an epidural block is good but a pudendal block, reinforced by a field block, is adequate for a low forceps delivery (Fig. 9.14).

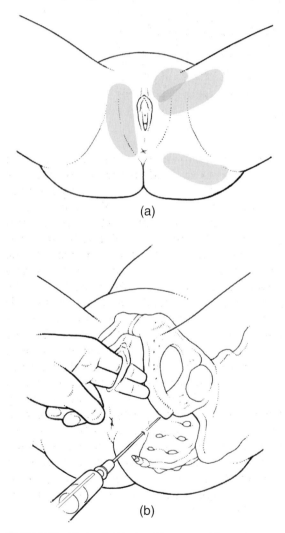

(a)

(b)

Figure 9.14 Pudendal block. **a** The areas of the perineum supplied by various sensory nerves. Block of the perineal nerve is not enough, and a field block must be done as well. **b** The siting of a pudendal block around the ischial spine.

It is usual to empty the bladder prior to a forceps delivery.

Delivery

Moderate traction with uterine contractions should be carried out in the axis of the birth canal. Once the occiput has passed beneath the symphysis, the face of the baby is swept across the posterior wall of the vagina in an upwards direction. In virtually all cases an episiotomy is necessary. Once the head is delivered the blades are removed, and the rest of the baby is delivered in the usual manner.

Complications

These may include:

- Tears of the labia and vagina or an extension of the episiotomy
- Cervical trauma, particularly if the cervix was not fully dilated at the time of application of the blades
- Disruption of the perineum, perineal body or sphincter, which occurs more often than previously thought, and minor degrees of flatal or even faecal incontinence may occur afterwards
- Minor abrasions to the skin of the infant, or cephalhaematoma or, very occasionally, intracranial trauma in the infant
- Urinary problems, but these are uncommon; where there is retention of urine, continuous bladder drainage may be necessary.

Ventouse delivery

The vacuum extractor consists of a cup with a suction outlet at the perimeter of the cup. A chain is attached to the centre, to which a handle is hooked. Suction tubing is applied to the outlet, and its other end attached to a suction apparatus, which can be either manual or electrical. The original cups were of metal in a number of sizes from 30 to 60 mm in diameter; more recently they have been largely replaced in the UK by silastic cups (Fig. 9.15).

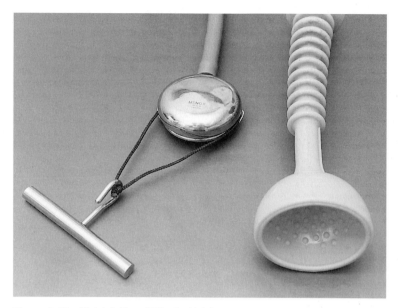

Figure 9.15   Metal (left) and Silastic (right) vacuum extractor cups.

The indications for ventouse delivery overlap with those for a forceps delivery. The ventouse, however, has the considerable advantage that it takes up little room within the vagina and can be used by fairly junior personnel without causing any major harm to the baby. Ventouse delivery is particularly useful where the head is lying in a transverse position, as rotational forceps deliveries are much more difficult. In addition, the ventouse can be applied when the cervix is not fully dilated, and there are occasions when fetal distress is so acute that it is quicker and safer to deliver a baby by ventouse, through an almost dilated cervix, than by caesarean section. However, the head must never be above the pelvic brim.

Complications

Maternal complications are few but will include vaginal and perineal lacerations. Fetal trauma is usually limited to a cephalhaematoma, which occurs in under 5% of cases.

Caesarean section

This operation is said to derive from an ancient Roman law (*lex caesaram*) requiring a child to be removed from a dead mother's womb before burial. The operation itself, although performed intermittently in history, did not become common until the introduction of general anaesthesia. Before 1940 a midline incision was performed both into the abdomen and into the upper segment of the uterus, the classical caesarean section. This enabled the baby to be removed in exceptionally fast times, in seconds rather than minutes. More recently, the operation has been considerably aided by the introduction of antibiotics, blood transfusions and, particularly, improved anaesthetic techniques. The lower segment operation, which was introduced to close off the peritoneal cavity from the intrauterine cavity with its potential infective content, gained popularity, and is now virtually the only approach made. The incidence of caesarean section has risen from about 5% in the mid-1960s to 17% at present (Fig. 9.16). Levels as high as 25% have been reported from the USA.

Indications

There are numerous specific indications for

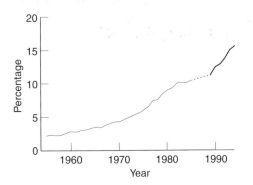

Figure 9.16 Rates of caesarean in the UK, 1954–94. The rise is documented well except for 1986–87.

performing a caesarean section, but they largely fall into two broad groups:

- *Elective caesarean section*:
  - As a repeat procedure where it is believed that vaginal delivery is unlikely to succeed
  - Where there is physical obstruction to the outlet of the birth canal such as placenta praevia or pelvic tumours such as fibroids of the uterus
  - Where the pelvis is untried and the baby is presenting by the breech
- *Emergency procedures:*
  - Obstructed labour where there is failure of progression either of cervical dilatation or descent of the presenting part due to pelvic or fetal problems such as malpresentation
  - Fetal distress.

There is an increasing demand for caesarean section by women, who see it as an atraumatic and simple way of delivery which avoids a prolonged labour and trauma to the birth canal. However, it is often forgotten that morbidity is higher with caesarean section, and this can be attributed to anaesthesia, pulmonary embolism, sepsis and haemorrhage. Most elective caesarean sections in the UK are conducted under regional block, with usually spinal anaesthesia being used. For emergency caesarean sections, epidural analgesia may be used if an indwelling epidural catheter has already been established. If not, where speed is needed, general anaesthesia is to be preferred.

Complications

During the procedure, haemorrhage is the major problem, and haemostasis must be secured adequately before closure of the abdomen. Postoperatively, bleeding can occur, and if this is the case re-exploration of the uterine wound must take place. Damage to the urinary tract is uncommon. The major postoperative problems are infection and thrombosis, with its ensuing danger of pulmonary embolism. It is normal to give antibiotic cover for all undergoing emergency caesarean section, and for thromboprophylaxis to be used during the operation, particularly the use of leg compression and, where possible, thromboembolic deterrent stockings. Subcutaneous heparin may also be used.

RECOMMENDED READING

Chamberlain G 1999 ABC of labour care. BMJ Books, London
Johnson F, Myerscough P 1998 Shoulder dystocia. British Journal of Obstetrics and Gynaecology 105: 811–814

Myerscough P 1992 Monro Kerr's operative obstetrics. Baillière Tindall, London
Spencer J, Ward H 1993 Intrapartum fetal surveillance. RCOG Press, London

10

The puerperium

During the puerperium the mother is recovering from childbirth. The various organs mostly return to their prepregnancy state, with the exception of the uterus and lower genital tract. The psyche will certainly have been altered by the pregnancy; it will probably never return to the prepregnancy state. The puerperium is also the time of establishing new relationships between the mother, the baby and the partner, all of whom have to make adjustments in their past behaviour patterns, the adults largely in psychology, the newborn in physiology. In this time, infant feeding patterns are established.

RESTORATION OF THE GENITAL TRACT

The vulva and vagina have been stretched in labour and probably will not go back to their previous state. There will be less fatty tissue in the labia, and the episiotomy or tear repair will leave a scar. If this heals well by primary intent, it will not intrude upon intercourse after the first few weeks, but infection, thrombosis or mal-aligned healing may lead to painful intercourse, sometimes permanently.

The uterus reduces in size by involution during the atrophy following the reduction of oestrogen levels, and becomes a pelvic organ again after about 10 days. The endometrium starts regenerating in 2–6 weeks, and menstrual periods may return by 6 weeks if the woman is not breast feeding. If she is, however, this may keep prolactin levels up, and follicle-stimulating hormone levels are depressed, so delaying the first period. The uterus is usually a bulkier organ than it was before the pregnancy, and remains so for the rest of the woman's reproductive life. The cervix has been stretched to allow the fetus to pass and no longer has a small central dimple-like external os but a split transversely across the cervix, and commonly the external os never reforms.

The pelvic floor muscles and fascia have been greatly stretched and may not return to the previous efficiency of the pelvic diaphragm. Hence, as well as laxness extending to uterine and vaginal prolapse in later life, the urethra and rectum which pass through the muscular pelvic floor are less well supported and their function is altered. Urinary and anal incontinence is common after childbirth, and recent evidence shows 10–20% of women suffer degrees of this in the months after birth. Although this is worse after long labours or operative vaginal deliveries, it is still found in a small number of women who had brief, apparently trouble free, births.

CARE IN THE PUERPERIUM

During the first 10 days the woman should be seen at least once a day by a qualified midwife, who checks for infection, uterine size and urine output; the haemoglobin level is rechecked on the second day. Afterpains vary enormously but analgesia is often needed in most women. The perineum may become oedematous; ice packs or hypertonic saline swabs are helpful. Any perineal skin sutures should be checked and if necessary cut. The majority of suture material used these days is man-made and absorbable, so the painful process of removing stitches is no longer necessary. Exercises taught by trained physiotherapists are helpful to restore muscle tone to stretched areas and maintain venous flow in the legs.

The psychological aspects of childbirth are only slowly being understood. There is a balance to be struck between the excitement of producing a new baby with the extra attention the mother receives on the one hand and the downside of anxiety and responsibility of looking after the child. In addition, there are the problems of physical discomfort after childbirth and the possibility of engorged breasts. 'Blues' after childbirth occur in many women, and are addressed by good pain relief and sleep.

RETURN HOME FROM HOSPITAL

An increasing number of women in the UK who deliver in hospital go home within 48 h (Fig. 10.1). It is hoped that they receive good community care, but this service is becoming overstretched. The woman who had a forceps delivery or one who had a caesarean section may stay in hospital for up to 5 days. By arranging for a woman to go home earlier she has more satisfaction and it reduces the possibility of hospital cross-infection in the baby. However, 5–10% of homes are unsuitable for the early reception of puerperal mothers and their babies. Going home may be wonderful for the first few hours but after that household duties may intrude. One of the finest gifts friends can give a newly delivered woman is to offer to do a day's work in her home, relieving her of domestic duties for that day.

Very few medical problems arise at this time and most of them can be detected and treated by the general practitioner and community midwives. Less than 1% of women have to be readmitted to the hospital after delivery for medical problems related to that delivery.

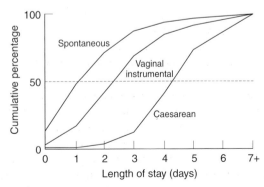

Figure 10.1 Cumulative distribution of postnatal hospital stay by method of delivery (England, 1994).

THE POSTNATAL VISIT

At about 6 weeks after delivery, the woman and her baby should be formally examined and assessed. The dedicated postnatal clinics held in hospitals have mostly been closed, and only those who had major problems in pregnancy or delivery are asked to come back. The other women visit their family practitioner's surgery and are seen by the general practitioner or the practice midwife.

Enquiry is made about any symptoms, specifically vaginal bleeding, discharge or pain in the genital tract. The blood pressure is checked, but if the woman is asymptomatic, a vaginal examination is not needed as this is not very useful. The baby is weighed and examined, and any problems are discussed. Appointments are made for immunization. An important area for discussion at the postnatal visit is further contraceptive plans (see Ch. 30). The woman is receptive to ideas at this stage, and contraception may usually be restarted from this visit.

PROBLEMS IN THE PUERPERIUM

A powerful measure of the potential hazards of the puerperal period is that over half of maternal deaths associated with childbirth occur in this time. Although deaths are rare, morbidity is commoner, and possibly this occurs in the same proportion.

Pyschiatric conditions

Many women are mildly depressed in the puerperium. The new baby gives rise to anxiety, and when the heady atmosphere of immediate postdelivery wears off, the woman may feel the attention of friends and family is past. Such 'blues' usually pass with supportive treatment. Prophylactic progesterone given either intramuscularly or in vaginal pessaries may be of assistance, but its value is unproven.

Real depression can develop, particularly amongst those where there may be a past history of depression. The borderline between treatable depression and the 'blues' is not easily defined, but when the woman starts expressing fantasies, extreme anxiety or guilt about her handling of the baby one should consider a new phase. Psychiatric help is useful, and supportive treatment with mild psychopharmacology will suffice. Should the condition worsen with rejection of the baby or with delusions and confusion, the mother should be admitted to a special mother and baby ward, which exist in the psychiatric services in each region in the UK. There she can have 24 h supervision and help with the baby as well as more effective psychotherapeutic drugs, or even possibly electroconvulsant therapy.

If the woman who has had depression becomes pregnant again, there is a high risk of reoccurrence of depression. This should be recognized in pregnancy long before the puerperium.

Thrombosis

After delivery there is increased haemoconcentration in the blood, which becomes more coagulable. Combined with stasis of blood in the leg veins, and damage to the venous endothelium, thrombosis may occur in the deep leg veins if the woman is immobilized. Clotting may also occur in the pelvis, where low-grade infection can track along the endometrial and uterine veins to the side walls of the pelvis. This can lead to a thrombophlebitis in the pelvic veins; such a clot is friable, so it may break off, allowing emboli to escape to the pulmonary system. A phlebothrombosis is found in superficial leg veins. It is a more stable clot and is less likely to embolize.

Clinical diagnosis

Leg thrombosis is associated with a history of calf pain and local tenderness of the calf between the muscular heads of gastrocnemius. The mother may have a tachycardia and a low-grade pyrexia. The diagnosis is confirmed by Doppler ultrasound, venography or radioisotope scanning. The first is the easiest and is readily available; with the addition of colour flow, the clot itself may be demonstrated.

Management

Prevention starts with early mobilization of the woman. Should a clot be suspected, full clinical anticoagulation with intravenous heparin through a continuous infusion is needed. This can be exchanged for longer-term anticoagulation with warfarin by mouth, although the dosage of this can sometimes be difficult to control in the puerperium.

Pelvic thrombosis is much harder to diagnose There may be low-grade pyrexia, and the woman may complain of dull pain in the abdomen, but this is common after most deliveries. Vaginal examination may show tenderness in one or other side of the pelvis. The treatment is with combined antibiotics and anticoagulation.

The most dangerous problem of peripheral clotting is that the embolus that may break off and go centrally to the pulmonary circulation: this is one of the major causes of maternal death. Undoubtedly microemboli do break off often, and diagnosis is not always made. This can lead to shortage of breath while there is little pleural pain. These areas of lung non-perfusion have few clinical signs, and the lesser ones probably resolve inside a week or so.

Severe cases follow from involvement of the leg veins in about a third of cases, and the pelvic veins in about 20%, but in about half no clinical signs are found in the periphery. The pulmonary embolism, a larger embolism lodging in the pulmonary arteries, produces acute shortage of breath with faintness and, a little later, chest pain. Physical signs are not usually found immediately after the embolism, but later on there is cyanosis and some right heart failure. When the affect has worked its way through the periphery of the lung to the visceral pleura, it may then affect the parietal pleura, which causes local chest wall pain and signs of collapsed lobe with sometimes a transient pleural rub. Investigations are not much help in the first few hours. Later on a radiograph will confirm the consolidation of the lung lobes. A VQ lung scan is probably the best acute test. It will show ischaemic areas, while pulmonary angiography may show clot. Left-to-right heart catheteriz-ation reveals reversal of pressures. Treatment must be prompt, starting on suspicion. Anti-coagulation should begin immediately, for to await results of sophisticated tests may be too late. Large doses of intravenous heparin and positive-pressure oxygen are the mainstay. Anti-coagulation must be continued, and thrombo-lytics such as streptokinase can be helpful, and their use is increasing. Embolectomy can only be done in a thoracic unit which is immediately available with fully staffed bypass facilities. It is only used for the life threatened who are fortunate (or unfortunate) enough to be in such a large hospital environment.

Puerperal pyrexia

This used to be defined as a temperature of 100.4°F on two occasions more than 4 h apart after the first 24 h of delivery. It used to be a notifiable disease, and a small fee was paid to the notifier by the public health authorities. Those financial incentives may not be unassociated with previous large numbers of reported out-breaks of puerperal fever.

The commonest infection is in the genital tract, although urinary and breast infections should be considered if there is no obvious infection in the pelvis. It is usually due to an ascending *Escherichia coli* or *Streptococcus faecalis* infection, which enters the placental bed and passes rapidly through the myometrium or along the fallopian tube.

Clinical course

Lower abdominal pain is accompanied by the return of either red lochia or frank vaginal bleeding. If the temperature is high enough, there may be systemic pyrexial symptoms of headache and shivering. The uterus is tender to examination, and there are often offensive lochia. High vaginal swabs should be taken, and treatment should be given with antibiotics. If the bleeding is of moderate level, a curettage may be required, but it is wise to await an effective level of antibiotics in the tissues before this is done (at least 8 h after the starting dose). If this precaution is waived, then one can spread infection, causing a systemic pyaemia and even worse effects.

Breast infection may be caused by *Staphylococcus aureus* entering through a break in the skin at the nipple. A painful area occurs in one breast lobule and, if allowed to proceed, may go on to form a breast abscess. The organism can be cultured in the milk from the infected breast. The woman should have a proper supportive brassiere and a broad-spectrum antistaphylococcal antibiotic, correcting this if the milk sample shows insensitive organisms. Should an abscess form, it needs an incision under general anaesthesia and dependent drainage of the offending part. However, it is not mandatory for breast feeding to cease.

Urinary infections

These are discussed in Chapter 5 on antenatal care.

RECOMMENDED READING

Howe P 1995 The puerperium and its complications. In: Whitfield C (ed) Dewhurst's obstetrics and gynaecology for postgraduates. Blackwell, Oxford

Hytten F 1995 The clinical physiology of the puerperium. Farrand Press, London

The baby

For hundreds of years the newborn baby was looked after by midwives and obstetricians. Paediatricians were only involved when a disease was diagnosed. In the last two decades, neonatal paediatrics has advanced enormously so that neonatologists not only care for sick babies but also are very good at looking after normal infants. In consequence, midwives' and obstetricians' roles have diminished in these fields, and most are now happy to work along-side the neonatal paediatricians and their team. However, not everywhere in the world is endowed with such experts, and all who deliver babies must be able to check a newborn child and look after that baby until neonatal help can be obtained. This section therefore is shorter than it would have been in a traditional textbook but contains the essence of neonatal care principles.

ASSESSMENT AT BIRTH

Most children start to breathe within 30 s of birth. In order to cry at an expiration, an inspiration must have occurred before, so the sound of the first cry is reassuring to both the parents and the professional attendants. Assuming the fetus is sufficiently developed to have normal lung physiology, the first inspiration is stimulated by:

- Removal from the gravity-free state inside the uterus
- Mechanical squeezing of vaginal delivery
- Skin touch stimulation on handling

- Temperature changes of the skin
- Stimulation of raised carbon dioxide levels
- Stimulation of reduced oxygen levels
- Pressure changes in the pulmonary circulation following the shutdown of the umbilical flow.

Most babies are pink with regular adequate respiration within minutes of birth. A small number have inadequate breathing which is either shallow or irregular, while an even smaller group are apnoeic and are white and floppy, making no attempt to breathe.

An Apgar score is performed usually at 1 and 5 min (Table 11.1). This scoring system is to check the condition of the baby at birth. It is only a guide to the present state of the baby and not one of prognosis; it is a mixture of one mathematical observation (heart rate) and four increasingly more subjective criteria. Most normal babies achieve a score of 8 or 9 by 1 min. Should there be any doubt about onset of respiration, a cord blood sample should be taken for pH and base deficit measurement.

If the baby has inadequate breathing, mucus and blood should be aspirated from the upper airway. The paediatrician should be summoned urgently, meanwhile the attendant should give oxygen to the baby using a well-fitting neonatal face mask and gently stimulate by stroking the soles of the feet (Fig. 11.1). More violent stimulation is ineffective and may be harmful. Pharyngeal suction through the nose will remove excess fluids and also provide some stimulus to the trigeminal nerve, which supplies the nasal mucous membrane. The baby should be kept dry and covered with warm towels. If by $1\frac{1}{2}$ min the baby is not breathing, a laryngoscope should be passed, and mucus in

the region of the cord aspirated under direct vision.

Intubation should be done by 3 min. This is a straightforward procedure, for the baby who needs it is flat and the cords stand out well. All who are practising active obstetrics and midwifery should be able to intubate a baby, and these skills should have been acquired and kept sharp. If pethidine or morphine has been given to the mother in the last 4 h, neonatal naloxone intravenously can help stimulate respiration if it is depressed.

Should the baby be in terminal apnoea, intubation should be done immediately after birth. Hand pressure on the oxygen supply bag can provide 20 breaths per minute, taking care not to exceed a pressure of $30\,mmH_2O$ (Fig. 11.1).

Once respiration is established, fuller examination of the baby is performed, usually with the mother watching. This is to detect congenital abnormalities which have not been diagnosed antenatally and to obtain an estimate of any pathological conditions which occurred *in utero*, such as infection or birth trauma. Ensure that the baby does not get cold during this examination.

The baby should be measured (length, head circumference and weight), and the mother should be kept informed of all points during the examination. Basically this consists of a general assessment of oxygenation and neurological

Table 11.1 Apgar score

Sign	0 points	1 point	2 points
Skin colour	Cyanosis pallor	Peripheral cyanosis	Pink
Muscle tone	Flaccid	Moves limbs	Good
Respiratory effort	None	Gasps	Good
Heart rate (beats/min)	None	<100	>100
Response to stimulus	None	Slight	Good

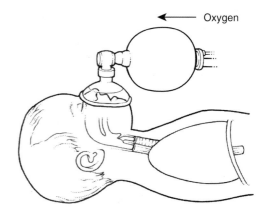

Figure 11.1 Positive pressure respiration with a well-fitting baby face mask, a springy bag and oxygen at 30 mm H$_2$O.

Table 11.2 Points to check on neonatal examination

Body area	Check
General	Cyanosis
	Breathing (Apgar score)
	Neurological behaviour
	Body weight
Head	Tension in fontanelles
	Ears – shape and position
	Eyes – position and epicanthal folds
	Lips – cleft lip and palate
Arms	Digits
	Palmar creases (Down's syndrome)
Chest	Respiration sounds
	Heart murmurs – only persistent ones are significant
Abdomen	Distension
	Umbilical cord has two arteries and one vein
	Exomphalos
	Check anal patency with thermometer
Genitalia	Female – clitoral size
	Male – hypospadias, descent of testicles
Back	Meningomyelocele
	Kyphosis or scoliosis
Legs	Digits
	Talipes
	Congenital dislocation of hips

behaviour and then, in order from the head down to the feet, a check of all the systems (Table 11.2).

INFANT FEEDING

The best food for a human baby is human milk. There may be reasons why breast feeding is not to be used when a substitute formula made from cows' milk is offered. Discussion about feeding usually takes place in the antenatal classes before labour. Figure 11.2 shows the rates of

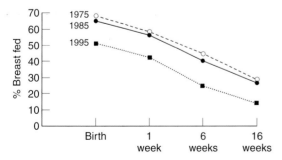

Figure 11.2 Incidence at birth and prevalence later of breast feeding in England and Wales.

breast feeding at various times after birth in the UK over the last 20 years. Whilst there was a considerable improvement between 1975 and 1985, increasing rates of breast feeding have not been maintained in subsequent years. It is wise to talk to parents about breast feeding and to deal with the myths that arise, particularly about the shape and size of a woman's breasts in future in relation to the method of feeding. A woman's breast shape and size is much more affected by the hormone changes of pregnancy than by subsequent breast feeding.

Breast feeding

The mother should be encouraged to put the baby to the breast very soon after delivery, preferably in the labour suite before transfer to the ward. At first the baby will get only a small amount of colostrum, but this is worthwhile for it stimulates the production of more colostrum and then milk; colostrum in its own right contains antibodies to prevent infection.

If breast feeding becomes established, the baby will obtain most of the milk required in the first 5 min, hence prolonged breast feeding is not particularly advantageous to the baby although it may be satisfying to the mother. Most babies are best fed on demand. Regimens laid down at set intervals of 3 or 4 h are doomed to failure; within a few weeks, demand feeding becomes a 3–4-hourly feed anyway.

It is difficult to overfeed a breast-fed baby. Conversely, if the mother's milk does not seem to be enough in the first week, breast feeding should be continued, with the mother increasing her own fluid intake to help produce the right amount of milk for her baby. If the baby needs supplementary feeding, then dextrose solutions can be used. Test weighing is not generally used now, for it is not held to be helpful to the management of the baby.

As can be seen from Figure 11.2, most people are starting to wean by 4 months, and breast feeding rarely continues after 6 months in the UK, although in parts of the world where continued lactation is used for contraception, breast feeding can continue for up to 2 years. As

a contraceptive, it has little effect after this.
The advantages of breast feeding are:

- It is the correct mix for the baby
- It helps with mother-to-baby and baby-to-mother bonding
- There are anti-infective agents in the milk
- It eliminates the risk of infection which may come from unclean bottles
- It aids uterine involution
- It is cheap

Breast feeding will be enhanced by:

- Advice and encouragement of the mother, preferably by one midwife – if several midwives are caring for her, they should all offer consistent advice and not give individual policies
- A well-fitting, properly selected brassiere
- Changing the baby's nappy before the feed so that the child is contented throughout
- Ensuring that the baby is awake and the mother is sitting comfortably
- Adequate fluid in the mother's diet.

Breast feeding may be hindered by:

- Conflicting advice given by different midwives
- The mother not really wanting to breast feed and only starting it to please others
- Retracted or inverted nipples which could not be corrected in the antenatal period
- Poor fixation of the baby on to the nipple
- Deformity of the lip or palate of the baby

- Inadequate stimulation of lactation when the baby is also having formula feed.

Bottle feeding

A substantial proportion of mothers in the UK do not want to, or cannot, breast feed. Formula feeds are of cows' milk with sodium and potassium concentrations reduced to those of the level of human milk. Many have added vitamins.

If the feeds are made strictly according to instructions, bottle feeding goes well. The bottles and teats need cleaning and sterilizing, usually with a hypochlorite solution. The milk will need warming before use. The advantage of bottle feeding is that people other than the mother can feed the baby, thus relieving her, for example, of some night feeds. Involvement of the partner may be beneficial to him as he may be feeling neglected and unwanted at this time.

The problems with bottle feeding are:

- It is not always the ideal mix for the baby
- There are no anti-infective properties as there are in breast milk
- Gastroenteritis can occur if the bottles are not sterilized properly
- The size of the hole in the teat has to be carefully adapted to the baby:
  - if too small the baby cannot get enough milk
  - if too large the baby will be overloaded and unable to cope
- It costs money

RECOMMENDED READING

Sinclair J, Bracken M 1993 Effective care of the newborn infant. Oxford University Press, Oxford

Statistics on childbirth

Long before audit was used in the rest of medicine, obstetricians, midwives and paediatricians were keeping and publishing good data on the events surrounding childbirth. Death is a firm diagnosis, and mortality figures have been kept efficiently in many parts of the world. Morbidity is harder to delineate and quantify; only recently have we been trying to measure the major problems of childbirth which are not associated with death.

MATERNAL MORTALITY

A maternal death is one that occurs during pregnancy, childbirth or the first 42 days of the puerperium. In the UK we still keep information up to 1 year after death, but 42 days is the internationally recognized puerperal time, and this definition allows comparison between one country and another.

Maternal death might be:

- *Direct* – the result of an obstetrical complication or its treatment, e.g. postpartum haemorrhage
- *Indirect* – previous existing diseases which deteriorate because of the pregnancy, e.g. mitral stenosis
- *Fortuitous* – when the death occurred in the pregnancy time period but was not related to the pregnancy, e.g. a road traffic accident.

In the UK, the proportions of maternal deaths in each group are respectively 50, 35 and 10%. When comparing different countries it is important to know whether the data on maternal mortality include all three of these group or, as

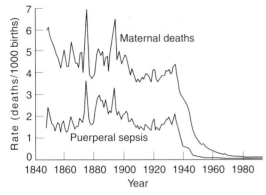

Figure 12.1   Maternal mortality (England and Wales, 1847–1993). Note how the total mortality rates mirror those of puerperal sepsis deaths.

is often done, only the direct deaths. Other variations arise from the inclusion of or omission of abortion and ectopic pregnancy. These occur in early pregnancy and sometimes are not included with maternal deaths.

Figure 12.1 shows the maternal mortality rate (MMR) for England and Wales over the last 150 years. They plateaued until about the mid-1930s, when they suddenly reduced.

Examination of Figure 12.1 also shows the deaths from puerperal sepsis, and gives clues about the major cause for this sudden reduction. Currently, in the UK the MMR is 9.8 per 100 000 maternities. There is an international move to change the denominator to 1 million. If this happens, the UK MMR will be 98/1 000 000 maternities.

In general, maternal mortality rates are improving in the world due to:

- Better nutrition of women
- Better health of mothers
- Change in reproductive patterns:
  - Smaller families
  - Fewer young mothers (< 16 years old)
  - Fewer old mothers (> 40 years old)
- Better education of women
- Improved communications and transport
- Improved antenatal and delivery care (both midwifery and medical)
- Wider use of antibiotics
- Wider availability of blood transfusion.

In the UK, details of maternal deaths are collected and published in the *Report of the Confidential Enquiry into Maternal Deaths*, produced by the Departments of Health, and to which most doctors are willing to submit their data. Every 3 years a new report is published, and is highly recommended reading for all who practice obstetrics.

Major causes of death in the UK are:

- Thrombosis
- Pulmonary embolism
- Haemorrhage (both antepartum and postpartum)
- Hypertensive disease.

Anaesthesia was associated with many deaths, often because it was attempted by inexperienced medical staff. In the UK, infection and abortion are both greatly reduced as causes.

The Confidential Enquiry scheme has allowed examination of all cases in detail. There is no judicial basis, and no blame is attached when the professionals assess their own work. In almost a half of the deaths reported, there was some diminution below acceptable standards of satisfactory care, and so the death may have been avoidable. Sometimes this was due to the patient not seeking medical advice or ignoring it when it was given; on other occasions it was associated with the use of too junior staff in the hospital performing or anaesthetizing for caesarean sections.

Probably the most efficacious ways of improving maternal death rates are by:

- Tailoring antenatal care to women who need it most and seeing that they have a more intensive system
- Improving women's education so that they are aware themselves of symptoms of impending problems.

A greater involvement of senior doctors in the labour ward, particularly in decision making and the practical performance of difficult procedures would help greatly.

Maternal mortality rates are now in the region of 9/100 000 in the UK, which means one might expect about 60 deaths a year. This, despite careful scrutiny, is a very small number, and once broken down for analysis is not so valid. Recently, numbers have increased slightly by examining maternal deaths in the whole UK together rather than just England and Wales or Scotland or Northern Ireland. One could also increase numbers by extending the time interval over which deaths are assessed, but since techniques in pregnancy and labour management are changing rapidly there is a limit to the length of the time period being examined. Currently it is triennial.

NEAR MISSES

Efforts have been made to widen the assessment of the morbidity of pregnancy by looking at women who have non-fatal episodes of the same conditions as the death enquirers examine. It is more difficult to create definitions, and the limits of the condition laid down must be strictly adhered to, but does give a larger database. For example, one could examine women who lose more than a measured 1000 ml of blood in a postpartum haemorrhage, thus giving between 10 and 20 times the number of cases to examine compared with the postpartum haemorrhage deaths. Similarly, analysis can be of women who have eclampsia and did not die or survivors of pulmonary embolism proven by a Xenon 133 ventilation lung scan. These near misses are now being assessed in several centres, and it is hoped soon that acceptable definitions of near misses may be formulated so that a national examination of this larger population can be made.

PERINATAL MORTALITY

Data on neonatal deaths, those babies who died in the first month of life, have been kept in the UK for over 100 years. Those on stillbirths, who are born dead in the viable period of gestation, have been collected since the 1920s. The definition of viability was moved in 1991 from 28 weeks to 24 weeks of gestation, because with much better neonatal care many smaller babies are surviving. Thus the neonatal death (NND) rate and stillbirth (SB) rates are

$$SB\ rate\ =\ \frac{SB}{1000\ total\ births}$$

$$NND\ rate\ =\ \frac{NND}{1000\ live\ births}$$

In the 1920s it was agreed in Europe to make use of a third definition, trying to relate events more to obstetrical pathology and management. The perinatal mortality rate (PNMR) was devised as a combination of the stillbirth and the first week of neonatal deaths, hence

$$PNMR\ =\ \frac{SB + \frac{1}{52}NND}{1000\ total\ births}$$

Currently the PNMR is about 8/1000 in the UK (Fig. 12.2).

Information is obtained from the stillbirth death certificates and neonatal death certificates filled in by the doctors or midwives who were involved in the case and handled by the Office of National Statistics, which used to be the Office of Populations, Censuses and Surveys. The range of death rates reported from most parts of the UK is wide (Fig. 12.3), considering that the country has a fairly uniform National Health Service. This is mostly due to variations in the standard of nutrition and education.

The factors that affect perinatal mortality are:

- The health of the mother
- The mother's past nutrition and diseases
- The mother's education
- The mother's age

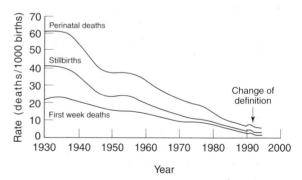

Figure 12.2 Perinatal mortality, stillbirths and neonatal death rates (England and Wales, 1930–94). Note the blip in 1991, when the definition of viability was reduced from 28 to 24 weeks of gestation.

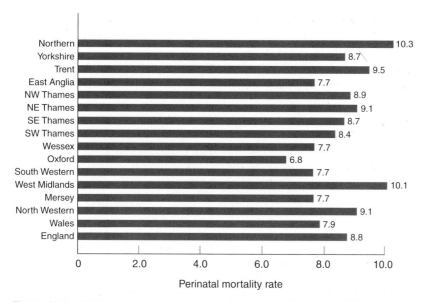

Figure 12.3   Relative perinatal mortality rates in regions of England and Wales.

- The mother's parity
- Services from midwives and doctors given at the appropriate place.

A new method of assay of UK perinatal deaths has started this decade. The *Confidential Enquiry into Stillbirths and Infant Deaths* (CESDI) is emulating the assessment performed on maternal deaths. At regional level all perinatal deaths are assessed in a confidential fashion, and from this conclusions are made. For example, in the most recent (1998) report, about half of the deaths of mature normal singleton babies which occurred in labour were considered to be associated with substandard care. This is an indictment on all who practice midwifery and obstetrics.

Causes of perinatal mortality in the West are:

- Small for gestational age:
  - Symmetrical: mature for age but born early – a miniature baby
  - Asymmetrical: inappropriately small for age – a baby with intrauterine malnutrition

- Congenital malformations, principally those of the central nervous and cardiovascular systems
- Asphyxia (hypoxia):
  - Before labour:
    Acute: abruption
    Chronic: placental malperfusion
  - In labour:
    Prolonged labour
    Fetal distress:
    Poor placental perfusion
    Cord entanglement

In the UK, birth injuries and infection are much less common as causes of death.

It is fortunate in the UK that maternal death information can be obtained from the *Report of the Confidential Enquiry into Maternal Deaths*. Unfortunately perinatal data, until the foundation of CESDI, has suffered from grave Governmental Statistical deficiencies – no data are available from 1986 to 1988 because of a change in computer systems, and even now the returns are patchy, with only 60% of regions producing satisfactory data.

RECOMMENDED READING

Department of Health 1999 Report of the confidential enquiry into maternal deaths in the UK 1994–1996. The Stationery Office, London

Department of Health 1999 Confidential enquiry into stillbirths and deaths in infancy. 6th annual report. The Stationery Office, London

Macfarlane A, Mugford M 1999 Birth counts – statistics of pregnancy and childbirth. The Stationery Office, London

Gynaecology

13

The gynaecological patient

It is impossible to gather precise data from nationally generated statistics on the involvement of primary or tertiary care doctors in gynaecological problems. Prevalence rates show an increase in consulting a general practitioner between 1981 and 1991 for genitourinary conditions of 30%. This is amongst the higher of the increases in consultations, but it shrinks in significance alongside female consultations for osteoporosis (214%), or benign neoplasms of the skin amongst women (185% increase). This is not reflected amongst females when examining hospital inpatient enquiry data, which show no great increase in hospital consultations for genitourinary problems on episode-based rates. It is probable that the average woman goes to a doctor 3.6 times a year, and about a tenth of these visits are for gynaecological causes, i.e. once every 3 years. All statistics certainly confirm that a woman will go to her doctor several times in her lifetime with gynaecological problems.

Initial consultation will be with the general practitioner and, often, it will stop there for he can nowadays diagnose and treat so many gynaecological conditions perfectly adequately. If the practitioner thinks it is necessary, the woman may be referred to a hospital gynaecologist, where she will be seen as an outpatient primarily, and may be admitted for further treatment. A parallel source of women requiring gynaecological assistance is from the Well Women Clinics. These have been formed in the last 20 years, and provide a centre where a woman can attend to discuss matters that relate to the pelvic organs. Some of these clinics take place in family-planning centres, others are free standing, while a third group is in the general practitioner's surgery. Additionally, cervical screening has been added, so that there is a move towards gynaecological problems at these Well Women Clinics. Women who are thinking of hormone replacement therapy attend, as do some who are concerned about their contraceptive practice. Whilst there is plenty of capacity for consultation in the primary and tertiary care system for these problems, it is to the Well Women Clinic that the women often turn. There they will get sympathetic attention from nurse practitioners as well as from doctors, and this is considered important by many women.

Typically, no woman wants to see a gynaecologist. Women will attend with various degrees of unwillingness, rather like we all go to the dentist, but they feel there may be some return from a pelvic examination which will help them in their lives. Hence the doctor who takes part in gynaecology must be sympathetic to the woman's feelings when she attends. A different attitude towards women is required from those doctors who attend to ear, nose and throat or orthopaedic problems.

CLINICAL GYNAECOLOGICAL ASSESSMENT

This starts when the woman enters the room: the way she walks and her demeanour are important features which the clinician should spot. Specifically a history should be taken, then an examination and investigations performed. All this will help to make a diagnosis.

History

The history is best done under a series of systematic headings, and often leading questions must be asked. The woman may be reluctant to mention certain matters relating to a previous termination of pregnancy or sexual activity, and therefore the questions should not follow a set order: she should be questioned as the practi-

tioner thinks fit, but the answers should be recorded in the notes in a systematic way.

In addition, the obstetrical history, menstrual history, details of vaginal discharge, micturition and sexual histories must be taken. A past history of major illnesses or major surgery is needed, and the social history and family history will be helpful.

The chief symptom must be examined with care: its duration, its relation to the menstrual cycle, and its description. There must be a note of all past drugs which have been taken.

At the end of the history, the practitioner should be in a position to make a working diagnosis. Probably two-thirds of gynaecological conditions can be suspected on history alone.

Examination

On examination, check the attitude of the patient and her demeanour, for a woman in acute pain will present in a different state from one with chronic pain or none at all. Anaemia must be assessed and the blood pressure taken.

The abdomen should be examined by inspecting from the costal margin down to the pubis, with the patient comfortably relaxed Fat or wasting should be noted, and previous scars recorded. The two commonest scars in gynaecology are the laparoscopy scar under the lower border of the umbilicus and the Pfannenstiel transverse scar in the lower abdomen. Light palpation to check for tenderness should be followed by deeper palpation to check for enlargement of the liver, kidneys, or ovaries and uterus. It is probably wise to use the left hand (for a right-handed observer) to examine the lower abdomen to check any pathology which rises up from the pelvis. Percussion may be required if ascitic fluid is thought to be present, and auscultation may reveal fetal heart sounds if the woman is pregnant.

Pelvic examination is essential in gynaecology. Conventionally it is a bimanual examination, where the index finger of the right hand is introduced into the vagina and the left hand gently palpates the abdomen above. Nearly all vaginal examinations should start with a single finger, although if the vagina is voluminous or particularly long, the middle finger may be required also. The woman should be asked if she would like a chaperone to be present; this is irrespective of the gender of the doctor. Some patients are comforted by the presence of another woman; others prefer the confidentiality of the doctor/patient relationship. The General Medical Council recommends that a chaperone should usually be present unless the patient specifically requests that she should not be.

After a full explanation and making the woman comfortable, the vulva is inspected for local lesions. The examination is usually performed using the dorsal position, although some prefer to assess a woman in the left lateral position with her face away from the examiner. A woman should be covered with a sheet or light blanket down to her knees, for once the vulva has been inspected, there is no need for it to be further exposed. With the lubricated finger or fingers in the vagina, the uterus is palpated through the abdominal wall with the examiner's other hand, noting its size, consistency and shape and the presence of any tumours. Tenderness will be noted, particularly on movement, and the mobility and position of the uterus will be tested. This is a bimanual examination, and the stereotaxic observations perceived by the observer will be from both hands, as much from the abdominal as the vaginal hand.

Once the uterus has been delineated, the fingers in the vagina are slipped into the right fornix, and the left hand is moved towards the right iliac fossa. By gentle palpation, the adnexa are found and then held between the examining fingers. Usually no ovarian or tubal swelling is felt. The fingers are moved across to the left fornix, and a similar examination performed on the left side. This is much harder to do. Then the fingers pass to the posterior fornix, seeking any swellings in the pouch of Douglas. On withdrawal of the fingers, check for any blood on the glove.

A rectal examination is rarely required unless the examiner may think there may be some problem with the uterosacral ligaments or the pouch of Douglas.

A speculum is passed to examine the cervix. It is better to do this after the bimanual examination, for the woman has a little more confidence then, rather than starting off with a metal instrument. Either a Cuscoe's speculum (Fig. 13.1) is gently passed when the woman is lying in the dorsal position, or a Sims's speculum (Fig. 13.2) if using the left lateral position. The latter is more commonly used when assessing a prolapse. Either gives a good view of the cervix and, if necessary, a cervical smear should be taken.

Investigations

It is probably wise to check the haemoglobin level if a woman is going to proceed to surgery, and other blood tests may be performed at the same time. Serum ferritin levels are useful in assessing the severity of bleeding problems. The urine should be checked for albumin and sugar. The cervical cytology may be investigated if the

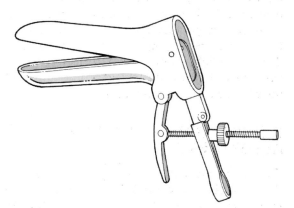

Figure 13.1   A bivalve (Cuscoe's) speculum.

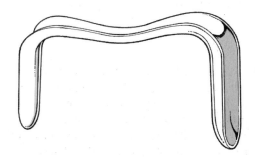

Figure 13.2   A Sims's speculum.

woman has not had a smear done in the last few years.

Hormone levels in the plasma are enormously wide ranged, depending on the stage of the woman's cycle and the phase of secretion of the hormone. However, in some instances, it may be specifically indicated, such as a luteal phase progesterone if pregnancy is considered. Ultrasound may detect and assess the existence of pelvic tumours, particularly those inside the uterus. Magnetic resonance imaging is being used more, particularly if there is some doubt about a mass inside the pelvis, and computerized tomography also gives good images of tissue changes.

Radiography is not so helpful in gynaecology now, but may still be used to look at gas and fluid levels in the gut when testing for intestinal obstruction. Further, they have a specific place when a tumour may contain calcium such as a dermoid of the ovary, which can show teeth. Intravenous urography may be helpful to check the renal tract, particularly if major surgery close to the ureters is planned; a barium enema can help the differential diagnosis of rectal conditions. Hysterosalpingography has a limited place. Endoscopy is very helpful in specific circumstances to examine the cavity of the uterus (hysteroscopy) or the pelvic cavity (laparoscopy).

Conclusion

After examination and the results of possible investigations, the doctor should have a differential diagnosis. He should discuss the likely diagnoses with the woman and her partner. Some will not require any treatment but reassurance. This is something which should not be dismissed, for it takes time and competence to put over. Others may require medical treatment with hormones, which should be described, and arrangements made to see the woman at appropriate intervals afterwards. It is not good enough to send her off next time to see somebody else in general practice, or a junior doctor, for she may require modification of the hormone therapy.

A small number of women will require surgery, and these women should be considered with special care. Details should be discussed of what the surgery might include, what may be removed and what is left. Complications, side-effects and, hopefully, good results should be talked about. Some idea of how long the woman will be in hospital, the degree of inconvenience to her then and later in life should be considered. Information leaflets are of considerable use, to allow the woman and her partner to learn more about her operation in the more relaxed atmosphere of her home. Ideally the surgeon should have an operations diary in the outpatients department in order to offer women a date for admission for surgery, even though it may be some months away. This allows for any essential rearrangement of business and household affairs. It is important that the practitioner keeps to these dates as far as possible: only major reasons should necessitate any cancellation.

RECOMMENDED READING

Royal College of Obstetrics and Gynaecology 1998 Intimate examinations. Report of a working party. RCOG Press, London

Miscarriage

The word abortion is used by the public to mean therapeutic abortion, i.e. an active termination of pregnancy. Miscarriage is a softer phrase for the spontaneous event – the expulsion or attempted expulsion of a fetus before the 24th week of gestation.

THREATENED MISCARRIAGE

The threatened miscarriage is designated as one where the pregnancy is continuing and the internal os of the cervix is closed. As might be expected, there is little bleeding or pain (Fig. 14.1).

If ultrasound shows a live fetus (with a heartbeat after 7 weeks) there is an 85% survival rate. Hospital admission is unnecessary, but most woman would expect the doctor to advise rest, avoidance of violent exercise and avoidance of sexual intercourse for the next few weeks. However, there is no evidence that any of these therapies actually affect the outcome.

INEVITABLE MISCARRIAGE

The woman has a greater increase of lower abdominal cramping, bleeding and the passage of clots. On examination, the internal os of the cervix is open. If all the products of conception have been expelled, the miscarriage is *complete*, an unusual occurrence before 14 weeks of gestation. Should there be retained products, pieces of membrane, decidua or placenta, the miscarriage is *incomplete*, and the woman might go on bleeding.

(a)

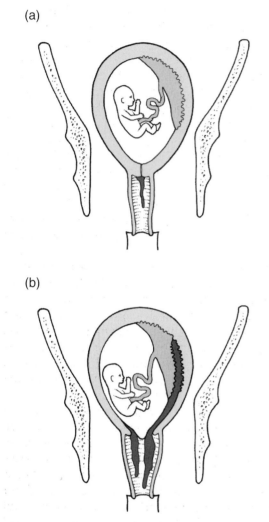

(b)

Figure 14.1 **a** Threatened miscarriage. Note that the cervix is closed and blood loss is slight. **b** Inevitable miscarriage. Note that the cervix has opened and much more blood is lost.

The treatment is evacuation of the incomplete miscarriage usually under general anaesthesia. The difficulty is deciding which of this group are going to be complete, so many hospital doctors perform an evacuation anyway if the pregnancy is before 16 weeks of gestation rather than waiting, for it is a more pragmatic use of hospital beds and may be more convenient for the woman.

SILENT MISCARRIAGE

This was previously called missed abortion. The

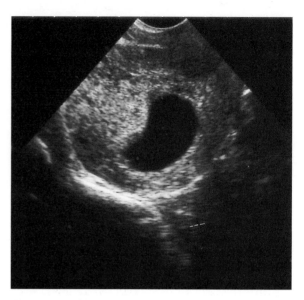

Figure 14.2 Silent or missed miscarriage.

fetus has died but no expulsion follows. It is hard to differentiate from a threatened miscarriage, but an ultrasound scan may well show the absence of a fetus who died earlier in pregnancy or that the fetus is smaller than the dates suggest and there is no fetal heart beat. Most women need an evacuation or a medical induction to complete the process (Fig. 14.2).

SEPTIC MISCARRIAGE

The woman may present with lower abdominal pain, pyrexia and vaginal discharge; on examination the uterus is tender. Traditionally these were suspected of being associated with attempted illegal interference, which assists the passage of bacteria up the cervical canal, but nowadays they are more likely to be associated with the presence of an intrauterine contraceptive device.

Evacuation should be performed under antibiotic cover with a high-dose of broad-spectrum antibiotic. Endometrial swabs are taken for bacteriological examination. A senior person should do the evacuation for in the presence of sepsis, perforation of the uterus is very easy, and the introduction of potentially septic matter into the peritoneal cavity is serious.

If the pyrexia goes within 24 h, the woman is considered to be recovering, but if it continues, specific antibiotics should be given, determined from sensitivities on the endometrial swabs. The use of intravenous heparin may be required at this point, for sepsis may have spread to the pelvic veins, causing a thrombophlebitis which could go on to a pulmonary embolism.

RECURRENT MISCARRIAGE

Roughly 15% of pregnancies end in a clinical miscarriage in women under the age of 35 years. The rate increases rapidly after this age, and for women over the age of 40 years, a rate of 25% can be expected. Recurrent miscarriage is defined as the loss of three or more consecutive pregnancies; the probability of three consecutive losses is near 1% of couples who suffer from recurrent miscarriage. This suggests that for some women there is a repetitive underlying cause for their pregnancy loss. The more common causes of recurrent miscarriage are:

1. *Thrombophilic defects*. It is now established that certain thrombophilic defects are an important cause of pregnancy loss. These are antiphospholipid antibodies, lupus anticoagulant and anticardiolipin antibodies. Treatment in those women with demonstrable antibodies has been with either low molecular weight heparin or low-dose aspirin or occasionally a combination of both. The live birth rate is increased from 40 to 70% in this group. For women with a history of second-trimester miscarriage, thrombophilic defects associated with activated protein C resistance and Leiden factor V have been implicated in up to 20% of cases, and thrombophilic defects such as lowered protein C, protein S and antithrombin III levels should be looked for in midtrimester loss.

2. *Genetic*. A parental chromosome abnormality is found in 3–5% of couples with recurrent miscarriage, the most common being a balanced reciprocal or a Robertsonian translocation. Blood from both partners must be taken, and if a genetic cause found, the couple should be referred for genetic counselling.

3. *Endocrine*. In the past it has been good practice to study both thyroid and carbohydrate dysfunction. However, these are uncommon causes of miscarriage nowadays. Twenty percent of women in their reproductive years are found to have polycystic ovaries, and among those with recurrent miscarriage over 30% have demonstrable polycystic ovaries on ultrasound, and hypersecrete luteinizing hormone (LH). Unfortunately, treatments that reduce LH levels do not seem to improve pregnancy outcome. High levels of LH may merely be a marker for some other endocrine pathology as yet unknown.

4. *Infection*. Many viral and some bacterial infections may cause a spontaneous miscarriage but are seldom a cause for recurrent loss. However, bacterial vaginosis appears to be an important cause of midtrimester loss and premature rupture of the membranes, although an association with first-trimester miscarriage has not been shown. Gram staining of a lateral vaginal wall smear for the presence of clue cells will confirm the diagnosis, and treatment with oral metronidazole or vaginal clindamycin (2% cream) will eradicate the infection.

5. *Anatomical*. It is interesting to note that the presence of recurrent miscarriage in women with uterine abnormalities is the same as in women without, so it is unlikely that corrective surgery will help. Cervical circlage (Shirodkar or MacDonald stitch) has been widely used for women with a previous midtrimester loss but following a Medical Research Council/Royal College of Obstetricians and Gynaecologists trial, a favourable outcome was only reported in one-third of cases.

6. *Immune*. The possibility of an immune basis to recurrent miscarriage is attractive, but a meta-analysis of recent trials has failed to show an association.

Of those women attending a recurrent miscarriage clinic where no cause for the problem has been found, over 65% went on to have a live child. The placebo effect is strong, and underlines the need for sympathetic and caring treatment for these women who are under considerable psychological strain.

15

Termination of pregnancy

Therapeutic termination of pregnancy is the medical or surgical interruption of a pregnancy; it has been legal in the UK since the passage of the 1967 Abortion Act, which was modified in 1991. Two registered medical practitioners have to be in agreement on one of the clauses in Box 15.1.

Box 15.1 Summary of the clauses in the Termination of Pregnancy Act

---

A. The continuance of the pregnancy would involve risk to the life of the pregnant woman greater than if the pregnancy were terminated.
B. The termination is necessary to prevent grave permanent injury to the physical or mental health of the pregnant woman.
C. The pregnancy has *not* exceeded its 24th week and the continuance of the pregnancy would involve risk, greater than if the pregnancy were terminated, of injury to the physical or mental health of the pregnant woman.
D. The pregnancy has *not* exceeded its 24th week and the continuance of the pregnancy would involve risk, greater than if the pregnancy were terminated, of injury to the physical or mental health of any existing child(ren) of the family of the pregnant woman.
E. There is a substantial risk that if the child were born it would suffer from such physical or mental abnormalities as to be seriously handicapped.

Approximately 85% of terminations are carried out before 12 weeks of gestation, most of the remainder being carried out between 13 and 24 weeks, the latter being the maximum gestational age allowed by law except under clause E, where there is no time restriction. Approximately 175 000 terminations are carried out per

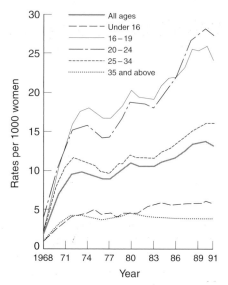

Figure 15.1 Reported termination of pregnancy (England and Wales, 1968–1991).

annum within the UK, of which approximately two-thirds are in women who are single and 10% under the age of 20 years (Fig. 15.1).

COUNSELLING

This should be impartial and non-directional; an adequate amount of time must be allowed. Two separate medical practitioners need to see the patient, and usually one of them is the gynaecologist who will carry out the procedure. It is important to take a full medical, social and contraceptive history, to discuss alternative courses of action, and, if required, to give information on the various methods of termination and their risks. It is important to allow the woman time to reach a decision although she may well have thought deeply about this decision while awaiting an appointment – 80% of women seeking a termination have. In cases where terminations are carried out for chromosomal or structural defects of the fetus, formal genetic counselling is wise.

For girls under the age of 16 years, consent from a parent or legal guardian is advisable although not an absolute necessity. In law, the procedure may be performed once two doctors have agreed to it provided that the girl fully understands the nature of the procedure and there are overwhelming reasons why the parent or guardian should not know of the intended termination.

When dealing with the mentally defective, consent of the legal guardian is required. If there is not one, then a judge in chambers should be consulted.

METHODS

First trimester

Medical

Antiprogestogens such as mifepristone in combination with prostaglandin may be used prior to the 9th week of pregnancy. A regime in which the antiprogestogen is taken on one day followed by the insertion of prostaglandin pessaries on the third day has a success rate of over 95%. Incomplete miscarriage occurs in 2–3% of cases, and there may be prolonged relatively light bleeding for up to a week following the procedure.

Surgical

Suction evacuation of the uterine contents under general anaesthesia is the most commonly used method in the UK, and can be carried out up to 12–14 weeks of gestation. It is usually performed as a day case procedure. Dilatation of the cervix is carried out followed by insertion of a suction curette. The uterine cavity is curetted gently at the end of the procedure to check that there are no remaining products of gestation. Priming of the cervix with a prostaglandin may be carried out before the procedure to facilitate dilatation and reduce trauma.

Second trimester

The use of intra-amniotic hypertonic solutions such as saline or urea has largely fallen into disrepute. An extra-amniotic prostaglandin infusion or, more commonly, vaginal prostaglandin pessaries are now the most widely used methods. The procedure is often lengthy, usually in excess of 8 h, and involves the woman going through a mini-labour with a vaginal delivery of the fetus and placenta. An epidural anaesthetic may be provided to cover the worst part of this.

Hysterotomy

This is a surgical procedure akin to a caesarean section. A vertical incision has to be made into the uterus as the lower segment is not formed, and this may have consequent problems for subsequent full-term pregnancies. The method is very rarely used in the UK.

MORBIDITY

Blood loss increases in first-trimester terminations with increased gestational age, and it is usual to give an oxytocic preparation with the procedure. Uterine perforation is a rare occurrence but it can occur, particularly with a retroverted uterus. In general, fundal perforation is not a problem, but when not recognized, bowel can be pulled down into the uterus and damaged. If there is any doubt, then laparoscopy should be undertaken to ascertain the severity of the perforation and damage to the intra-abdominal contents. Repair may need a laparotomy.

The incidence of chlamydial infection prior to the procedure can be as high as 25% in single women. For this reason it is advisable to give prophylactic antibiotics from the time of the procedure onwards, and endocervical swabbing prior to termination of pregnancy is advisable. The rate of postoperative sepsis is dependent upon the presence of retained products and untreated pelvic inflammatory disease.

Long-term complications are fortunately few. Some women develop feelings of guilt and depression following the procedure which may last for years, but serious psychiatric disturbance is rare provided the woman entered into the termination voluntarily.

Infertility is similarly rare, while cervical incompetence, although reported, is not a problem, especially when cervical softening agents are used. Rhesus iso-immunization is prevented by routinely giving anti-D immunoglobulin to susceptible patients.

FOLLOW-UP

Because of the social circumstances of the termination, this is often very difficult. However, it is essential that adequate contraception is provided for the woman prior to her discharge from the hospital environment. This should be followed up either by the general practitioner or in a family planning clinic.

RECOMMENDED READING

Cameron S, Baird D 1997 Implications for gynaecological service of new medical methods of therapeutic abortion. Contemporary Reviews in Obstetrics and Gynaecology 9: 121–127

Gold M, Luks D, Anderson M 1997 Medical options for early pregnancy termination. America Family Physician 56: 533–538

Grimes D 1997 Medical abortion in early pregnancy. Obstetrics and Gynaecology 89: 790–796

Murry S, Muse K 1996 Mifepristone and first trimester abortion. Clinical Obstetrics and Gynaecology 39: 474–485

16

Infections

VULVAL AND VAGINAL INFECTIONS

In the reproductive years the most common vaginal infection is thrush caused by candida, which typically presents with intense pruritus and a thick creamy discharge, often likened to cottage cheese. When removed from the vaginal wall there is an erythematous patch beneath it which may bleed. There are numerous anti-fungal agents on the market, most of which are given vaginally, but some may be adminstered orally. It is important to treat the patient's partner even though most men remain asymptomatic.

In the postmenopausal patient, atrophic vaginitis will lead to a thin greyish watery discharge which may cause pruritus. It is due to a lack of lactobacillus in the vagina as a consequence of oestrogen deprivation. Bowel bacteria, particularly *Escherichia coli* and *Streptococcus faecalis*, invade the vagina and lead to the discharge. The most effective treatment is re-oestrogenization of the vagina with topical creams or oral preparations.

Sexually transmitted infections are listed in Table 16.1.

Table 16.1 Sexually transmitted infections

Bacterial	Viral	Other
Gonorrhoea	Human	Trichomonas
Syphilis	papillomavirus	Pediculosis pubis
Chancroid	Herpes simplex	
β-haemolytic	Molluscum	
streptococcus	contagiosum	
Bacterial vaginosis	HIV	
Chlamydia		

Less common is bacterial vaginosis (also known as anaerobic vaginosis), which leads to a profuse often frothy discharge with a characteristic fishy smell. Diagnosis can be made by performing a Gram stain on an air-dried vaginal wall smear. This shows the presence of characteristic clue cells, mature epithelial cells covered with mixed bacteria. The most common bacterium is *Gardnerella vaginalis*. Treatment is with a week's course of metronidazole.

Chlamydia infections are common and are dealt with later in the section on pelvic inflammatory disease. The infection seldom leads to a significant vaginal discharge but may occasionally lead to intermenstrual or postcoital bleeding.

Trichomonas vaginalis is an uncommon cause of a vaginal discharge nowadays. It leads to a profuse green, frothy and highly offensive discharge. The diagnosis can be made by a wet-slide preparation in which the trichomonads can be easily seen. Treatment is with metronidazole.

Other local infections are considered in Chapter 7.

PELVIC INFLAMMATORY DISEASE

Pelvic inflammatory disease (PID) has become a major problem both in the developed and in developing countries, where it is a leading cause of infertility. Although associated with an incomplete miscarriage and retained products of conception, it is classically a sexually transmitted disease.

The main vector of infection is seminal fluid, and PID is therefore an ascending condition, affecting first the endometrium and parametrium and later the tubes (salpingitis), the ovaries (oophoritis) and eventually the peritoneum.

The incidence of the condition varies in different parts of the world; estimates of a rate of 2% per year amongst sexually active women being quoted both for the USA and western Europe. In parts of Africa it is even more common. It is known that 20% of women seeking termination of pregnancy under the age of 18 years harbour *Chlamydia*, one of the major causes of PID.

Aetiology

For infectious agents to ascend through the genital tract they must first pass through the cervix. For much of the menstrual cycle the cervical mucus provides a relatively strong barrier to the ascent of infection. However, this is absent at the time of ovulation, in the menses and during pregnancy, and is particularly deficient with miscarriage or therapeutic termination of pregnancy. The quality of cervical mucus can be altered by hormonal therapy, and progestogen-only preparations lead to a thick mucus plug which is inhospitable both to sperm and infection. Similarly the combined oral contraceptive acts on the cervical mucus, reducing its effectiveness as a barrier to infection. Young women who take the contraceptive pill and are having intercourse with a new partner are advised to use barrier methods as well. Any instrumentation through the cervix such as the insertion of an intrauterine contraceptive device, evacuation of retained products of conception, or even hysterosalpingography may introduce infection into the uterine cavity.

Causes

In the past the most common cause of pelvic inflammatory disease has been gonorrhoea, caused by the bacterium *Neisseria gonococcus*. However, in western Europe and the USA the most common organism now is *Chlamydia tracomatis*, although this is usually associated with the presence of other organisms including *Bacteroides*, *Gardnerella*, *E. coli*, *streptococci*, *Mycoplasma* and *Ureaplasma*.

Signs and symptoms

The condition usually presents as bilateral lower abdominal pain, dyspareunia and often irregular menstrual bleeding. A vaginal discharge is not necessarily present, especially with chlamydial infections. An acute peritonitis may develop, and this may be associated with abscess formation. Occasionally patients may present with acute right upper abdominal pain, which can be easily confused with cholecystitis. The pain is due to a chlamydial infection leading to adhesion formation between the peritoneum of the underside of the diaphragm and the liver, the Fitz–Hugh–Curtiss syndrome.

The patient may be pyrexial, particularly with gonococcal infections. On examination of the abdomen there is often evidence of pelvic peritonitis with guarding and rigidity, although in milder cases there may just be bilateral tenderness on deep palpation.

On pelvic bimanual examination there is bilateral adnexal tenderness, and movement of the cervix will exacerbate the pain. In severe cases a pelvic mass may be palpable, and in chronic cases the uterus may be fixed by adhesions in retroversion. At the time of the initial examination a bivalve speculum should be passed to expose the cervix. Both high vaginal and endocervical swabs should be taken for pathogens, the latter being for detection of *Chlamydia*. An air-dried smear of the vaginal discharge for Gram staining is also taken.

Diagnosis

Because of the serious consequences of the condition, many cases are diagnosed purely on the signs and symptoms and treated accordingly to prevent the development of tubal occlusive disease. However, there are cases where the pain and tenderness may be predominantly unilateral, and a diagnosis of ectopic pregnancy or appendicitis will be considered. The former may be excluded by measuring the β-human chorionic gonadotrophin level in the serum, but when a mass is present laparoscopy may be needed to make a diagnosis.

Treatment

This should be instituted as soon as possible after the investigations have been performed. It is usual to commence therapy with oxytetracycline 250 mg four times a day for 10 days, combined with metronidazole 200 mg three times a day for 7 days. Doxycycline or erythromycin may be substituted for the tetracycline. If *Neisseria* is isolated from the bacteriological swabs, then penicillin therapy is to be preferred. Sexual partners should be treated even if they are asymptomatic. If there is no response within 72 h and a pelvic mass is present, laparoscopy and perhaps laparotomy is required. One tube or an ovarian mass may need to be removed.

Long-term sequelae

In mild forms of salpingitis there may be intratubal adhesion formation without blockage, and these women are therefore susceptible to ectopic pregnancy. In more advanced stages of the disease, clubbing of the fimbriae may follow, leading to fimbrial occlusion by adhesions and the development of a hydrosalpinx. Ovarian adhesions are common, and in cases where there is pelvic peritonitis there may be omental adhesions to the tubes and ovaries and between the posterior surface of the uterus and the pouch of Douglas. Multiple blockages of the fallopian tubes may occur, salpingitis isthmica nodosa.

The success of surgery to restore fertility is dependent upon the severity of the disease and the amount of tissue handling that is required. Unless the fimbrial end of the tube is mobile, patent and free of fimbrial adhesions, successful results are unlikely. Even with successful reanastomosis and demonstration of tubal patency at operation there remains a much increased incidence of ectopic pregnancy.

A woman with a history of salpingitis, or even with an unproven history of salpingitis, should not be fitted with an intrauterine contraceptive device because of the risks of reactivating the condition.

RECOMMENDED READING

MacLean A 1995. Pelvic infection. In: Whitfield C (ed) Dewhurst's textbook of obstetrics and gynaecology. Blackwell, Oxford, pp 562–576

Mundy P 1994 The management of gynaecological infections. In: Jarvis G (ed) A critical approach to clinical problems in obstetrics and gynaecology. Oxford Medical Publications, pp 115–184

Menstrual disorders

PHYSIOLOGY OF MENSTRUATION

In the early menstrual cycle, follicle-stimulating hormone (FSH) is produced by the anterior pituitary in ever increasing amounts (Fig. 17.1). This in turn leads to an increase in oestrogen production from the ovary, and thence stimulation of the growth of endometrium (the proliferative phase). At the same time, primordial follicles in the ovary start developing. At around about day 10, one of these becomes dominant, releasing an inhibiting hormone which leads to atresia of the remaining follicles.

The increasing levels of oestrogen lead to a fall in FSH levels until a still higher level of

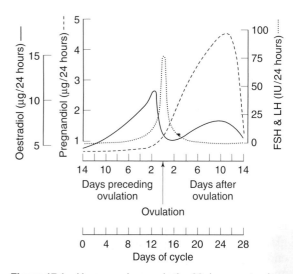

Figure 17.1   Hormone changes in the 28 day menstrual cycle.

oestrogen triggers off a surge of luteinizing hormone (LH) from the pituitary. This causes rupture of the dominant follicle with the release of the ovum. The collapsed follicle becomes a corpus luteum, which produces progesterone in the second half of the cycle, levels remaining constant for 14 days. The effect of progesterone is to convert the endometrium from proliferative to the secretory phase in preparation for nidation of a fertilized ovum. In the absence of pregnancy the corpus luteum starts to degenerate with falling oestrogen and progesterone levels. This in turn leads to the onset of menstruation and, once again, an increase in FSH levels with the start of another cycle.

The relationship of ovulation to menstruation being relatively constant means that ovulation will only take place at midcycle in a 28 day cycle. In a woman menstruating every 34 days it is on day 20 (Fig. 17.2).

Normal menstrual loss is approximately 30–40 ml, and only 10% of women will have losses greater than 80 ml per period. It is difficult to make objective measurements of blood loss in routine clinical practice, and therefore menorrhagia, in practical terms, is what the woman herself considers to be excessively heavy periods, particularly if heavier than in the past.

In the absence of ovulation, menstruation may still occur if the graafian follicle produces oestrogen, but the bleeding may be irregular and can often be prolonged. This form of anovulatory bleeding is most common at either extreme of reproductive life. It is associated with amenorrhoea of 6 weeks or more followed by heavy continuous loss.

Treatment is with a suitable progestogen (e.g. norethisterone 5 mg twice daily for 7 days) but the patient must be warned that following cessation of the hormone, there will be a further short bleed. Cyclical progestogens (days 15–26 inclusive) are given for the next three cycles (or longer). In the older patient, endometrial biopsy is usually performed. Histology shows cystic glandular hyperplasia – the classic *Swiss cheese* endometrium. This condition of prolonged anovulatory bleeding is known as metropathia haemorrhagica.

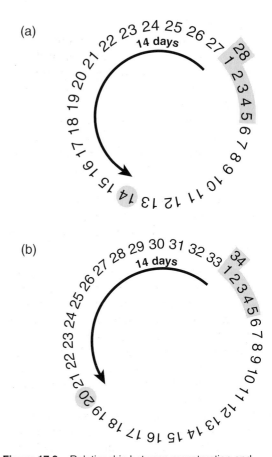

Figure 17.2   Relationship between menstruation and ovulation: **a** with a 28 day cycle, ovulation is 14 days before the onset of the next period, i.e. on day 14: **b** with a 34 day cycle, ovulation is still 14 days before, i.e. on day 20.

INTERMENSTRUAL BLEEDING

A careful history taken from the woman with irregular vaginal bleeding will help to find a cause. It is first necessary to establish whether the intermenstrual bleeding is regular or irregular. Should it be regularly around midcycle, it is usually at the time of ovulation, and, following a normal pelvic examination, the woman can usually be reassured, for the cause is a surge of oestrogens at ovulation. Any other form of intermenstrual bleeding requires careful assessment, for it implies some pathology of the surface of the genital tract.

Visualization of the vagina and cervix may show a local cause:

- Infection by *Monilia*
- Trauma from an ill-fitting diaphragm
- Cervical polyps, which are common and benign and can be removed by the general practitioner in the surgery by twisting them off their pedicle
- Cervical neoplasia, which is the most important cause of irregular bleeding – as well as cervical cytology if there is an obvious lesion on the cervix, biopsy must be undertaken
- Ectopy (previously called cervical erosion) – does not lead to spontaneous bleeding.
- Corrosive agents (used in the past) to procure an abortion

Patients taking oestrogen/progestogen preparations such as the combined oral contraceptive pill may have breakthrough bleeding. A young woman on the pill only needs an increase in the oestrogen dose or a change in the progestogen to stop the bleeding. In a woman who is on hormone replacement therapy, irregular bleeding must be considered as postmenopausal bleeding and investigated accordingly.

Even if a local cause for irregular intermenstrual bleeding is found, it is essential that an endometrial biopsy is undertaken. This can be an outpatient procedure using an endometrial sampler (Fig. 17.3) or by hysteroscopy. Ultrasound examination of the endometrial cavity is a useful adjunct.

Treatment is obviously dependent upon the cause, but where none is found, cyclical hormonal therapy with either progestogens or a combined oestrogen–progestogen will usually solve the problem.

POSTCOITAL BLEEDING

Vaginal bleeding after intercourse is unusual. It may be a variant of intermenstrual bleeding, the investigation and treatment of which has been described. It is more commonly seen with cervical malignancy and occasionally with cervical polyps. More thorough examination under anaesthesia with formal cervical biopsy may be necessary.

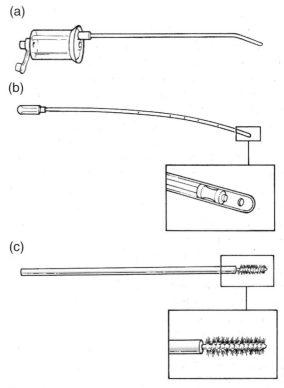

(a)

(b)

(c)

Figure 17.3   Outpatient endometrial sampling. **a** Vabra curette – suction removes the sample down the tube into a bottle when connected to the central vacuum. **b** Pipelle – suction removes the sample when the plunger is withdrawn. **c** Endometrial brush – this is passed into the cavity and rotated to gather the sample on the brush.

POSTMENOPAUSAL BLEEDING

Vaginal bleeding more than a year after the last menstrual period requires investigation, with a full history and clinical examination of the pelvis. The most common cause is atrophic change in the vagina and cervix with a superimposed vaginitis. Even in the presence of an obvious cause, endometrial sampling must be undertaken, for in this age group, endometrial carcinoma is an important cause and must be excluded, although malignancy is relatively uncommon As with intermenstrual bleeding, hysteroscopy and ultrasound are useful diagnostic tools.

In the event of the cause being atrophic vaginitis, topical oestrogen preparations are of use. Alternatively the woman may be given systemic hormone replacement therapy, either orally or transdermally.

MENORRHAGIA

Menorrhagia is excessive regular menstrual loss. It is one of the most common conditions referred to gynaecological clinics, and it is the main presenting problem among half the women having hysterectomies performed in the UK.

A measurement of the haemoglobin level is rarely helpful, but serum ferritin levels may reflect blood loss; levels below 20 µg/ml suggest recurrent heavy blood loss. In a recent national survey, 31% of women described their blood loss as heavy whilst 40% of those with objectively heavy losses (over 80 ml) considered their periods to be moderate or light. The aims of treatment are, therefore, to control the menstrual loss and to improve the quality of life for the woman.

Causes (Table 17.1)

Any condition that increases the surface area of the endometrium will lead to heavier periods. *Intramural* or *submucous* fibroids represent the most common pathological cause for menorrhagia. Extrauterine causes such as *pelvic inflammatory disease* and *endometriosis*, which significantly increase the blood flow to the pelvis, may also lead to menorrhagia and secondary dysmenorrhoea. *Adenomyosis* is endometriosis involving the myometrium, more commonly seen in multiparous patients, and leads to an enlarged

Table 17.1 Some causes of menorraghia

Pathological	Other (less easy to document)
Fibroids	Multiparity
Adenomyosis	Obesity
Endometriosis	Psychological disorders,
Pelvic inflammatory disease	including stress
Hormonal (including thyroid disease)	
Iatrogenic: intrauterine contraceptive devises	
Anticoagulation	

tender uterus. This condition is commonly associated with an increase in menstrual loss. Confirmation of the diagnosis can only be made following hysterectomy and histological examination of the whole uterus.

Metabolic disorders such as *thyroid disease* must also be considered. Of the iatrogenic causes, an *intrauterine device* is the most common, and effective treatment is simply removal of the device.

Anticoagulation for most patients is temporary, usually following a deep-vein thrombosis, but for some who are on long-term therapy, menorrhagia can exacerbate a problem.

Sterilization has been widely and incorrectly cited as a cause of increasing menstrual loss. With the almost universal use of occlusive methods of sterilization using clips or bands, there is no evidence derived from large multicentre trials to support the view that there is an increased menstrual flow following the procedure. Sometimes the previously used method of family planning was the oral contraceptive pill, which suppressed menstrual loss. With the termination of this method at the time of sterilization, the menses seem heavier. The probability is that women, having finished their reproductive life and undergone sterilization, become less tolerant of their menstrual flow and are more likely to complain. Objective measurements of flow do not support that there is an increase at this time.

Emotional stress is a common cause. Should the cause be resolved, then the menstrual disorder improves dramatically. Such remedies are often beyond the control of the clinician.

Where no gynaecological or systemic cause for the heavy bleeding can be found, the condition is labelled *dysfunctional uterine haemorrhage*, and probably represents the largest single group for the condition. An excess of oestrogen leads to overstimulation of the endometrium.

Diagnosis

The mainstay of diagnosis has traditionally been dilatation and curettage of the uterus, a procedure of limited diagnostic value and of no therapeutic value whatsoever. It is no longer recommended for women under the age of 40 years, as the possibility of serious pathology such as endometrial cancer is extremely remote.

For those over the age of 40 years, outpatient endometrial sampling is preferred. This is a procedure that does not require any dilatation of the cervix (Fig. 17.3). A narrow plastic cannula (diameter approximately 2.5 mm) is passed into the uterine cavity, suction is applied, and endometrial samples obtained. The procedure is acceptable to patients having a low complication rate, and does not require admission or general anaesthesia.

If the procedure proves unsatisfactory, or there are other symptoms present such as intermenstrual or postcoital bleeding, hysteroscopy is preferred. Again this can be carried out as an outpatient procedure, and endometrial sampling carried out under direct vision.

Where fibroids or polyps are suspected, transvaginal ultrasonography is of considerable use, and can be combined with outpatient hysteroscopy. There are significant cost savings to the health service where outpatient procedures are carried out in preference to admissions for diagnostic curettage.

Management

The menstrual history is, of course, of paramount importance in making an attempt to assess a woman's menstrual loss. The duration of bleeding and the length of the cycle are key issues. An idea of the heaviness can be ascertained by asking about the passage of clots, flooding and the use of pads or tampons.

The last obviously depends upon how fastidious the patient is. Enquiry can be made about any increased use of protection, and women who need double protection (i.e. both internal tampons and sanitary towels) are likely to be having heavy periods. A menstrual diary kept by the woman with examples of menstrual loss is sometimes helpful.

Treatment

The majority of patients can be treated by their

> **Box 17.1**   Drugs used in the treatment of menorrhagia
>
> - Non-hormonal:
>   - Anti-fibrinolytics: tranexamic acid
>   - Non-steroidal anti-inflammatory drugs (NSAIDs): mefanamic acid
> - Hormonal:
>   - Progestogens: norethisterone or medroxyprogesterone acetate
>   - Combined oestrogen/progestogen preparations: combined oral contraceptive pill combined sequential hormone replacement therapy
>   - Levonorgestrel intrauterine system
> - Antigonadotrophins: danazol
> - Gonadotrophin-releasing hormone (GnRH) analogues: goserilin, buserilin or leuprorelin

---

general practitioner prior to any diagnostic procedure. The drugs used to treat menorrhagia are detailed in Box 17.1.

Antifibrinolytics

Tranexamic acid produces up to a 60% reduction in menstrual blood loss, and has the advantage over the NSAIDs that the woman does not need to take it prior to menstruation but can be used when the patient feels there is a need (when she is bleeding very heavily). It has very few side-effects and should be used as the first-line treatment for menorrhagia.

Non-steroidal anti-inflammatory drugs

Mefenamic acid has been shown to decrease menstrual blood loss by 20–40%. It needs to be given for at least 3 days prior to the onset of menstruation, has few side-effects when taken with food, and offers the advantage of alleviating menstrual pain. Other NSAIDs such as naproxen and ibuprofen are of similar proven efficacy.

Hormones

Progestogens. Norethisterone in the second half of the cycle has been the most popular drug prescribed for menorrhagia by general practitioners but there is no evidence to support its continued use. Randomized controlled trials have failed to show any decrease in menstrual blood, and in one trial there was a 20% increase in the loss. Prolonged use at high doses throughout the menstrual cycle may lead to a reduction in flow, but doses of 15 mg or more a day are not recommended for long-term use. Medroxyprogesterone acetate and dydrogesterone have similarly been shown to have little effect except in regularizing the cycle. The real use for progestogens is in the treatment of frequent periods, when the cycle can be regularized.

Combined oestrogen–progestogen preparations. The combined oral contraceptives have long been known to reduce menstrual flow, and remain the drug of choice in the younger woman. However, the majority of women complaining of menorrhagia tend to be in the fourth or fifth decade of life and they, or their partners, have often been sterilized. At this age they usually decline the oral contraceptive because of the perceived dangers, although with the use of low-dose third-generation progestogens these are minimal. For women approaching the menopause (45 years old or more), and particularly those with vasomotor symptoms, continuous sequential preparations of hormone replacement therapy should be tried. Those preparations containing levonorgestrel or norethisterone are particularly useful in providing a regular cycle, but the effect on flow is variable.

Antigonadotrophins. Danazol has a direct effect on gonadotrophin secretion. It has androgenic properties, and amongst these are weight gain, greasy skin and hair, facial acne and, occasionally, an increase in facial and body hair. A dose of 200 mg a day is sufficient in reducing menstrual flow, but in practical terms persuading a woman to take an effective medication which is likely to increase her weight can be difficult. Paradoxically, slim patients are less likely to gain weight on therapy.

Gonadotrophin-releasing hormone analogues. Following an initial flare of activity, these analogues depress secretion of FSH and LH. The consequence is cessation of ovarian function (medical castration), and the patient becomes acutely menopausal and menstruation ceases.

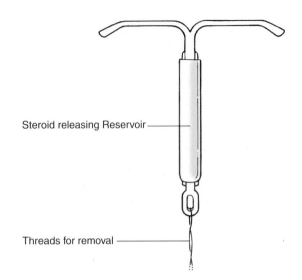

Steroid releasing Reservoir

Threads for removal

Figure 17.4 The levonorgestrel-releasing intrauterine system. It may be inserted in outpatients with a twist into the myometrium from a transcervical inserting rod.

Therapy is very expensive, but may be used in the treatment of fibroids. It otherwise has little place in the management of menorrhagia except for preparation of the endometrium prior to resection or ablation techniques.

The levonorgestrel intrauterine system. A plastic T-shaped device is now manufactured with a semipermeable rate-limiting membrane containing levonorgestrel (Fig. 17.4). Twenty micrograms of the hormone are released each day. It is like the copper intrauterine contraceptive device with progestogen in place of the copper windings on the main stem. At present the system has no licence for the treatment of menorrhagia, but a number of reports show a decrease in menstrual loss of 75% within the first 3 months and up to 95% after 6 months. The major side-effect of the system is unscheduled bleeding occurring in the first 2–3 months after fitting. Despite the initial high cost, this treatment is more economic than it first appears as the system has a life span of 5 years.

Surgical treatment

Techniques to remove or ablate the endometrium have become popular over recent years. A number of methods are available, all of which have similar results. They are:

- Laser ablation
- Endometrial resection
- Cryosurgery
- Microwave techniques
- Thermal coagulation.

In the last technique, a balloon catheter is inserted into the uterine cavity, and inflated to above systolic blood pressure. Water at 85–90°C is then circulated for 8 min, leading to coagulation.

All the endometrial ablative techniques can be carried out as day case surgery. There is a very low rate of immediate postoperative complications, although uterine perforation, fluid overload, haemorrhage and bowel perforation have been reported with endometrial resection (Table 17.2). Microwave techniques have led to fistula formation.

The effects of the procedure on menstrual symptoms vary, but between 13 and 20% of patients have no menstrual bleeding, and up to 80% of patients have light flow only. However, menstrual blood loss and menstrual pain may increase with time, and there are relatively high rates of reoperation after 5 years. The techniques are therefore best used in women who are aged 45 years or more and approaching the menopause.

Table 17.2   Some advantages and disadvantages of endometrial resection

Advantages	Disadvantages
Minor surgery	Menstruation persists for 80%
Suitable for women unfit for general anaesthesia	Not suitable for a grossly enlarged uterus
No scars	Abdominal contents cannot be inspected
Short hospital stay (day case)	Other surgery not possible
Rapid convalescence	Risk of subsequent uterine or cervical malignancy persists
Possibility for repeat procedure	Risk of uterine perforation and/or bowel injury
Uterus retained	Risk of fluid overload

Hysterectomy

Hysterectomy can be carried out by either the abdominal or vaginal route (Fig. 17.5). Total abdominal hysterectomy involves the removal of the body of the uterus and the cervix. The advantages and disadvantages of this procedure are listed in Table 17.3. Subtotal hysterectomy is an easier operation, leaving the vaginal portion of the cervix. This was thought to increase the incidence of malignancy of the cervix, but there is no evidence to support this. It has been suggested, perhaps owing more to popular perceptions than to medical texts, that leaving the cervix behind may enhance orgasm, and this has led to an increased demand for subtotal hysterectomy. The operation is certainly easier, has less morbidity and will return to popularity with time.

Oophorectomy is often performed at the same time as abdominal hysterectomy to eliminate the risk of ovarian cancer. It is difficult to justify this practice in women under the age of 40 years when hormone replacement therapy must be given at least until the age of 50 years. Unfortunately, compliance with long-term hormone replacement therapy is not good, and the routine removal of healthy ovaries in women who are not at high risk of ovarian cancer is difficult to justify.

Vaginal hysterectomy is increasingly popular, although many surgeons are reluctant to perform the procedure if there is no uterine descent. The stay in hospital is considerably shorter and there is a high level of patient satisfaction.

Laparoscopically assisted vaginal hysterectomy has become more popular in the 1990s. It has the advantages of a short stay in hospital and less postoperative analgesia. However, it requires a fully trained and experienced surgeon and specialized instruments. Morbidity, at present, is higher than other approaches, and the supposed reduction in cost is open to debate. A small incision does not mean a small operation, and real recovery times are similar to conventional surgery.

AMENORRHOEA AND OLIGOMENORRHOEA

Amenorrhoea is the absence of periods for at

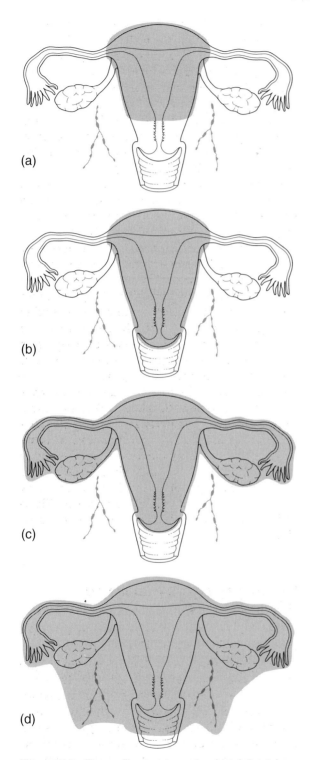

(a)

(b)

(c)

(d)

Figure 17.5 Types of hysterectomy: 1, subtotal; 2, total; 3, total with bilateral salpingo-oophorectomy; 4, Wertheim's radical hysterectomy.

Table 17.3 Some advantages and disadvantages of total abdominal hysterectomy

Advantages	Disadvantages
Amenorrhoea certain	Major surgery with its problems
Suitable for any size of uterus	Requires general anaesthesia usually
Abdominal contents can be inspected	Abdominal scar
Other surgery possible (e.g. oophorectomy)	Hospital stay of 4–6 days
No risk of uterine or cervical malignancy	Prolonged convalescence
	Depression possible
	Psychosexual problems possible
	Earlier menopause
	Functional bowel and bladder problems

least 6 months; the most common causes, which are all physiological, are the menopause, pregnancy and lactation, and the prepubertal state. By convention, amenorrhoea is divided into primary and secondary causes, although this is probably an unhelpful categorization for there is considerable overlap between the two groups.

Oligomenorrhoea implies prolonged menstrual intervals, usually between 6 weeks and 6 months.

Primary amenorrhoea

A failure to menstruate by the age of 16 years is the arbitrary age for defining amenorrhoea, although a small proportion of normal girls will not menstruate until 17 or 18 years old. The differential diagnosis is dependent upon the presence of secondary sexual characteristics such as breast development and axillary and pubic hair. Likely diagnoses include cryptomenorrhoea (haematocolpos), an absent vagina or uterus with normal functioning ovaries, or, very occasionally, polycystic ovaries, or pregnancy. When secondary sexual characteristics are absent, then the cause may be simply that the patient is still prepubertal. Otherwise the most likely diagnosis is a primary gonadal failure or, less commonly, a hypothalamic/pituitary disorder.

Investigations

A careful history and examination is, of course,

a primary necessity. Haematocolpos is dealt with elsewhere (see Ch. 27). In this condition there is occluding membrane of the vagina above the hymen. Where an absent vagina is suspected, examination may be very difficult in the out-patient department, and may be best performed under general anaesthesia. If haematocolpos is excluded, the basic investigations are:

- *Karyotyping.* This is of particular importance where ovarian failure is suspected, as in Turner's syndrome (45XO) or androgen insensitivity (testicular feminization), where the karyotype is 46XY.
- *Endocrine.* The gonadotrophin levels of FSH and LH are important. Similarly, tests of thyroid function and prolactin levels may be of use. Testosterone and 17α-hydroxyprogesterone levels may be elevated, the latter particularly where congenital adrenal hyperplasia is present.
- *Ultrasound.* This non-invasive test will demonstrate the ovaries, if present, and also the uterus. It in no way replaces laparoscopy, which is more informative in the pelvis.
- *Laparoscopy.* Obviously, this investigation is invasive and requires a general anaesthesic. However, there are occasions when it might be necessary to delineate the pelvic anatomy precisely, particularly of the uterus.

Treatment

Only a few of these will be considered here, for only basic conditions are needed by most in gynaecology: experts should be consulted early in the diagnostic programme.

Absent vagina. Plastic operations to construct a vagina are possible although the results may be disappointing. The use of vaginal dilators on the perineal dimple and repeated attempts at vaginal intercourse will often lead to con-siderable stretching of the vaginal skin, leading to a reasonably good lumen, and is the preferred course of action.

Turner's syndrome. Sexual development is considerably retarded because of gonadal dysgenesis. Affected individuals are of short stature and have, classically, webbing of the neck, a low hair-line, cubitus valgus, pigmented naevae and cardiovascular anomalies. It must be stressed that there is no intellectual impairment in these children, and if treated at an early age with growth hormone they regain a normal stature. Treatment with oestrogens with cyclical progestogens will lead to normal sexual dev-elopment and cyclical blood loss in imitation of menstruation. Those affected are permanently infertile, but pregnancy is possible with *in vitro* fertilization involving donor eggs.

Androgen insensitivity. These girls present a dilemma. Their chromosome sex is male with a normal 46XY complement but because their end organs are totally insensitive to androgens the external genitalia of the female persist and there is sufficient oestrogen activity for normal breast development. However, the uterus and vagina are absent, and the gonads are testes. Because these remain undescended and either lie within the inguinal canal or within the pelvis; there is a theoretical danger of malignancy developing in later years. It has been general advice to remove them, although this may prove to be un-necessary, especially if annual ultrasound scans can be performed to check. Because these individuals are phenotypically female they are brought up as girls, and are therefore psycho-logically female. It is incumbent upon those who care for these girls that they should not be told of their karyotypic or gonadal sex as this may lead to grave psychological disturbance. These girls remain infertile and unable to bear children.

Secondary amenorrhoea and oligomenorrhoea

Over 85% of cases of secondary amenorrhoea are due to disorders of the hypothalamic–pituitary–ovarian axis. The causes of oligo-menorrhoea and amenorrhoea are therefore usually the same. Rarer causes for secondary amenorrhoea are primary hypothyroidism, which can be diagnosed on clinical grounds and by thyroid function tests. Anatomical problems are extremely rare. In developing countries, tuberculosis still remains one of the more common causes. Asherman's syndrome is seen a little more frequently, with intrauterine adhesions caused by traumatic curettage following pregnancy. It may also arise following endometrial ablation techniques used for therapeutic treatments of menorrhagia.

Causes of secondary amenorrhoea

Hypothalamic. Hypothalamic disorders are most commonly caused by emotional problems, particularly those associated with weight loss due to anorexia or to strict dieting for cosmetic reasons. It would appear that it is the weight lost rather than the absolute weight that is important in causing amenorrhoea; for example, a rapid loss of 10 kg almost inevitably leads to menstrual disturbance. The body mass index (the weight in kilograms divided by the square height in metres) may also be useful, and figures below 19 are commonly associated with amenorrhoea. This may be seen not only in anorectics but also in elite athletes, such as long-distance runners and ballet dancers.

Rapid and repeated changes of time zones, as experienced by air-hostesses for example, may also lead to temporary menstrual cessation. These women often have oestradiol levels in the postmenopausal range and are susceptible to osteoporosis and vertebral crush fractures, even though they are young and often physically very active. The mechanism of their amenorrhoea is hypothalamic suppression of GnRH, which in turn leads to gonadotrophin deficiency and ovarian inactivity. It follows that FSH and LH levels are usually very low.

Pituitary disorders. Large tumours of the pituitary may lead to amenorrhoea. Such tumours nearly always lead to a rise in prolactin levels, and therefore this is a useful screening test. The most common tumour of the pituitary is the prolactin-secreting adenoma of the anterior pituitary. Surprisingly, galactorrhoea is not a common associated symptom. If the tumour should grow significantly it will press on the optic chiasma, causing lateral visual field defects. Where the prolactin levels are in excess of 1000 IU/l, visual fields should be tested, and

computerized tomography or magnetic resonance imaging of the pituitary fossa performed. Pituitary tomography is no longer considered a relevant investigation. Treatment is either by the use of dopamine agonists such as bromocriptine or, occasionally, by surgery, where the anterior pituitary is removed by a transphenoidal approach.

DISORDERS OF THE OVARIES

Ovarian failure can occur at any time during a woman's reproductive life because of a depletion of ovarian follicles. The average age of women at the menopause is 51 years, but it can occur prematurely anytime after the menarche. Rarely, an autoimmune condition may lead to ovarian failure. However, iatrogenic causes such as surgery, radiation or chemotherapy are common reasons for premature ovarian failure. In all cases the gonadotrophin levels, particularly of FSH, are elevated into the menopausal range, and there is a concomitant fall in oestradiol levels to postmenopausal levels. Because of the risks of osteoporosis and cardiovascular disease, it is important that hormone replacement therapy is given at least up to the age of a natural menopause. Rarely, some of the women with premature menopause will spontaneously ovulate again whilst on replacement therapy.

Polycystic ovaries

This occurs in over 20% of women during their reproductive lives. It is the major cause for oligomenorrhoea, and accounts for about 30% of cases of amenorrhoea. The polycystic ovarian syndrome is associated with obesity, hirsutism and subfertility. Polycystic ovarian disease is characterized by hyperandrogenaemia. This may vary from very mild to severe, and its symptomatology is dependent upon end organ response. The condition is characterized by numerous follicles arrested in their maturation and clustering around the periphery of the ovaries. This gives a characteristic ultrasound

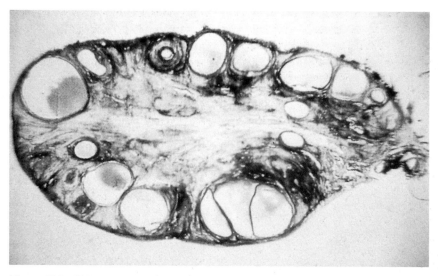

Figure 17.6 Polycystic ovary.

appearance known as the pearl necklace sign (Fig. 17.6). On visual examination the ovaries appear to have a smooth irregular and thickened surface with no evidence of follicular or luteal activity.

Each follicle will produce small amounts of oestrogen, and because there are so many the patients have raised oestrogen levels. The other typical feature is a raised serum LH level. This is usually in excess of three times the FSH level, and is often over a level of 12 IU/l. When blood is taken on day 5 of the cycle for those who have a cycle.

The condition is associated with a hyper-secretion of androgens from the ovary which inhibits follicular maturation. On the occasion when ovulation takes places and fertilization occurs, there is an increased risk of miscarriage. Hyperinsulinaemia leads to an increase in triglyceride levels and a reduction in HDL_2 cholesterol levels. There is often impaired carbohydrate tolerance. The underlying problem of insulin resistance leads to an increased risk of diabetes mellitus, hypertensive disease and cardiovascular disease. In addition, the persist-ent high levels of oestrogen may lead to hyper-plastic changes of the endometrium, which in turn can lead to malignant change.

Treatment

As these women are usually hyperoestrogenic, there is no need for hormone replacement therapy, but because of the risk to the endometrium, a regular withdrawal bleed, at least on a 3 monthly basis, is necessary; this can be provided with medroxyprogesterone acetate 10 mg for 5 days.

If the woman is anxious to become pregnant, then treatment with clomiphene citrate 50 mg for 5 days following the withdrawal bleed is safe and often effective. Increasing doses up to 200 mg for 5 days may be given safely. Monitoring should be carried out by measuring a midluteal progesterone level. Failure to ovulate following this regime will necessitate referral to a specialist clinic where gonadotrophin therapy can be administered.

Recent work shows that metformin (an oral hypoglycaemic) at a dose of 500 mg twice a day is effective in the treatment of the obese patient with oligo- or amenorrhoea. The effect is to reduce weight and to sensitize the ovaries to clomiphene. Often the patients will start menstruating spontaneously.

Laparoscopic multiple diathermy punctures of the ovary restores ovulatory cycles in many for up to a year. The procedure has replaced wedge resection of the ovary.

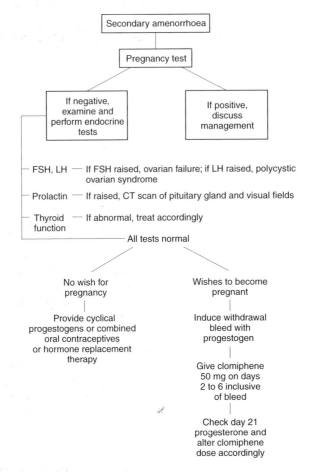

Figure 17.7 Management of secondary amenorrhoea.

SUMMARY

All women presenting with amenorrhoea and oligomenorrhoea should have a careful history taken and a full examination performed. This alone will often lead to the correct diagnosis. The most important investigations are serum gonadotrophin levels, thyroid function tests and serum prolactin levels. In addition, ultrasound scanning of the pelvis is often very helpful, and karyotyping of the patient with primary amenorrhoea may also be of use. A simple approach to secondary amneorrhoea is shown in Figure 17.7.

RECOMMENDED READING

Dramusic V, Yang M, Ratham S, Rajan U 1995 Reproductive chances after persistent menstrual disorders. Contemporary Reviews in Obstetrics and Gynaecology 7: 230–238

Duckett K, Shaw R 1998 Is medical management of menorrhagia obsolete? British Journal of Obstetrics and Gynaecology 105: 569–572

Sherman R (1995) Primary and secondary anenorrhoea. In:

Whitfield C (ed) Dewhurst's textbook of obstetrics and gynaecology. Blackwell, Oxford, pp 24–42

Sturridge F, Guillebaud J 1997 Gynaecological aspects of the levonorgestrel releasing intrauterine system. British Journal of Obstetrics and Gynaecology 104: 285–289

Wood C, Mahev P 1997 (eds) Hysterectomy. Clinics in Obstetrics and Gynaecology 11: 1

Benign lesions

SOLID TUMOURS OF THE VULVA

Tumours of epidermal origin include condylomata, skin tags, hydradenomata, sebaceous cysts and basal cell carcinomata; those of mesodermal origin include fibromata, lipomata and neurofibromata.

A urethral caruncle is an adenomatous growth of the external urethral meatus. It is exquisitely tender, and will often bleed with minor trauma. It is often confused with the much more common postmenopausal urethral prolapse, which presents as a reddened urethral meatus but is usually non-tender.

CYSTIC LESIONS OF THE VULVA AND VAGINA

These include epidermal inclusions cysts, cysts of the urogenital sinus, cysts of the canal of Nuck and pilonidal sinus, which can occur just lateral to the labia majora.

Both Bartholin's duct and gland can become cystic if there is an obstruction. This presents as a soft non-tender cystic lesion at the introitus. Infection is common, leading to a Bartholin's abscess. Treatment of this is incision and marsupialization. Excision of the gland is a difficult and bloody procedure which should only be tried in cases of recurrence.

A Gärtner's cyst is an embryonic remnant found in the lateral walls of the vagina, and is usually asymptomatic. These can be marsupialized.

A suburethral cyst is usually of Skene's duct,

and can become infected, as can small urethral diverticula.

TUMOURS OF THE CERVIX

The most common of these is the Nabothian follicle or mucus retention cyst. This is commonly seen in women who have had a previous vaginal delivery. They present as hard raised circular lumps on the surface of the cervix, usually about 2–3 mm in diameter, containing mucus. They are caused by squamous epithelium growing over the glandular ducts of the columnar epithelium, thus leading to retention of the cervical mucus. Such follicles are entirely harmless, but sometimes give cause for concern when a woman inadvertently finds them herself and, very occasionally, can reach a diameter in excess of 1 cm, when they may need rupturing and draining.

Endometriotic deposits on the cervix are rare but occasionally give rise to atypical endometrioma containing dark altered blood. They can easily be removed by simple diathermy.

UTERINE FIBROIDS

Uterine fibroids, leiomyomata or myomata, are benign growths of uterine muscle. They are usually round in shape and firm in consistency; when cut, fibroids have a characteristic white whorled appearance. They may occur as a solitary growth, but much more commonly are multiple, varying in size from significant masses to tiny growths. They are classified according to their site of origin (Fig. 18.1).

Subserous fibroids are beneath the serosa of the uterus, and distort the shape of the uterus considerably, for they project outwards. Very occasionally they become pedunculated, and may become adherent to surrounding tissues such as omentum or bowel, seeking to develop an alternative blood supply. Occasionally they project laterally from the uterine body between the two leaves of the broad ligament.

Intramural fibroids lie within the wall of the uterus and are the most common. They may vary considerably in size. The growth of

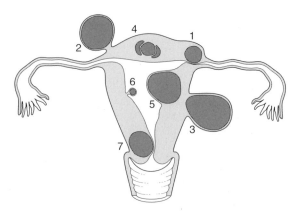

Figure 18.1 Sites of fibroids (see text). 1, subserous; 2, pendunculated; 3, broad ligament; 4, intramural; 5, submucous; 6, polyp; 7, cervical.

intramural fibroids often distorts the body of the uterus considerably and can increase the surface area of the uterine cavity.

Submucus fibroids are found just beneath the endometrium, and cause considerable distortion of the uterine cavity although the body of the uterus may not appear to be enlarged. They may become pedunculated, and appear at the cervical os as a fibroid polyp.

Cervical fibroids are less common. If large they can cause problems in labour, and later in life may be difficult to remove because of poor access.

Signs and symptoms

Most fibroids are discovered by chance, but when they do present clinically it is either because of their direct effect on the uterine cavity or their effect on surrounding structures.

Menorrhagia

Menorrhagia is a common symptom where the uterine cavity is enlarged. Fibroids do not cause irregular cycles or intermenstrual bleeding except in the rare instance of an ulcerated fibroid polyp. The increase in blood loss associated with fibroids may also be due to changes in the uterine circulation or increased prostaglandin synthesis in addition to the simple mechanical effect.

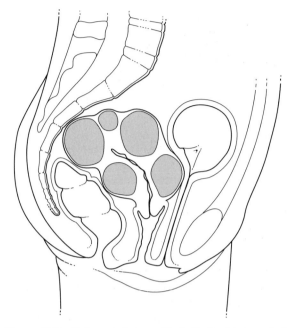

Figure 18.2   Retroverted uterus filled with fibroids impacted in the pelvis causing dislocation of the bladder into the abdomen, stretching the urethra and causing retention of urine.

Large fibroids, like a pregnant uterus, fill the pelvis and press upon the bladder and bowel, leading to urinary frequency and nocturia. In addition they may lead to constipation. Very rarely, a large fundal fibroid in a retroverted uterus can become incarcerated in the pelvis, leading to acute urinary retention (Fig. 18.2).

Pain

Pain is not usually a feature of fibroids unless a pedunculated fibroid undergoes torsion, or red degeneration occurs during pregnancy. Fibroid polyps may give rise to primary spasmodic dysmenorrhoea as the uterus attempts to expel the fibroid through the cervix.

Histology

Fibroids consist of smooth muscle bundles mixed with connective tissue, and generally have a poor blood supply. Their rate of growth is variable, and is probably under the control of oestrogen. Because of the poor blood supply, large tumours may undergo *hyaline* degeneration in the centre, and liquefaction may occur. In post-menopausal women the process of degeneration may lead to *calcification*, and the formation of womb stones. In pregnancy the fibroid may undergo *red degeneration*, which leads to acute pain and tenderness, for the tumour is filled with extravascular blood.

Incidence

By the end of reproductive life about one in five women will have fibroids, although, for the majority, these will be small and asymptomatic. There is no evidence of a genetic cause but there are definite racial differences. West African and Afro-Caribbean women are at considerably greater risk of developing fibroids. Their formation among Europeans is associated with nulliparity or low family size. However, whether this is a cause or effect is uncertain. It does seem that delaying reproduction leads to a higher incidence of fibroids, but there is a lower inci-dence in long-term users of the combined oral contraceptive pill.

Diagnosis

Fibroids may present as a lower abdominal mass with little in the way of symptoms. A diagnosis can usually be made by bimanual pelvic exam-ination, when movement of the abdominal mass causes a reciprocal movement of the cervix, and the mass is felt to be in continuity with the body of the uterus. Smaller fibroids may present as simple uterine enlargement or give the uterus an irregular contour when palpated.

Although the diagnosis may be fairly obvious, it is important to carry out an ultrasound investigation to confirm the nature of a pelvic mass. Large fibroids may compress the ureters, and it is therefore important to visualize the kidneys at the same time. When conservative management is adopted, serial ultrasound is a useful tool to monitor the size of fibroids. Laparoscopy is occasionally undertaken, par-ticularly when fibroids are small, but usually as part of investigation of subfertility. Hysteroscopy is useful in assessing a patient with menorrhagia, and operative intervention may be undertaken at the same time.

The best treatment for symptomatic women is surgery. This may be either removal of the uterus or removal of individual fibroids.

Treatment

Hysterectomy

This should only be carried out in the symptomatic patient who has completed her family. It is usually a simple procedure with low morbidity, although adhesions may be encountered if there is endometriosis or pelvic inflammatory disease. Occasionally problems are encountered if there is a large fibroid in the cervix or broad ligament.

Myomectomy

For those who wish to retain their reproductive capability, the operation of choice is myomectomy. This operation is usually carried out at laparotomy, but smaller fibroids may be removed through the laparoscope or hysteroscope. Myomectomy is a relatively easy procedure as the fibroids are simply enucleated from their false capsule. However, the procedure is often accompanied by brisk haemorrhage, and it is useful to apply a tourniquet or clamp around the lower part of the uterus to reduce blood loss during surgery. In the case of multiple fibroids, patients should be warned that hysterectomy may have to be undertaken, although this, fortunately, is a rare occurrence.

The major postoperative problem is adhesion formation. To reduce this, as many fibroids as possible are removed through a single uterine incision, and a hood formed to cover the incision (Fig. 18.3). Plication of the round ligaments is often undertaken to prevent the uterus becoming fixed in retroversion.

Medical management

A number of hormonal preparations have been

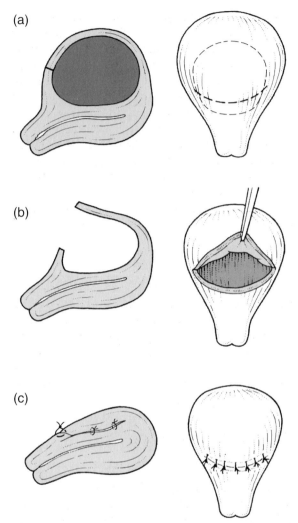

(a)

(b)

(c)

Figure 18.3 A Bonney hood used after a problem myomectomy: 1, a curved incision is made below the meridian of the fibroid; 2, the fibroid is shelled out, with haemostasis of fibroid bed; 3, space obliterated with buried sutures with the flap resutured low down the anterior wall to reduce adhesions.

tried to reduce either the blood flow or the size of the fibroids but, in general, they are disappointing. Combined oral contraceptives containing levonorgestrel have been shown to reduce blood flow and prevent further growth of fibroids, and may be useful in young women who are not yet ready to start a family and do not want to undergo surgery.

The only preparations that have been shown to be of real use are gonadotrophin-releasing hormone (GnRH) analogues. The use of agonists leads to pituitary down-regulation and suppression of ovarian activity. This creates a pseudo-menopause, and 6 months of treatment can lead to a reduction in fibroid volume by as much as 50%. This may make surgery considerably easier, or for those with smaller fibroids it may provide a sufficient time to attempt pregnancy. Unfortunately, within 6 months of ceasing treatment the fibroids will regrow.

Arterial embolization under radiological control has been reported to be successful.

Subfertility

Endometrium over a fibroid may be thinner and less receptive to an implanting ovum. Intramural fibroids, particularly in the fundus, may occlude the transmural portion of the fallopian tubes. In addition, irregularities of the uterine cavity can lead to recurrent miscarriage while changes in uterine blood flow may not favour successful implantation.

Fibroids in pregnancy

The effect of fibroids on pregnancy

This is dependent upon the site and size of the fibroid. Fibroids that distort the uterine cavity are liable to increase the incidence of spontaneous miscarriage. Low-lying fibroids may remain within the pelvic cavity and thus prevent engagement of the presenting part. In these circumstances a caesarean section should be undertaken. It is mandatory that fibroids are not removed at the time of caesarean section because of the risk of uncontrollable haemorrhage.

The effect of pregnancy on fibroids

The major complication during pregnancy is red degeneration of the fibroid. The inner portion of the fibroid becomes haemorrhagic and undergoes necrosis. This procedure causes acute pain and can be confused with placental abruption, although red degeneration typically occurs in mid-pregnancy, and abruption later. The patient usually requires hospital admission and may be pyrexial. Strong analgesia is usually required, and the pain settles after 2 or 3 days. Fibroids tend to become softer and often smaller as a consequence of pregnancy.

ENDOMETRIOSIS

Endometriosis is a very common condition, affecting as many as 25% of women in their reproductive years. Many are asymptomatic, the diagnosis only being made during laparoscopy for other reasons such as sterilization. Tissue histologically similar to endometrium is found outside the uterus, usually within the pelvic cavity. When endometrial tissue is found deep within the myometrium, the condition is known as *adenomyosis*.

To confirm the diagnosis histologically there must be the presence of glands, stroma and evidence of past bleeding such as haemorrhage or haemosiderin staining. The most common sites of endometriotic deposits are over the uterosacral ligaments and the ovaries. However, deposits are often widespread throughout the pelvic peritoneum, especially in the pouch of Douglas and over the sigmoid colon and rectum. Very occasionally they may be seen at distant sites within the peritoneal cavity, and extremely rarely at other sites, particularly the lungs, presumably as a result of venous embolism. The lesions characteristically undergo histological changes similar to endometrium throughout the menstrual cycle, and at the time of menses they bleed. This leads to them becoming discoloured, initially brown and later as black deposits. When occurring on the ovary, cyst formation is not uncommon; the cysts contain dark viscous altered blood with the consistency and colour of melted plain chocolate, and it is this characteristic appearance that gives them the name of chocolate cysts.

Aetiology

Retrograde menstruation and implantation

There have been numerous theories as to the

origins of endometriosis, the first formulated by Sampson as long ago as 1927. He noticed that at the time of menstruation there is a flow of menstrual fluid along the fallopian tubes and into the pouch of Douglas. He postulated that this fluid contained endometrial cells which became fixed on structures in the pelvis and later proliferated and reacted to circulating hormones. Since the widespread introduction of laparoscopy, retrograde menstruation has been confirmed and is probably normal. However, the development of endometriosis may only occur in susceptible individuals.

Endometriotic deposits can be found in surgical incision sites, particularly following operations where the endometrial cavity is opened, such as hysterotomy and caesarean section. Presumably endometrium is transported from the uterine cavity to the wound during the procedure, implantation occurs and the endometrioma then responds on a cyclical basis to the circulating hormones.

Lymphatic or venous embolization

Because endometriotic deposits have been found in distant sites such as the lung, kidney and joints, it is postulated that venous or lymphatic embolization may occur.

Coelomic metaplasia

It has been proposed that the coelomic epithelium, which forms structures such as the peritoneum and the müllerian system, can undergo changes back to its primitive origin and then transform to endometriotic deposits. Why this should happen remains unknown, but it may be due to abnormal hormonal sensitivity.

Genetic theory

There is a higher incidence of endometriosis in first-degree relatives, and there may therefore be a genetic basis. There are also racial differences in the occurrence of the disease.

Immunological causes

There is evidence of decreased cellular immunity to endometrial tissue in the majority of women with endometriosis. Antigens have been identified, which may stimulate an immune response of the peritoneum in the form of fibrosis.

Symptoms

The symptoms of the condition bear little relationship to the size of the lesions, particularly in the pelvis. The most common symptom is one of pain usually associated with menstruation and the immediate few days before it. The pain is dull, continuous and is often accompanied by low back pain. It is the most common cause of secondary dysmenorrhoea.

The second most common symptom is of dyspareunia, presumably due to stretching of the lesions over the uterosacral ligaments in the pouch of Douglas. Occasionally endometriosis is sufficiently widespread to fix the uterus in retroversion, and this leads to more severe dyspareunia. Menstrual loss is said to be heavier, but this is not always the case. Changes in bowel habit are relatively common, and when the rectum is involved, cyclical rectal bleeding and tenesmus may occur. Where implantation endometriomata exist in scars, then there is cyclical enlargement of the endometrioma, with tenderness and occasional bruising.

Infertility

Endometriosis is commonly diagnosed at laparoscopy, particularly in patients who are undergoing fertility investigations. Where there is disruption of tubal patency or the ovaries are severely damaged, there is an obvious cause for infertility, but many patients who are infertile appear to have scattered small deposits, and the relationship between them and the fertility problem is still unknown.

Signs

A diagnosis of endometriosis should be considered when any patient presents with the above symptomatology. Examination of the abdomen usually fails to reveal any obvious pathology, but on bimanual examination tender nodules can often be found in the uterosacral ligaments. Alternatively the uterus may be found to be fixed in retroversion or there may be evidence of ovarian enlargement. However, a definite diagnosis can only be arrived at by direct visualization of deposits by laparoscopy. The classical laparoscopic appearance is that of a powder burn in the peritoneum. There is an area usually a few millimetres across containing spots of brown or black discoloration due to deposition of haemosidrin. These lesions can be red or pink if seen at an earlier stage.

Even earlier stages of endometriosis are now recognized where there may be red flare-like lesions, café au lait spots or glandular blebs on the peritoneum. Alternatively, old burned-out endometriosis will leave white scar-like areas. Because of repeated haemorrhagic episodes there may be intense adhesion formation, particularly between the bowel and the posterior aspect of the uterus and also the ovaries and the lateral pelvic wall.

Treatment

Medical treatment

The principle of medical treatment is to induce prolonged amenorrhoea. It has been shown that pregnancy and subsequent amenorrhoea induced by breast feeding induces a remission. The following hormonal therapies have therefore been used with varying success.

Progestogens. Amenorrhoea can be induced using relatively high doses of medroxy-progesterone acetate or dydrogesterone. These two progestogens have fewer side-effects than the 19-nor-testosterone derivatives but are still associated with weight gain, breakthrough bleeding and, occasionally, androgenic effects such as acne. Treatment should continue for at least 6 months and possibly longer.

Combined oral contraceptive pill. Monophasic contraceptive pills can be given on a continuous basis so that there is no withdrawal bleed. Side-effects such as breakthrough bleeding, breast tenderness and weight gain may occur. The usual contraindications to the combined pill apply.

Danazol. This is a testosterone derivative with androgenic and anabolic properties. It has been the most widely used medical treatment of endometriosis for many years. It suppresses the hypothalamic pituitary axis and also has a direct effect on ovarian steroidogenesis. Amenorrhoea is easily induced and it is highly effective in suppressing the symptoms of endometriosis and affecting resolution of deposits.

Unfortunately danazol has a number of side-effects which are largely androgenic; the most common of these are weight gain and acne, but also fluid retention, oily skin, muscle cramps, unwanted body and facial hair and, very occasionally, voice changes have been reported. These side-effects make the treatment less popular nowadays.

GnRH analogues. The GnRH agonists, when given for a prolonged period of time, induce amenorrhoea by causing a medical menopause. This down-regulation of the pituitary leads to a rapid development of amenorrhoea together with side-effects such as hot flushes, vaginal dryness and other menopausal symptoms. The most important long-term problem has been bone loss, and treatment is not advised beyond a period of 6 months unless the agonist is combined with a period-free preparation of hormone replacement therapy. Such add-back therapy is very effective for long-term use.

Medical treatment alone will provide symptomatic relief for many patients, and is most useful as a preoperative treatment for patients in that it will reduce the size of an endometrioma and decrease the vascularity of lesions.

Surgery

Conservative surgery aims at freeing organs which are adherent and destruction of endometrial deposits by coagulation or laser therapy. The aim is to restore pelvic anatomy, usually to improve fertility.

Radical surgery is reserved for those women with severe problems who have either abandoned hopes of having a child or who have completed their family. In these circumstances a total abdominal hysterectomy and bilateral oophorectomy is carried out.

Hormone replacement therapy is offered to these premenopausal patients, but it is essential that it is opposed with a continuous progestogen to prevent a recurrence of endometriosis.

BENIGN TUMOURS OF THE FALLOPIAN TUBE

Embryonic remnants of the epoophoron are common as hydatids of Morgagni. These are small pedunculated cysts that arise from the fimbrial end of the tube, and are an incidental finding at laparoscopy. Occasionally large cysts within the mesosalpinx occur. They also arise from embryological remnants, are unilocular, and present in the same way as an ovarian cyst. Simple drainage via the laparoscope may be all that is necessary.

BENIGN TUMOURS OF THE OVARY

Benign tumours of the ovary are a common occurrence. In most cases they are asymptomatic, and may be found coincidentally on routine pelvic examination. Many will resolve spontaneously. However, those that are persistent raise the possibility of malignant change, and further investigation is warranted.

Types

The benign tumours of the ovary are outlined in Box 18.1.

Physiological cysts

Functional cysts can be either follicular or luteal. They are merely an exaggeration of the graafian follicle or the corpus luteum, and may occur as a result of ovulation induction.

Luteal cysts are more commonly seen associated with adhesions of the ovary. They are most often found in young people, in early

---

Box 18.1 Benign tumours of the ovary

- *Physiological cysts:*
  - Follicular
  - Luteal
- *Epithelial tumours:*
  - Serous cystadenomata
  - Mucinous cystadenomata
  - Endometrioid cystadenomata
  - Brenner tumours
- *Germ cell tumours:*
  - Dermoid cysts
- *Sex cord stromal tumours:*
  - Granulosa and theca cell tumours
  - Fibromata
  - Sertoli–Leydig cell tumours

---

pregnancy, and usually regress spontaneously. Their maximum diameter seldom exceeds 3 cm although occasionally they may reach up to 10 cm. In the event of them failing to regress, aspiration under laparoscopic or ultrasound guidance may be required.

Epithelial tumours

Serous cystadenomata. Occurring most commonly in women in their later reproductive life, the most common epithelial tumour is the serous cystadenoma. This presents as a unilocular cyst, often with papilliferous processes on the inner and occasionally outer surface. The fluid is thin and serous, and embryologically they represent fallopian tube epithelium. They are bilateral in 10% of cases.

Mucinous cystadenomata. These are usually larger than serous cysts, are multiloculated and contain thick mucinous fluid. They represent approximately 20% of all ovarian tumours. Histologically they are similar to cervical columnar epithelium.

Very occasionally pseudomyxoma peritoni may be associated with the cyst. In this condition the peritoneal cavity contains mucinous fluid derived from seedlings on the peritoneum. This may later lead to massive intra-abdominal adhesion formation.

Endometrioid cystadenomata. Presentation is in a similar fashion to the serous cystadenoma but these tumours contain not only serous fluid but altered blood. Histologically the lining resembles endometrium.

Brenner tumours. These tumours are rare and are usually found in association with other benign tumours. They consist of nests of transitional epithelium in a dense fibrotic stroma. Although most are benign, they can occasionally be malignant, and they are usually no more than 2–3 cm in diameter.

Germ cell tumours

Dermoid cysts are common in young women, and may occasionally be bilateral. They are unilocular and usually about 8–10 cm in diameter. They classically contain thick sebaceous material and hair, but the epithelial lining may contain a variety of tissues such as bone (which shows up on radiographs), nervous tissue, muscle and, very occasionally, thyroid tissue (stroma ovarii).

Benign sex cord stromal tumours

These can occur at any age, and represent about 5% of all ovarian tumours. Many of them will secrete hormones. *Granulosa cell tumours* are more often of very low malignancy and do not necessarily produce oestrogen. *Theca cell tumours* are nearly always benign, produce oestrogen and may lead to systemic effects. *Fibromata* are more common in postmenopausal women. They are derived from stromal cells and are similar to thecomata, but are hard, mobile and lobulated. Classically they can cause peritoneal irritation leading to ascites, which may, on occasion, be associated with pleural effusions, Meig's syndrome. *Sertoli–Leydig cell tumours* are very rare, small and usually unilateral. They are classically associated with androgen production but can produce oestrogens. They are of low-grade malignant potential.

Presentation

The majority of benign ovarian tumours are asymptomatic and are found at routine pelvic examination, on ultrasound scan or laparoscopy.

However, because they have a pedicle (the ovarian ligament) and are round, they are able to roll within the pelvic cavity and therefore may undergo torsion. This gives rise to extremely sharp pain which may be intermittent as the cyst twists and untwists. More often, however, it increases in intensity and becomes constant. Haemorrhage may occur within the cyst. Unless prompt surgical action is taken, the ovary may undergo necrosis and be lost.

The pelvis and abdominal cavity are capacious areas, and it is not until the cyst reaches a large size that it presents as an abdominal swelling. Often the tumours can be extremely large but may not be diagnosed because of obesity or a woman attributing the swelling to middle age spread. Very occasionally, pressure symptoms may develop, and can be similar to those in pregnancy such as oedema, varicose veins and haemorrhoids. Uterine or vaginal wall prolapse may be caused by large ovarian cysts.

Differential diagnosis

Acute pain because of haemorrhage or torsion of the cyst may be similar to either an ectopic pregnancy or appendicitis. Careful pelvic and abdominal examination, ultrasound examination and estimations of serum β-human chorionic gonadotrophin levels will usually lead to a correct diagnosis.

Other masses arising out of the pelvis include a fibroid or pregnant uterus and a full bladder. Careful bimanual examination should differentiate these, but ultrasound examination may be necessary to confirm the clinical diagnosis. Pressure symptoms such as frequency of micturition and constipation occur later with larger cysts.

Investigation

As always, history and examination are of paramount importance. Gentle abdominal palpation may reveal areas of tenderness and peritonism. Where a mass is present, the radial border of the left hand should be used to examine the patient's lower abdomen, starting from above and working down in the midline towards the pelvis. A bimanual examination is essential. It is important to ascertain whether the mass is in continuity with the uterus or separate from it. Other important features will include its consistency, its mobility and smoothness of the surface. The presence of nodules, particularly in the pouch of Douglas, and fixity of the mass make it more likely to be malignant. Ultrasound examination has now become a standard procedure in the diagnosis of the pelvic mass.

Management

In the case of a young woman, under 35 years of age with a small unilateral tumour less than 10 cm in diameter, observation is probably all that is necessary over a period of 6–8 weeks unless there is clear evidence of a dermoid cyst. Larger asymptomatic cysts can be aspirated using ultrasound guidance, or under direct vision through the laparoscope when the fluid can be sent off for cytology.

In older women the cysts tend to be larger, and must be presumed to be malignant until proven otherwise. Essentially this means removal. Whenever a cyst is larger than 10 cm or where there are symptoms, particularly of pain, surgery should be considered. Laparoscopy may be of some value when there is uncertainty about the nature of the mass but, in general, laparotomy needs to be undertaken.

In the older woman with a large cyst, a midline incision is mandatory so that the omentum can be sampled and a proper laparotomy performed. In a younger woman an ovarian tumour is most unlikely to be malignant and, in these circumstances, it is probably justifiable to perform a small suprapubic transverse incision which can be extended laterally if necessary. Efforts should be made to enucleate the cyst from the ovary, and the ovary reconstituted to reduce adhesion formation.

RECOMMENDED READING

Dmawski N, Braun D 1995 Immunological aspects of endometriosis. Contemporary Reviews in Obstetrics and Gynaecology 7: 167–171
Hutchins F 1995 Uterine fibroids; diagnosis and indications for treatment. Obstetrics and Gynecology Clinics of North America 22: 659–665
Rock J, Schweppe K 1997 Recent advance in the management of endometriosis. Parthenon, Carnforth

Premalignant lesions

Premalignant disease is reported more commonly in the UK than it was 20 years ago. This may not be a real increase: but better diagnostic techniques may be picking up conditions which were missed previously.

THE VULVA

Premalignant disease of the vulva is mostly squamous vulval intraepithelial neoplasia (VIN). A small number of adenocarcinoma *in situ* (which used to be called Paget's disease) does occur, usually associated with adenocarcinoma of the underlying sweat glands.

VIN presents with pruritus vulvae and leukoplakia, although about a third of women are asymptomatic and the condition is found at a routine examination. Biopsies should be taken and reported before a final diagnosis is made or treatment considered.

The management of VIN is not easy, for some of the women are young and the condition is asymptomatic. Further, even after histological examination, the malignant potential is uncertain. The least active end of the treatment spectrum is to observe women closely with repeated biopsies of the areas of leukoplakia or where the skin may heap up or bleed. Excision biopsy may be used for small single lesions, or laser can be used to destroy the area. A local vulvectomy may be required with the older woman but not the younger, for the malignant potential of VIN is uncertain.

THE VAGINA

Premalignant lesions are termed vaginal intra-epithelial neoplasia (VAIN). This is similar to cervical intraepithelial neoplasia in that it is confined by the basement membrane but the vagina has no crypts, so the lesion remains more superficial until it becomes malignant and spreads with invasion.

Usually VAIN is a vaginal extension of cervical lesions and is not found in isolation. Colposcopy to confirm the diagnosis is difficult because of the oblique angle which the colposcope can bear on the vaginal walls. A biopsy is required to exclude invasive disease, and then a laser is a satisfactory way of treating VAIN. Excision of the vault and the vagina is difficult, particularly if there has been a previous hysterectomy, pleating and tacking up the upper end of the vaginal tube.

THE CERVIX

The major lesion is cervical intraepithelial neoplasia (CIN), although a small number of adenocarcinomata *in situ* are found. The diagnosis is made by biopsy, commonly one that has been colposcopically directed. Changes are limited by the basement membrane, and three degrees are commonly recognized (Table 19.1).

The depth of penetration into the surface layers is one feature, but others are important, such as nuclear abnormalities, the nuclear/cytoplasmic ratio, the nuclear size and variation of density of the nucleus. If there is invasion through the basement membrane, then the woman has a microinvasive lesion. If the penetration is more than 3 mm, the lesion needs to be assessed in the same way as invasive carcinoma of the cervix. However, CIN can travel along the crypts of the glands although it is still topographically on the surface. All these histological changes can vary from one part of a sample to another, and it is important to consider the imprecision of the grading of CIN via the microscope. About a quarter of those diagnosed with CIN I will progress to CIN III, while about a third of those with CIN III will go on to invasive disease.

The diagnosis of this condition often starts with abnormalities of cytology on a smear, known as dyskaryosis, and continues with colposcopic biopsy (dysplasia).

A population of women properly selected and adequately treated should have a 95% 5 year follow-up with no recurrent CIN. Hence, annual or maybe 2 yearly cervical smears should be performed for about 10 years after treatment. Any variation of these from the normal will lead to further biopsy.

THE OVARY

With ovarian tumours appearing so late, it is difficult to make any real comment on pre-malignant disease of the ovary. About 10% of all the epithelial tumours (serous, mucinous and cystadenocarcinoma) are considered to be *borderline*, showing various degrees of mitotic activity with multilayering of the neoplastic cells, but no invasion of the stroma. These tumours usually remain confined to the ovaries but can metastasize locally and are of low malignant potential.

In serous cystadenomata, papillomatous areas can be found in which some parts contain undifferentiated cells, a move towards malignancy, while others are perfectly normal. Often all grades of differentiation are seen in the same tumour.

RECOMMENDED READING

Singer D, Monaghan J 1994 Lower genital tract precancer. Blackwell, Oxford

Table 19.1 CIN classification based on adequate biopsy. Grading is at the discretion of individual histologists

Grade	Degree of dysplasia	Surface signs	Deep signs
CIN I	Mild	Outer two-thirds stratified squames	High nucleocytoplasmic rates Pleomorphic nuclei
CIN II	Moderate	Outer one-half stratified squames	Basal cells occupy lower half
CIN III	Severe	Outer two-thirds of stratified squames only	Immature cells with large nuclei. Many mitoses

Malignant lesions

The increase in background rates of some cancers is reported widely, but the lay press rarely mention lessening rates, as in lung cancer in men, and in stomach cancer in both sexes. Similarly, treatment of cancer is a highly emotive subject, fuelled by the media. Each time there is a recall of women for cervical smears after inefficient cytology reporting, there is intense media interest. Perhaps these emotions should be turned around and considered more of a benefit resulting from increasing vigilance and high standards for the vast majority.

The recent Department of Health Advisory Group report on the management of cancer which was backed by the Royal College of Obstetricians and Gynaecologists has focused gynaecologists' attention very much on the future care of women with cancers of the pelvis. Here were outlined the principles of equity and access to higher standards irrespective of where women lived, with care concentrated in centres of experience.

THE SIZE OF THE PROBLEM

Table 20.1 shows that about half the deaths amongst women in the UK in recent years were due to circulatory diseases and only a quarter from all neoplasia. Figure 20.1 and Table 20.2 respectively give the relative incidence and mortality of the commonest cancers amongst women in recent years. Breast, colorectal and lung are the major sites, with the ovary and cervix involved less commonly. Cervical mortality rates have been reported as reducing

Table 20.1 Major causes of death in females (England and Wales, 1992)

Cause	Number	Percentage
Circulatory disease		46
Ischaemic heart disease	23 000	
Cardiovascular and hypertension	15 000	
Malignant disease		24
Breast	12 000	
Lung	10 000	
Ovary	4 000	
Respiratory disease		7
Accidents		2
Infections		0.4

Table 20.2 Mortality rate for females with certain common cancers (England and Wales, 1991–92)

Site of cancer	Average deaths/year
Breast	11 761
Lung	9 958
Colon and rectum	6 764
Ovary	**3 625**
Stomach	2 851
Oesophagus	1 708
Cervix	**1 612**
Leukaemia	1 503

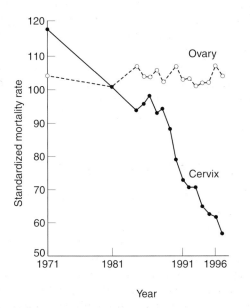

Figure 20.1 Standardized mortality ratios (based on 1981–82 = 100) for cancer of the cervix and ovary (England and Wales, 1971–97).

much more sharply than those for ovarian cancer.

THE OVARY

Primary carcinoma of the ovary is the commonest gynaecological malignant tumour, accounting for twice as many deaths than cancer of the cervix.

When carcinoma of the ovary is examined by age group over the last 20 years in the UK, there is a diminution in the younger age groups but no change in the commonest age group, 50–69 years; there was even an increase by 20% for the ages 70–84 years. Ovarian cancers, both by incidence and mortality, are related to parity, and it may well be that the wider use of oral contraception in reproductive years will be associated with reduction in carcinoma of the ovary in the older age group who have used this method in the past.

Risk factors

The risk factors relate to the activity of the ovarian germinal epithelium. There is a decreased risk after many pregnancies or the use of oral contraception. Conversely, there is an increased risk in a woman who has no pregnancies, with regular monthly ovulation causing monthly disruption of the germinal epithelium and also those having induction of ovulation.

Types

The tumour may be cystic, containing mucinous fluid (mucinous cystadenocarcinoma) or serous fluid (serous cystadenocarcinoma). There may be papillary areas in either, and these cystic tumours make up 80% of ovarian carcinomata. Of the rest, the tumour may be solid with no cystic areas (approximately 10%) or may arise from special ovarian tissue such as a granulosa cell tumour or a disgerminoma.

The grading of ovarian carcinoma depends upon the spread of the tumour and its staging is shown in Box 20.1. Most spread is transcoelomic through the peritoneal cavity to

---

Box 20.1	Staging and spread of ovarian cancer
Stage I	Tumour limited to the ovaries
IA	Tumour limited to one ovary
IB	Tumour limited to both ovaries
IC	IA or IB with capsule ruptured, surface involvement, malignant cells in ascites or peritoneal washings
Stage II	Tumour involves one or both ovaries with pelvic spread
IIA	To tubes or uterus
IIB	To other pelvic tissues
IIC	IIA or IIB with malignant cells in ascites or peritoneal washings
Stage III	Tumour involvement of abdominal cavity
IIIA	Microscopic peritoneal metastasis beyond pelvis
IIIB	Macroscopic peritoneal metastasis ≤ 2 cm diameter
	Involvement of retroperitoneal or inguinal nodes
IIIC	Tumour in pelvis with involvement of small bowel or omentum
Stage IV	Distant metastases
	Liver
	Bowel
	Pleural fluid with malignant cells

---

the structures in the pouch of Douglas, the omentum and the small bowel. Malignant cells travel easily to other intra-abdominal sites. This leads to ascites. Ovarian cancer may spread along the lymphatics to the para-aortic glands, but blood spread is late.

The ovary may be the seat of secondary carcinoma, particularly from adenocarcinoma of the large bowel, breast or stomach leading to Kruckenberg tumours.

Presentation

Most women with an ovarian carcinoma present late. General ill health, cachexia, anaemia and loss of weight all may be presenting symptoms. Some women come to their doctor because of a swelling in the abdomen; vaginal bleeding or pain are late symptoms.

The tumour may be felt abdominally or bi-manually, and ascites may be detected clinically. Magnetic resonance imaging or computerized tomography give an accurate representation of

tumour size and spread. Serum levels of the carcinoembryonic antigen (CA-125) reflect only coarsely the progress of the growth. They may be of use in following the progress of ovarian cancer after primary treatment but are not of much help in the original diagnosis.

Treatment

The primary treatment of ovarian tumours is surgical. If possible, the tumour and areas into which it has spread locally are removed at total hysterectomy, bilateral salpingo-oophorectomy and omentectomy. If the tumour has spread further, an attempt must be made to remove as much of the malignant tissue as possible by excision if necessary and by bowel or urinary tract reanastamosis. The best chance of cure is radical surgery by a competent oncology surgeon who is not just accomplished in gynaecological surgery but also in dealing with the ureters and bowel. Hence, ovarian cancer should be dealt with in special centres where such surgeons and their teams work.

Radiotherapy is used rarely for ovarian cancer since it affects the bone marrow of the lumbar vertebrae and thus lead to intractable anaemia. Further, the liver is very intolerant of radiation and is in the field of therapy for any ovarian cancer spread, and intestinal complications are likely at the doses required.

Chemotherapy gives variable results. The commonest used is cisplatin or carboplatin (Box 20.2), either alone or in combination with other cytotoxic agents such as actinomycin D, methotrexate or taxol.

Prognosis

Carcinoma of the ovary has a poor prognosis, with less than 30% of women surviving for 5 years. The variations within this rate depend upon the stage at which the disease is diagnosed, the extent of the first treatment, the differentiation of the tumour, and how much tumour tissue has to be left behind at the first debulking operation. Of these variables, the first is the one that oncologists are currently

Box 20.2 Some of the cytotoxic agents used in the chemotherapy of ovarian cancer

- Akylating agents:
  - Cyclophosphamide
  - Chlorambucil
  - Melphalan
- Platinum agents:
  - Cisplatin
  - Carboplatin
- Combinations:
  - Platinum agents with cyclophosphamide
  - Platinum agents with cyclophosphamide and doxorubicin
  - Platinum agents with taxol

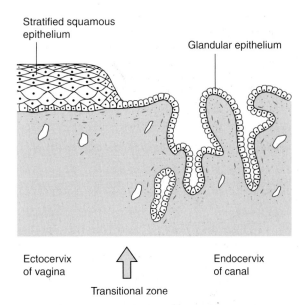

Figure 20.2   The quite sharp transitional zone at the squamocolumnar junction where stratified squamous epithelium of the surface of the cervix gives way to glandular epithelium of the cervical canal.

emphasizing. Earlier diagnosis including an effective screening method would lead to more early stage tumours being treated with improved results.

THE CERVIX

Expressing the data for gynaecological cancers by age, then those of the cervix show striking associations. They have mostly been declining, excepting in the age group of 15–34 years, which showed a rise in the 1970s but now is diminishing. This was not unique to the UK. With the wider spread use of the oral contraceptive pill accompanied by a decrease in use of barrier methods, many young people are exposed to greater risks of sexual transmitted infection along with herpes transmissions.

Nearly all malignant disease of the cervix (85%) is squamous carcinoma from the epithelium at the junction of the ectocervix and endocervix (Fig. 20.2). A few tumours may be adenocarcinoma from the columnar cells in the cervical canal.

Risk factors

Cervical cancer is extremely rare in virgins; the act of coitus seems to have associated factors which probably act on the squamocolumnar junction at some fragile time in its history. These include coitus starting very early in life or occurring close to recent pregnancies. Multiple partners increase the risk, and it is probable that

the wart virus (types 16 and 18 particularly) and certain herpes viruses are the triggering agents. Attempts made to implicate sperm with its proteins or prostaglandins in the semen have not been successful.

Types

The majority of growths of the cervix are squamous carcinomata arising at the squamocolumnar junction. These commonly, but not inevitably, follow carcinoma in situ. The growth spreads in flat sheets and downgrowths into the substance of the cervix, invading lymphatics and veins as it goes.

The disease spreads mostly in the lymph glands and by direct spread; it is staged according to the clinical estimation of its spread (Box 20.3).

Cervical intraepithelial neoplasia is considered in Chapter 19.

Presentation

Cervical cancer has symptoms when the surface

Box 20.3   Staging of cancer of the cervix

Stage 0   Carcinoma *in situ*. The growth remains within the epithelial layer of the cervix

Stage 1   Cancer clinically limited to the substance of the cervix

Stage 2   Growth has spread to the upper two-thirds of the vagina or into the parametrium but not to the pelvic wall

Stage 3   The growth has spread to the lower one-third of the vagina or into the parametrium to the lateral pelvic wall

Stage 4   Metastases beyond the pelvis or the bladder or the rectum

---

of the epithelium becomes ulcerated, producing a watery, offensive, or even blood-stained discharge. Later comes contact bleeding at coitus or insertion of a diaphragm. Later still in stage III, continuous severe bleeding can occur. Pain is a late symptom, implying involvement by secondary growth.

The cervix feels hard, and, on speculum examination, ulceration or even a cauliflower growth may be seen. In extreme cases, the whole vault is filled with an ulcerated mass, and pieces of growth come off on the examining finger. If the growth is an adenocarcinoma in the cervical canal, the cervix is expanded into a barrel-shaped mass.

The diagnosis should always be confirmed by biopsy, combined with curettage of the uterine cavity and canal to see how far the growth has moved up in the genital tract. Smaller tumours may be diagnosed at colposcopy. A Schiller's test, where the cervix is painted with an iodine solution, does not stain brown in malignant areas where glycogen is not being metabolized. Care should be taken to differentiate carcinoma of the cervix from other chronic granulomatous infections such as tuberculosis, especially in tropical parts of the world.

Treatment

The major treatments of cervical cancer are either by surgery or radiotherapy. The former is probably best for stage I and some stage II cases. It depends upon the age and condition of the patient and the extent and histology of the lesions. If surgery is agreed upon, then a Wertheim's radical abdominal hysterectomy is performed. This removes the uterus, tubes, parametrium and the upper third of the vagina, along with regional lymph glands of the iliac and obturator groups (see Table 17.3). The ovaries may rarely be conserved in a young woman with early disease. If the tumour extends into the bladder or rectum, an exenteration may be needed, removing one or other of those organs *en bloc*.

Radiotherapy is the first line of choice with more disseminated tumours, or with women at poor medical risk for other reasons. However, it is unwise to use it when the bladder is already involved because of the risk of fistula formation. Radiation involves the loading of caesium into capsules in predetermined sites in the canal of the cervix and the fornices. Usually two or three applications are given, each of about 22 h duration. Some units use a cathetron, whereby an empty container is clamped into position and high-intensity cobalt sources are after loaded by remote control, eliminating the risk of radiation to the staff.

Cavity radiation is often used as a preliminary to surgery to shrink the tumour. A gap of about 6 weeks should take place between the two treatments.

Later stages of carcinoma of the cervix are best treated by radiotherapy alone, either using a cobalt bomb or a linear accelerator for external radiation of the side walls of the pelvis and the para-aortic regions.

Prognosis

Five year follow-up of those in stage I usually gives a cure rate of 80%, whereas the rate is 10% for stage IV. The wideness of this range underlines the value of early diagnosis. If nothing active can be done to treat the tumour, palliation is used. Pain in the later stage of the disease must be avoided by liberal use of analgesics, or even intrathecal injections of alcohol; chordotomy has the same affect. Both morphia and heroin are of great use here, and should be used liberally. Death is usually from uraemia because of involvement of the renal tract or from local haemorrhage.

THE ENDOMETRIUM

Carcinoma of the endometrium is a less common condition than that of the ovary. It is comparatively slow-growing and has a reasonable prognosis.

Risk factors

Most women with endometrial cancer are postmenopausal. It is associated with hyper-oestrogenic states in obesity or oestrogen-producing tumours; other aetiological factors are low parity, late menopause, and the prolonged use of unopposed oestrogen.

Types

Usually carcinoma of the endometrium is an adenocarcinoma which is fairly well differentiated. There may, in addition, be squamous metaplasia, which can lead to an adenoacanthoma. Spread is by invasion of the myometrium, and later along the lymphatics, either along the round ligaments to the inguinal region, or the cervical lymphatics to the internal and common iliac nodes. Bloodstream spread can occur later, often to the lungs.

Presentation

The commonest symptom is postmenopausal bleeding. Most doctors would consider this to be a symptom of malignancy until proved otherwise. There may, however, be just a blood stained discharge. Often there are no physical signs. CA-125 levels may be raised.

Ultrasound can help assess the dimensions of the tumour, and endometrial biopsy as an outpatient procedure can provide material for histological examination. Hysteroscopy should be done with care, for perforation of the uterus may occur.

The *staging of the carcinoma* depends on clinical

Box 20.4	Staging of cancer of the endometrium

Stage 0	Histology suspicious of invasive cancer
Stage 1	Carcinoma confined to the body of the uterus
Stage 2	Extension to the cervix
Stage 3	Extension outside the uterus but within the pelvis
Stage 4	Involvement of the bladder and rectum, and extension outside the pelvis

examination before and at operation (see Box 20.4).

Treatment

The best treatment of endometrial carcinoma is surgical, with removal of the uterus and bilateral salpingo-oophorectomy. The tumour is often at stage I, and so this operation removes the involved area. At operation it is wise to open the uterus immediately after removal and check the spread of the tumour. If this goes into the lower third of the cavity or penetrates over halfway into the myometrium, a block dissection of the paracervical and lymphatic nodes should be performed, for these are the ones at risk of spread to the lymphatics. Radiotherapy is not very helpful alone, but is used as an adjunct to invasion of more than a half of the myometrium or evidence of node involvement.

Treatment with progestogens is not useful but may be used in the palliation of advanced disease.

THE VULVA

Vulval carcinoma is less common than other gynaecological cancers, occurring mostly in older women, the peak incidence being at 65 years. Spread is by direct extension into the adjoining vulval tissues; it may also cross the introitus to produced a lesion on the other labium. Secondary spread is by the lymphatics, with which the vulva is amply supplied. Whilst this is on the same side as the lesion at first, it can spread to the contralateral side as well as to the inguinal, femoral and, later, iliac nodes.

Risk factors

The association with poor vulval and vaginal hygiene is notable. An association with cigarette smoking occurs, but whether this is causal or an association of other life factors is uncertain. There is a strong association with vulval intra-epithelial neoplasia and vulval dystrophies.

Types

Vulval carcinoma is nearly always a squamous carcinoma, although very rarely, in the younger age group, melanoma may be found, noticeably among those who have had some exposure of the area to the sun in childhood and youth.

Presentation

There may be a small nodule in the vulval region, possibly on the inner surface of the labia minor which is unnoticed. This can develop into an ulcer which produces an offensive discharge or bleeding. A biopsy should always be taken before treating carcinoma of the vulva, for other ulcerations can occur, particularly among those living in tropical parts of the world.

Treatment

The primary treatment of carcinoma of the vulva is radical vulvectomy, which includes removal of the area concerned and bilateral dissection of the superficial and deep inguinal and femoral nodes. If spread has gone beyond the uppermost femoral node (checked by frozen section biopsy in theatre) then more radical dissection should take place up into the side walls of the pelvis. A large area of skin is removed, and relieving incisions may be required to reduce tension to assist healing. Sometimes skin grafts are done, again if there is too much tension.

Radiotherapy and chemotherapy are not commonly used for carcinoma of the vulva, although the latter may be helpful if there is spread to the anus.

Prognosis

Surprisingly, carcinoma of the vulva has a very good prognosis, with a 5 year survival of 70% overall; the degree of lymph node involvement is probably the major variable feature. The low-grade nature of the squamous carcinoma helps. Melanomata have a worse prognosis, for they have a more multifocal spread, with patchy involvement of the lymphatic chain.

RECOMMENDED READING

Macleod A, Kitchover H 1995 A review of prognostic factors in cervical carcinoma. Contemporary Reviews in Obstetrics and Gynaecology 7: 106–112
NHS Centre for Reviews 1999 Management of gynaecological cancers. Royal Society of Medicine Press 5(3): 1–2
Shepherd J, Monagham J 1990 Clinical gynaecological oncology. Blackwell, Oxford

21

Screening for cancer

Cancer screening is the investigation of a population of apparently well people to test for cancer at a preinvasive or very early invasive stage. It should provide benefit much greater than any potential harm, hence tests of low specificity which give many false positives would be less useful. Similarly those tests with a low sensitivity will miss many cases, offering too many false-negative results. There must be a balance between these two: if the cut-off point is made too low then sensitivity may improve but specificity would decrease, so there would be more false positives; conversely, if it is set too high, while specificity would improve, sensitivity would be lower, giving more false negatives. It must be remembered that screening is different from diagnosis; in practice, screening at best circumscribes a subset of the population who deserve more thorough diagnostic investigations.

In gynaecology, the cervical smear has been in use for many years, having been first devised by Papanicolaou in the 1940s. Carcinoma of the vulva and endometrium tends to produce early symptoms of bleeding, and so screening programmes have not been developed for them. The major problem is the lack of good screening tests for carcinoma of the ovary, the most common and least easy to treat gynaecological cancer.

CARCINOMA OF THE VULVA

About 600 new cases of carcinoma of the vulva occur in England and Wales annually, almost all in older women. Symptoms of bleeding, ulceration or irritation are early signs in this condition, and no screening programmes exist.

CARCINOMA OF THE CERVIX

Exfoliated cells from the junction of the ecto-cervix and the cervical canal – the squamo-columnar junction – are easy to obtain if the tester is skilled in the use of the vaginal speculum and performing a vaginal examination.

The programme of cervical screening, however, was introduced haphazardly and done opportunistically wherever women appeared and were having vaginal examinations. Hence many women at antenatal and family planning clinics were screened merely because they were there, yet these were an inappropriate age group to whom cervical screening should be offered. These women are nearly all young (mostly under 35 years of age), while the best results come from cervical screening of women between the ages of 35 and 64 years.

In counties where the screening programmes were in the hands of the public health departments, they were better organized rather than done as an ad hoc part of the clinical gynaecologists' work load. Effective screening programmes have led to a reduction in both death rates and incidence of cervical carcinoma in countries such as Finland and Iceland. This improvement was not observed in the UK until a well-organized GP screening service was implemented more recently.

Management

Women are now invited to their family practitioner's surgery for screening at intervals. Whilst annual screening is the norm in the USA, a 3–5 year interval is more usual in this country. As well as the differences produced by the fee-for-service payment method in the USA compared with the salaried service in the UK, an annual appointment is easier to remember. Table 21.1 shows the percentage reduction in the risk of a carcinoma of the cervix by the number of tests needed. This indicates that a 3 yearly programme would be the most cost-effective.

Table 21.1 Potential cervical screening programmes for women aged 35–65 years

Frequency of screening (years)	Percentage reduction of risk of carcinoma of the cervix	Number of tests that will be required
1	93.3	30
2	92.3	15
3	91.4	10
5	83.9	7
10	64.2	4

On reception, women are seen by the trained practice nurse or the general practitioner. An explanation of the examination is given, and the woman prepared on a couch. Either the left lateral or the dorsal position may be used according to the preference of the woman and the examiner. A bimanual examination first is vital, for it tells the position of the cervix and any tilt of the uterus as well as some idea of any other gross pathology in the pelvis, such as fibroids or ovarian masses. The finger should not be rubbed over the surface of the cervix, because this could interfere with, but not negate, the obtaining of a reasonable sample of cells. A speculum is now passed, a Cusco bivalve speculum if the woman is in the dorsal position, or a Sims's speculum if she is in the lateral position. When the cervix is exposed, it should not be cleaned or prepared in any way, but a spatula should be passed around the full circumference of the cervix (Fig. 21.1). Despite the invention of other devices, such as

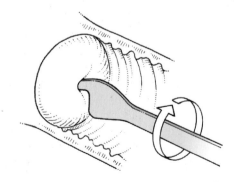

Figure 21.1 Taking a cervical smear. The beak of the spatula goes up the cervical canal and the stem is rotated through 360° to scrape all of the squamocolumnar junction.

(a)

(b)

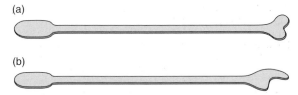

Figure 21.2   **a** The Ayre's spatula. **b** The Aylesbury spatula.

Christmas tree-shaped brushes and aspiration pipettes for the posterior fornix, the spatula with a long lip that goes up the cervical canal is still the most frequently used in the UK (Fig. 21.2). When the smear has been taken it should be spread rapidly on a dry clean microscope slide. The woman's name and identification number should have been entered on the frosted end of the slide before the smear. Once a layer of the material removed has been made, it should be fixed rapidly before it can air dry, as this distorts the cells and causes difficulties for the histologist. Once fixed there is then no hurry for it to get to the laboratory, and it may be sent at a convenient time.

At the laboratory the slide is stained and examined by cytology laboratory workers. It is good practice in the UK that two technicians scan each slide, which, if not perfectly normal, is put to one side for further examination by a histocytologist. Most slides are considered normal, but about 5% of the total show some abnormality of the cells, including obvious inflammation. These are reported to the family doctor.

The report can take several forms. Of late, laboratories are reporting cervical intraepithelial neoplasia (CIN) at various degrees of severity. This was originally a description of tissue, not of individual cells, and could only be given after a biopsy tissue specimen has been examined. The cells are best considered in their own right. They are usually considered to be dyskaryotic to a mild, moderate or severe degree, and whilst there is a loose correlation between an underlying histology (CIN I, II or III) this is not always so.

Normal cervical epithelial smears show regular orderly London pavement cells in sheets of surface squamous epithelium. Four abnormalities describe dyskaryosis in various degrees:

- Increased mitotic activity
- Nuclear abnormalities
- Lack of differentiation
- Increased nuclear: cytoplasmic ratio.

Inflammation may flood the slide with leucocytes while stained bacteria or microorganisms may be seen. Columnar cells from the endocervix are a normal finding; indeed, their absence is considered to be an indication that the spatula has not gone far enough up the canal.

Management of the woman with an abnormal smear

Some clinicians consider that every woman with an abnormal smear should be examined with a colposcope. Others only examine those with moderate and severe dyskaryosis, asking the woman with the mild condition to return for a repeat smear in 6 months time (Table 21.2). Colposcopy is best learnt about in practice, and most colposcopic clinics will welcome practitioners to attend and see this very visual subject. The colposcope is a field microscope with magnifications ranging from ×4 to ×25, with ×10

Table 21.2   Cervical abnormality pathology related to cervical smear reports

Reported	Prevalence of abnormal tissue	Possible action
Normal cytology	0.1% CIN	Repeat 3 years
Borderline cells	9% CIN	Repeat 6 months
Borderline nuclear change	37% CIN	Repeat 6 months Colposcopy if 2 abnormal smears
Mild dyskaryosis	50% CIN	Repeat 6 months Colposcopy if 2 abnormal smears
Moderate dyskaryosis	70% CIN	Colposcopy
Severe dyskaryosis	90% CIN 5% Invasive carcinoma	Colposcopy
Invasion suspected	50% Invasive carcinoma	Urgent colposcopy

After Soutter 1994.

being used by most practitioners for scanning the cervix.

After positioning the patient comfortably in the dorsal position with her legs supported in lithotomy poles, a warmed Cuscoe speculum is gently introduced, and the cervix is cleaned. Weak acetic acid is painted on to the surface to allow identification of areas of abnormal cells, which show up white. The transformation zone between the columnar and squamous epithelium should be carefully examined, as it is the most likely site of problems.

If abnormal tissue is sighted, a biopsy can be removed with an ethmoid punch without general anaesthesia. If the transformation zone cannot be seen, then the woman should be admitted for a formal cone biopsy to allow examination of the hidden canal to take place. This is unusual, for most women attending for colposcopy are multiparous, and the zone can usually be made visible.

Treatment of local lesions can be by electrical diathermy or the paradoxically called cold diathermy (which only heats to 95°C). Alternatively, cryosurgery or a carbon dioxide laser may be used. These techniques should destroy the entire transformation zone down to 6 mm. Local treatment avoids cone biopsy, which is a much bloodier and complex proceeding. Cryosurgery can be done without anaesthesia, for the cold numbs the nerve endings. Laser vaporization has come into its own over the last 20 years. Although the capital outlay on equipment is expensive, it has a precision much greater than any other technique, and it is again an outpatient procedure. Once diagnosed it is best to treat lesions soon and surgically. Hysterectomy is often unnecessary. Cone biopsy is effective in removing the tissues. (Fig. 21.3), provided both the upper and lower ends of the lesion can be seen at colposcopy. General anaesthesia is required for a cone biopsy, and the patient may have to stay in hospital for a day or two.

If wide excisional therapy is to be done, as an alternative to a knife cone, a large loop excision of the transformation zone (LLETZ) can be performed with a diathermy loop of very thin stainless steel wire, making the treatment

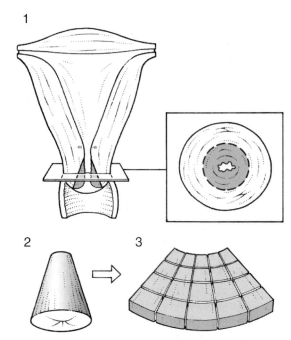

Figure 21.3 Surgical conization; 1, the area of invasion; 2, the cone; 3, the cone opened out showing the 20 blocks that will be examined. Clinically, it is important that blocks 1–5 and 16–20 are clear of growth.

quicker (Fig. 21.4). This is done as an outpatient procedure at the colposcopy clinic, although the bleeding may occasionally result in the patient being kept in hospital.

Cryosurgery was popular but there was some fear that this would seal in deeper CIN lesions at the base of crypts of the glands in the cervical canal. However, cryotherapy is easy to do and is precise; furthermore it avoids hospital admission. While surgical biopsy makes for a more precise pathological opinion, primary or secondary bleeding or infection may follow.

CARCINOMA OF THE ENDOMETRIUM

Whilst several trials of screening for carcinoma of the endometrium have been carried out, there is no established national programme at the moment. Usually the lesions are on the surface of the endometrium and bleed early in the progress of the disease. Attempts with fine

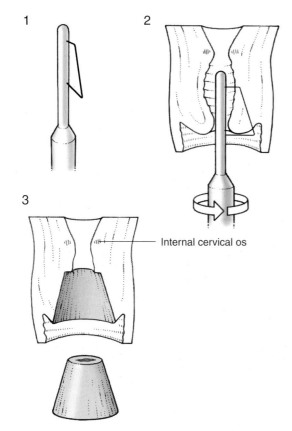

Internal cervical os

Figure 21.4 LLETZ loop biopsy: 1, the gib sail shape of the biopsy cone; 2, cutting through the cervical canal; 3, what is removed and what is left.

brushes and aspirations of the cavity have been made, but the pick-up rate has been low. The introduction of outpatient hysteroscopy has put a better tool in the hands of gynaecologists, although this, in itself, is not a screening device.

CA-125 serum levels are often raised in endometrial cancer, and may act as a pointer, but the correlation is not good enough as the basis of a reliable screening programme.

OVARIAN CANCER

Had we a good screening test, it would be hoped that patients with earlier malignant disease of the ovary would be detected. In this it would imitate mammography used for breast cancer screening, rather than cervical cytology which looks for premalignant conditions. While the 5 year survival rate of all ovarian cancer is about 20%, the cure rate for stage 1 is 90%. Hence there are many who are seeking a good screening programme. Early detection is limited because:

- The tumour is tucked deep in the peritoneal cavity
- There is no well defined premalignant state
- There is poor knowledge of cancer spread.

Clinical examination is probably the most widely practised method, but as a screening technique it is not especially sensitive nor specific for asymptomatic ovarian cancer. Further, it is probably only the more skilled observers who would detect early stages of change in the ovaries.

The most commonly used ovarian *tumour marker* is CA-125, a glycoprotein shed by cancer cells derived from the peritoneum. However, the serum levels are increased in many other irritant conditions of the peritoneum, such as inflammation and fibroids. If used as a preliminary screen and backed up with ultrasound, then CA-125 elevation has a positive prediction rate of about 25%. Combining it with other tumour markers such as CA-123 or M-CFS does increase the specificity somewhat, but large studies are still awaited. It is probable that CA-125 by itself used as a screening test on a low-risk population is not much help in trying to predict who is going to get carcinoma of the ovary or even those who have it at an early stage.

Transvaginal ultrasound used alone has a low prediction value but, in combination with tumour markers, this can be improved. In women who have a family history or some other significant aetiological feature, it helps to localize a smaller population on whom further studies should be performed. Since this usually means an invasive operation such as laparoscopy or laparotomy, the false-positive rate is important to consider.

Abdominal *colour Doppler imaging* can be used to improve specificity, but this remains low, and gathers in a rather larger population than that of vaginal ultrasound. For example, one large review showed that Doppler imaging would lead to 17 laparotomies to detect one stage 1 cancer (Jacobs et al 1993).

Work is still proceeding, but there is currently not much evidence to support widespread cancer screening in the general population of women who have no familial or historical risk. Even amongst those at higher risk, the increased morbidity that would come from the result of unnecessary surgery must be considered as well as the patient anxiety that the result of a positive test would generate. For those with a family history of cancer there are networks which store essential genetic data. All relevant families should be indexed there. It is probable that genetic testing will be available in the near future.

BREAST CANCER

In the UK, breast diseases are not usually investigated by gynaecologists, but some women expect the gynaecologist to examine their breasts along with the genital tract. Mammography has been introduced this decade, and women between the ages of 50 and 65 years are offered screening every 3 years. This can reduce breast cancer mortality by up to 40%. Unfortunately, below this age, while the woman is in a more active hormonal phase, breast tissue is much denser and so lesions are less readily spotted. It should always be remembered that the lesion looked for by mammography is an early carcinoma of the breast whereas in cervical screening it is precancerous states that are assessed.

RECOMMENDED READING

Jacobs H et al 1993 Prevalence screening for ovarian cancer in postmenopausal women by CA-125 measurement and ultrasonography. British Medical Journal 306: 1030
NHS Centre for Reviews 1999 Management of gynaecological cancers. Royal Society of Medicine Press 5(3): 1–12
Soutter P 1994 Cervical screening in the UK. Contemporary Reviews in Obstetrics and Gynaecology 6: 208–213

22

Premenstrual syndrome

The premenstrual syndrome (PMS) is a cluster of physical, emotional and psychological symptoms with a fixed relationship to the onset of menses occurring in the second half of the menstrual cycle. The symptoms disappear immediately after the onset of menstruation. Virtually all women will experience some PMS, and up to 40% will seek medical advice sometime during their reproductive life, with about 5% being incapacitated.

PMS is most common in the fourth decade of life, when symptoms may become most acute, but it can be at any age in the reproductive life. Over 150 symptoms have been described; the most common of these are shown in Box 22.1.

Box 22.1 Some common symptoms of PMS

- Physical:
  - Breast swelling and tenderness
  - Abdominal swelling
  - Weight gain
  - Acne
  - Backache
  - Headache
  - Gastrointestinal disturbance
- Emotional and behavioural:
  - Aggression
  - Irritability
  - Lability of mood
  - Anxiety and depression
  - Poor concentration
  - Fatigue
  - Change in libido

CAUSE

The cause of PMS is unknown. Psychological factors are important, but hormonal events during the luteal phase of the cycle contribute. The measurement of hormone levels such as serum progesterone or follicle-stimulating hormone are so variable as to be of no help. No consistent disturbance in any system has yet been observed.

DIAGNOSIS

Most important is the timing of symptoms in relationship to menstruation; whilst some commence 14 days prior to the onset of menses, for most they are only severe for 2 or 3 days before bleeding starts. The diagnosis becomes obvious in most women after taking a careful history, but when there is doubt, a menstrual calendar with a concurrent record of symptoms may be useful.

MANAGEMENT

An understanding and sympathetic doctor who will take the patient's symptoms seriously is often all that many patients will require. An explanation that the symptoms, although uncomfortable and often disabling, will not impair future fertility and that no long-term harm will come to them may suffice. Traditionally, exercise has been recommended, but for many this is often the most difficult time of the menstrual cycle for them to undertake such activities.

Because of the multifactorial nature there are many treatments; some of these will work for individual patients.

Dietary advice aims to maintain a steady blood glucose level; this certainly helps some. For those with fluid retention, a reduction in fluid intake and a restriction of salt may help, but there is little convincing evidence that this is effective. Vitamin B_6 (pyridoxine 100 mg/day) has been popular for many years. The vitamin alters dopamine and serotonin concentrations, and is held by many to be effective although controlled trials have failed to show any significant improvement. A governmental restriction

in the dose used in the UK (50 mg is adequate) has recently been rescinded.

DRUG TREATMENT

Virtually all well-controlled drug trials have shown an initial placebo effect of over 50%. This will usually last for the first three cycles but then wears off. Some of the therapies are listed in Box 22.2.

Evening primrose oil

This is useful for premenstrual breast pain but often does not help other symptoms.

Prostaglandin synthetase inhibitors

Mefenamic acid is the most widely used, and helps generalized aches, pains and headache. It may also improve some mood symptoms. Other non-steroidal anti-inflammatory drugs will have a similar effect.

Diuretics

These are useful for fluid retention with bloating and weight gain. Spironolactone has been associated with an improvement in mood.

Antidepressants

Fluoxetine has been widely used, particularly with those with depression as a major element

---

Box 22.2   Drugs used in PMS

- Evening primrose oil
- Vitamin B_6
- Prostaglandin synthetase inhibitors
- Diuretics
- Antidepressants
- Bromocriptine
- Danazol
- Progestogens and progesterone
- Oestrogen
- The combined oral contraceptive pill
- Gonadotrophin-releasing hormone (GnRH) analogues

in their syndrome. Amitriptyline may also be of use.

Bromocriptine

This relieves breast symptoms, but is commonly associated with nausea and gastrointestinal upsets. In general it is not very helpful.

Danazol

This synthetic steroid depresses gonadotrophin secretion and leads to anovulation often with amenorrhoea. It is highly effective in suppressing many PMS symptoms. Unfortunately, the drug itself is commonly associated with weight gain and androgenic side-effects which may outweigh the advantages.

Progestogen and progesterone

These have been widely used in the belief that there may be a faulty luteal phase associated with the syndrome. There is no consistent evidence that progesterone levels are altered in women with PMS. There are many advocates of the use of progesterone given vaginally in doses

of 800 mg/day, but there are no properly controlled trials to show any benefit. Synthetic progestogens, particularly dydrogesterone, have been widely used but are of little benefit. Norethisterone may actually cause symptoms of PMS.

Oestrogens

The use of natural oestrogens either by subdermal implantation or transdermal oestradiol patches has some merit although to work most effectively, circulating levels of oestradiol in excess of 1000 pmol/l are usually required. Because of the effects of oestrogen on the endometrium, cyclical progestogens are needed to promote a withdrawal bleed, and this may have the disadvantage of recreating some of the premenstrual symptoms.

The combined oral contraceptive pill is useful in younger women, particularly those needing contraception. Because it leads to a constant hormonal level there is some reduction in symptoms, and this has been shown in retrospective studies. However, some women continue to have severe PMS even when taking the combined pill.

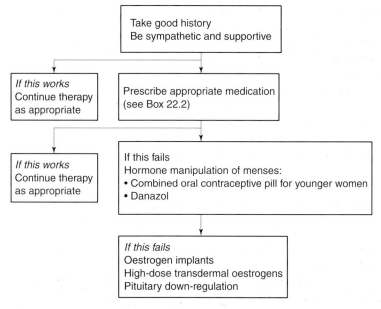

Figure 22.1 Management of PMS.

GnRH analogues

These may be administered as a subdermal implant (goserelin), an intramuscular injection (leuprorelin) or as a nasal spray (naferelin/ buserelin). Following an initial flare-up there is then down-regulation of pituitary function, leading to cessation of ovarian function. In effect the patient becomes menopausal and amenorrhoeic. The side-effects are those of the menopause, and they can be avoided by giving add-back therapy with a continuous combined form of hormone replacement therapy which is not associated with bleeding. This treatment is extremely effective and may be the most logical in the very worst of sufferers. However, it has the distinct disadvantage of being relatively complicated to use and very expensive.

MANAGEMENT

Management is summarized in Figure 22.1.

RECOMMENDED READING

Zamblera D, Studd J 1993 Treatment of mild premenstrual syndrome. Contemporary Reviews in Obstetrics and Gynaecology 5: 214–220

The menopause

The diagnosis of the menopause can only be made in retrospect, 1 year after the final menstrual period. For some time preceding this there is a decline in ovarian function, and many patients develop a number of symptoms attributable to a lowering in oestrogen levels. This perimenopause is referred to as the climacteric.

The menopause occurs naturally around the age of 50 years; this is independent of geography, state of nutrition, race or age of menarche. The menopause will also follow surgical removal of the ovaries, radiotherapy or chemotherapy.

Some physiological changes associated with the climacteric and menopause are shown in Table 23.1.

OSTEOPOROSIS

Patients at increased risk of osteoporosis include those with a family history of osteoporosis, fair-skinned people, those on steroid therapy and those who lead a sedentary life. Fifty per cent of women will have developed some osteoporosis by the age of 70 years compared with 8% of men. However, it is difficult to identify a more precise at risk population. Dual X-ray absorptionometry (DEXA) is available in a number of centres; this gives a reasonable prediction of bone density, and should be employed in those who are at risk. Hormone replacement therapy (HRT) not only has an anticatabolic effect, i.e. it stops bone loss, but it also has a mild anabolic effect. There is up to a 3% increase in bone mass per annum in patients taking HRT. Although there are no randomized controlled trials with

Table 23.1 Changes associated with the menopause

Early changes	Intermediate changes	Long-term problems
Hot flushes	Loss of skin elasticity	Osteoporosis
Night sweats	Vaginal dryness and dyspareunia	Cardiovascular disease
Insomnia	Urinary symptoms of stress and urge incontinence,	Alzheimer's disease
Palpitations	frequency, nocturia and urgency	
Loss of concentration		
Loss of short-term memory		
Lability of emotions		
Irritability		
Loss of libido		
Decline in orgasm		
Loss of vaginal lubrication		
Depression		

fractures as an end-point. It is probable that HRT should be used in the treatment of those who are at increased risk of developing osteoporosis.

CARDIOVASCULAR DISEASE

Following the cessation of menstruation, the incidence of myocardial infarction and stroke rapidly increases in women to levels similar to those in men. It is considered that this does not occur before the menopause because of the protective effect of oestrogens which have been shown to increase favourably the high-density to low-density lipoprotein ratio (HDL/LDL), to prevent atherogenesis and also to improve blood flow through the coronary and cerebral arteries. As a consequence, some studies have shown that the incidence of myocardial infarction and stroke is almost halved in women on HRT compared to those who are not on treatment. Prospective controlled trials are being carried out to confirm these studies, but at present women who smoke heavily, or have strong family history of cardiovascular disease, should be encouraged to take HRT.

PSYCHOLOGICAL AND NEUROLOGICAL EFFECTS

It is known that oestrogen enhances mood and well-being. It has also been shown in randomized controlled trials that oestrogen-treated women who have had their ovaries removed perform better in various psychometric tests than a placebo-treated group, especially for verbal memory. Any intervention with HRT that would delay the onset of symptoms of Alzheimer's disease by 3–5 years would reduce the number of affected people by a third to a half.

Recent studies have suggested that women on HRT have a 30% decreased incidence of developing Alzheimer's disease. Those with Alzheimer's disease also evince better cognitive skills if given HRT.

Women weighing over 63 kg have an estimated risk of developing Alzheimer's disease 30% lower than women weighing less than 56 kg (body fat is an endogenous source of oestrogen).

Some of these positive effects may be mediated through an increase in cerebral blood flow and enhanced cerebral metabolism, but there is also a direct effect on the hippocampus and on neurotransmitter systems.

HORMONE REPLACEMENT THERAPY

Most HRT preparations include natural oestrogens derived from vegetable sources such as yam, cactus and soya; they include oestradiol, oestrone and oestriol. Conjugated equine oestrogens are obtained from pregnant mares' urine. The synthetic form of oestrogen (ethinyl oestradiol) is available but not used in HRT. Tibilone, a gonadomimetic, is a synthetic preparation that has proven useful for treatment of post-menopausal women.

The progestogens commonly used are derived

from 17-hydroxyprogesterone (dydrogesterone and medroxyprogesterone acetate) or 19-nortestosterone (levonorgestrel and norethisterone).

HRT can be given either systemically or topically. Traditionally it was given orally, but the transdermal route has become increasingly popular, using matrix patches or by rubbing in an oestrogen-containing gel. Oestradiol transdermal preparations can cause local skin reactions, but since the wide introduction of matrix patches this is less of a problem. Subcutaneous implants of oestrogen are used, particularly in patients who have undergone hysterectomy, while topical administration of oestrogens to the urogenital tract is by vaginal creams, rings, tablets or pessaries. The progestogens used in HRT are usually administered orally, but a number of skin patches containing a progestogen are also becoming available, allowing transdermal administration. The use of continuous oestrogen without a progestogen can lead to endometrial hyperplasia. This could eventually become malignant, and for this reason a progestogen is given in the second half of the cycle to prevent further endometrial proliferation and induce a withdrawal bleed after 28 days of administration. These are combined sequential preparations.

After a minimum of 1 year from the menopause, either a continuous combined preparation of oestrogen/progestogen or tibolone can be given. The effect of these is to prevent any endometrial growth; therefore, there is no shedding and so no period, although up to 50% of patients will have some light unscheduled bleeding in the first year of therapy.

Lack of compliance has been a major problem in the maintenance of therapy: with combined sequential preparations, over 60% of patients cease therapy after 1 year. The major reason for this is cited as being a continuation of periods. Thus, *period-free* products are a major advance, and compliance is much improved. A progestogen is not needed for patients who have had a hysterectomy unless they have a previous history of endometriosis, when continuous combined therapy is advisable.

As with the combined oral contraceptive pill, breakthrough bleeding may occur. This is usually due to insufficient absorption from the gastrointestinal tract, and so a different route of administration should be tried. However, certain drugs have enzyme-inducing actions within the liver, such as phenytoin and carbamazepine, and these patients may have to take relatively higher doses of HRT orally or else use a transdermal route.

Oestradiol implants are placed in the subcutaneous fascia of the anterior abdominal wall or buttock. They need to be replaced every 6 months, the dose being adjusted according to the circulating level of oestradiol. Their use is almost entirely confined to those who have undergone hysterectomy. Some patients may experience a return of menopausal symptoms, particularly vasomotor symptoms, whilst their oestradiol levels are high, over 500 pmol/l. This has been termed tachyphylaxis. The situation may be overcome by providing the patient with small doses of transdermal oestrogen until the next implant is due or suggesting that she might change to a different route of administration.

Prescribing HRT

It is important to establish with the patient why she wishes to commence HRT. Most usually it is for the control of the short- and medium-term problems, but occasionally it may follow peer pressure or because of magazine articles. However, increasing numbers of women require HRT for the prevention of long-term problems such as cardiovascular disease, osteoporosis and Alzheimer's disease.

Oestrogen therapy rapidly relieves the vasomotor symptoms and may also improve mood changes and changes in the libido. Problems with the urogenital tract will respond but over a longer period of time.

Contraindications

These are undiagnosed irregular vaginal bleeding, pregnancy and patient refusal. There are a number of relative contraindications, of which oestrogen-dependent tumours are the most important.

Side-effects

The side-effects of HRT are somewhat dependent upon the time the patient starts treatment. If she is perimenopausal it is unlikely that she will suffer much in the way of side-effects. If therapy is started, however, after the menopause, when oestrogen levels are low, it is likely that the patient will develop the mild side-effects of any oestrogen therapy – breast tenderness and swelling, an increase in vaginal discharge, possibly some abdominal bloating and, if she is on a cyclical regime which induces withdrawal bleeding, symptoms similar to the premenstrual syndrome. Weight gain is a constant worry of patients, but in a trial of a matched group of women between the ages of 45 and 55 years taking and not taking HRT no significant increase in weight in either group was noted. It is an unfortunate fact that women of this age group tend to gain weight, and HRT is blamed wrongly. Careful counselling of the patient is therefore necessary.

Breast cancer

For a woman who starts HRT at the age of 50 years there is a minimal increased risk of breast cancer in the first 5 years of therapy. However, observational studies suggest that if HRT is taken for 10 years, the relative risk of developing breast cancer is increased by 5/1000 cases. However, the breast tumours that develop on HRT appear to be better differentiated with less nodal involvement. There is a better prognosis for patients taking HRT compared with those who are not. Paradoxically, in a matched age group there are more deaths from breast cancer in those not taking HRT. However, further prospective trials are still needed, and the long-term safety in relation to breast cancer has still not been clearly elucidated. There is no good evidence that HRT has any disadvantages among those postmenopausal patients taking tamoxifen, a selective oestrogen receptor modulator, who develop menopausal symptoms.

Cancer of the uterus

The incidence of cancer of the endometrium is not increased providing the patient is taking additional progestogen. In those taking prolonged unopposed therapy (as often used to be the case in the USA) the relative risk is increased sixfold.

For both endometrial and breast cancer patients, topical vaginal applications can be given with safety.

Thromboembolism

The risk of developing a venous thromboembolism on HRT is at least three times that of women not on HRT. However, compared with women who are still menstruating, the increase is very little and the overall risk is very small (about 3:10 000 patients per year). For those patients with a history of deep-vein thrombosis which occurred whilst taking the combined oral contraceptive pill or during pregnancy, or those who have a family history of deep-vein thrombosis, a full thrombophilic screen should be performed before contemplating HRT therapy. This includes protein C, protein S, antithrombin III and activated protein C resistance (Leiden factor V).

RECOMMENDED READING

Boaji I, Djahanbathch O 1996 What is the optimum duration of hormone replacement therapy. Contemporary Reviews in Obstetrics and Gynaecology 8: 109–114
Godfree T, Whitehead M 1999 HRT – your questions answered 2E. Churchill Livingstone, Edinburgh
Studd J, Whitehead M 1998 The menopause. Blackwell, Oxford

Urogynaecology

Urinary symptoms are extremely common amongst women, but a large proportion consider them to be a consequence of growing old or having children. Probably as many as 50% of women who reach the age of 80 years suffer from some degree of incontinence. Frequency and nocturia are so common that for the post-menopausal woman she might consider it entirely normal.

URINARY SYMPTOMS

Incontinence

There are different types of urinary incontinence, of which the most important are:

- *Stress incontinence* – the involuntary loss of urine with a sudden rise in intra-abdominal pressure when laughing, jumping, dancing, running or sneezing. It is characterized by a short spurt of urine which is then controlled by the patient; a urethrocele or cystocele is often present.
- *Urge incontinence* – the loss of urine which accompanies a strong desire to pass urine. It may well be triggered by coughing or sneezing, but control is more difficult than with stress incontinence, and there is often dribbling.
- *Overflow incontinence* – loss of urine when the bladder is overfilled.
- *True incontinence* – loss of urine at any time, a consequence of fistula formation.

Irritative symptoms

- *Frequency* is usually complained of when the patient has to pass water more than 10 times a day.
- *Nocturia* implies awakening two or more times during the night to pass urine.
- *Urgency* is the sudden desire to micturate which becomes overwhelming, and, if impossible to control, leads to *urge incontinence*.
- *Dysuria* implies pain whilst passing urine.

Problems of voiding

- *Poor stream* is self-explanatory and usually implies an outlet obstruction.
- *Hesitancy* occurs when there is difficulty at the commencement of micturition.
- *Straining to void* is associated with an outlet obstruction.
- *Incomplete emptying* often occurs following operations on the urethra, and is temporary; when it is a chronic problem, intermittent self-catheterization is needed.

CAUSES OF INCONTINENCE
Genuine stress incontinence

This occurs when the pressure within the bladder exceeds the maximum urethral closure pressure in the absence of any bladder activity. Aetiological factors are multiparity, oestrogen deficiency, obesity and other causes of raised intra-abdominal pressure (e.g. ovarian cyst). Continence of urine is maintained by the proximal portion of the urethra and the bladder neck being intra-abdominal. In these cases the same pressures that apply to the bladder also apply to the proximal urethra and maintain it in the closed position. If the bladder neck descends, and with it the proximal urethra, the pressure on the bladder will exceed that within the urethra, and incontinence results (Fig. 24.1).

Surgery for genuine stress incontinence is based upon the principle of the restoration of the

(a)

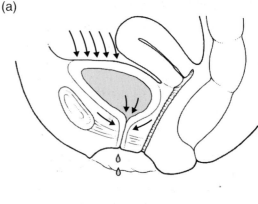

(b)

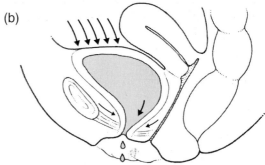

Figure 24.1   The mechanism of stress incontinence; **a** In the normal woman, when the intra-abdominal pressure is raised (↓↓↓↓↓), the levator ani muscles and rest of the pelvic diaphragm contracts, tending to close off the urethra and counter the pressure. **b** If the pelvic floor is deficient, there is less muscle effort, and the closure is less effective.

intra-abdominal position of the bladder neck and proximal urethra.

Detrusor instability

This condition, otherwise known as irritable bladder, occurs when the detrusor muscle contracts either spontaneously or following a sudden rise of intra-abdominal pressure. It is entirely involuntary, and leads to the symptoms of frequency, urgency, nocturia and then urge incontinence or nocturnal enuresis.

The causes are often not found, but there may be an association with recurrent urinary tract infections, the postmenopausal state, poor patterns of voiding earlier in life, urethral stenosis and, occasionally, as a consequence of incontinence surgery.

Overflow incontinence

This follows excessive bladder filling associated with poor bladder sensation. It is seen in the elderly, but can also follow bladder neck surgery and the use of regional analgesia such as epidural and cordal block.

True incontinence

A leak of urine will follow fistula formation. It is unfortunately common in countries where there is poor obstetric care so that fistulas may occur between the bladder and vagina following prolonged obstructed labour. In the UK they more commonly follow malignancy or its treatment by surgery or radiotherapy.

DIAGNOSIS

History

A relatively accurate diagnosis can be made on seeing a patient, but patients with pure stress incontinence or pure detrusor instability are not so common, and a mixed picture is more general. There may be chronic bronchitis or constant straining through constipation. While faecal or flatal incontinence is a common accompaniment of genuine stress incontinence, it is often not mentioned spontaneously by the patient since she finds it embarrassing, but tactful questioning will reveal it. Diabetes mellitus and neurological disorders are also of importance.

In the elderly, medication may be important, particularly diuretics. The obstetric history may be relevant, especially the size of their babies, the mode of delivery and if obstetric intervention was necessary.

Examination

Examination of the patient must include the abdomen to exclude an intra-abdominal mass or a distended bladder. Initial pelvic examination is usually carried out in the dorsal position, when most menopausal atrophic changes can be easily seen. It is common practice to examine for prolapse in the left lateral position, although stress incontinence may be difficult to demonstrate. Ideally this should be done in the standing position with a moderately filled bladder, but this often causes extreme embarrassment to the patient and is best attempted initially in the dorsal position.

Investigations

For all patients who have evidence of bladder irritability, bacteriological examination of a midstream specimen of urine is essential.

Frequency/volume charts are increasingly used in the assessment of patients' urinary symptoms. They determine the intake and output of the patient, frequency and when she wets herself.

Using preweighed pads, patients perform various exercises with a moderately filled bladder. The pads are then weighed to assess the amount of leakage, and an increase in weight of 1 g in 1 h is considered to be significant.

Urodynamic investigations

Flow rate is defined as the volume of urine expelled from the bladder per second. The most important measurements are the maximum flow rates and the total volume voided. Rates of below 15 ml/s are considered abnormal in women, and the total volume voided should exceed 150 ml for a test to be reliable.

Bladder pressure measurement (cystometry) involves pressure readings inside the bladder during filling and voiding, and is the most useful test of bladder function. Urethral pressure measurements are usually carried out as well. It is essential that urethral pressure is above bladder pressure, to maintain continence. It is of particular use in patients with a mixed picture of urge and stress incontinence, and in those who have had unsuccessful incontinence surgery. Normal cystometric findings include:

- An initial desire to void, with filling volumes of 150–200 ml
- A capacity of around 500 ml
- Detrusor pressure rise on filling

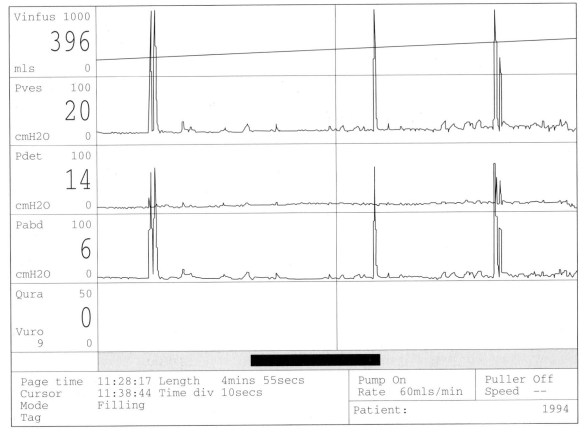

Figure 24.2 A normal cystogram: Vinfus, rate of infusion of fluid into the bladder; Pves, intravesical pressure; Pdet, detrusor pressure (Pves – Pabd = Pdet); Pabd, intra-abdominal pressure (measured rectally); Qura, urine flow (none as this was not a voiding cystogram). The spikes are cough-induced pressure rises.

- No leakage with straining or coughing
- A maximum voiding pressure of below 70 cmH$_2$O
- A residual urine volume of 50 ml or less
- An ability to stop micturition on command.

Figure 24.2 shows a normal cystogram.

Cystometry assesses the function of the bladder and urethra, including measurements of flow rate and bladder and urethral pressure profiles. They are specialized tests carried out in secondary or tertiary referral centres, and are a necessity where there is any ambiguity about the diagnosis. Many now favour urodynamic studies in all patients with urinary symptoms who are going for surgery, as it is important to determine the degree of detrusor instability in addition to genuine stress incontinence (Fig. 24.3).

Intravenous urography, electromyography studies, ultrasound and magnetic resonance imaging may also prove useful in the more difficult cases.

TREATMENT

Genuine stress incontinence

For the milder cases, initial treatment should aim at improving the pelvic floor musculature. Simple exercises, as taught in the postnatal period, involve the contraction of the levator ani, and may be all that is necessary. However, where there are moderate degrees of stress

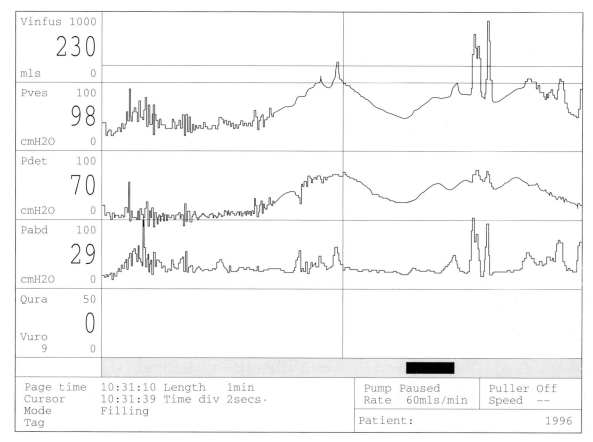

Figure 24.3 Cystogram showing detrusor instability: high intermittent detrusor pressures (Pdet) irrespective of abdominal pressures (Pabd).

incontinence, then active physiotherapy is necessary, and weighted vaginal cones may be used (Fig. 24.4). These are in graded weights which are inserted and held in the vagina for 15 min at a time, which encourages contraction of the levator ani. As the weights increase, the strength of the pelvic floor contractions improves.

Faradic stimulation or interferential therapy

This utilizes an electric current to the pelvic floor, leading to pelvic floor contractions. They have the advantage that they teach the woman which muscle groups to contract during pelvic floor exercises, and therefore should be carried out in conjunction with supervised exercises.

Operative procedures

There are a number of possible approaches:

- *Anterior colporrhaphy* was the mainstay of therapy in the past. It is suitable only for those with anterior vaginal prolapse. Urethral buttressing should be carried out with the repair, and success rates are approximately 50%.
- *Marshall–Marchetti–Kranz procedure.* This is a retropubic operation in which the bladder neck is suspended to the periostium at the back of the pubic bone (Fig. 24.5). It will not cure prolapse but the success rates for incontinence are reasonable and exceed 70%.
- *Colposuspension* is another retropubic procedure in which the vault of the vagina is attached to the ileopectineal ligament on each

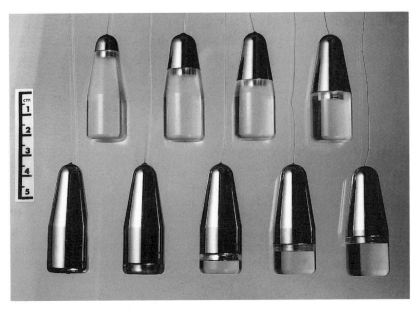

Figure 24.4 A set of graduated Peattie cones to assist pelvic floor exercises. (Courtesy of A. Peattie.)

side (Fig. 24.5). Voiding difficulties are common in the immediate postoperative period, but success rates are usually in excess of 80%. The operation can be performed laparoscopically, but at present success rates are not as great.

- *Sling procedures* are usually used for recurrent incontinence problems, and are performed using either strips of rectus sheath or synthetic materials. The sling is usually inserted from above through an abdominal incision and placed suburethrally (aided with manoeuvring from below through a vaginal approach). Voiding problems are common postoperatively, and intermittent self-catheterization may be necessary for sometime afterwards. However, success rates in terms of incontinence are as great as 95%.

- *Injectables*. A variety of substances have been injected around the bladder neck to produce outflow obstruction. Initially Teflon was used, and later collagen, and the results seem to be encouraging.

- *Artificial sphincter*. This involves the insertion of a cuff around the bladder neck connected to a pump. It is a complex and expensive procedure, and only used in the most extreme cases where other surgery has failed.

Detrusor instability

For patients with mild symptoms, an adjustment in their fluid intake may be all that is necessary. However, for the more severe cases a number of options are available:

- *Bladder training*. This is usually performed in hospital and carried out at home if there is good motivation. Initially the patient is instructed to empty her bladder every $1\frac{1}{2}$ h. She should have a normal fluid intake and should keep a fluid balance chart. The voiding interval is then increased by $\frac{1}{2}$ h when the initial goal is achieved. This is repeated day by day with an increase in the time intervals of a $\frac{1}{4}$ or $\frac{1}{2}$ h until she is able to retain urine for 4 h.

- *Drug therapy*. Anticholinergic drugs may be of use but often lead to unacceptable side-effects, with a dry mouth, tachycardia and heartburn. The most effective drug available at present is tolterodine – an initial dose of 5 mg twice a day may be increased to as much as a total of 20 mg/ day. Other drugs such as imipramine may be used, particularly with nocturia and enuresis. Hormone replacement therapy helps with sensory urgency.

(a)

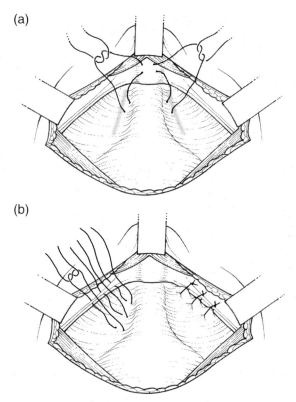

(b)

Figure 24.5 Operations to deal with true stress incontinence; **a** Marshall–Marchetti–Kranz operation – sutures alongside the vesicourethral junction hitch it to the periosteum over the back of the symphysis pubis. **b** Burch's colposuspension – the fascia alongside the lower bladder and upper urethra is sutured to the ileopectineal ligament. **c** Stamey colposuspension – the fornices of the vagina.

• *Surgical techniques* are of very little use, although augmentation cystoplasty in which the bladder capacity is enlarged by the grafting of a portion of an ileum on to the bladder has a very limited place. There is, however, concern that this may lead to possible malignant change.

RECOMMENDED READING

Casement M 1997 Conservative treatment of urinary incontinence. Contemporary Reviews in Obstetrics and Gynaecology 9: 149–155

Cardozo L, Staskin C 2000 Textbook of female urology and urogynaecology. Isis Medical Media, Oxford

Kutar V, Cardozo L 1997 The use of ultrasound in detrusor instability. Contemporary Reviews in Obstetrics and Gynaecology 9: 129–135

Prolapse

Genital prolapse implies protrusion of either the vaginal wall or the uterus from its normal anatomical position. Although most patients believe that it is the uterus which is involved in prolapse, anterior vaginal wall prolapse is far more common. Indeed, after pregnancy a mild degree of anterior wall prolapse is almost the norm.

The following classification is used depending upon the organ involved (Fig. 25.1):

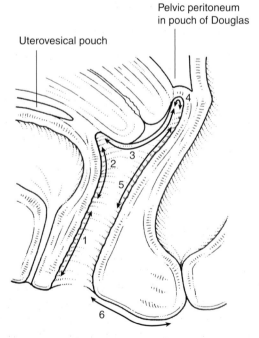

Figure 25.1 Elements of a vaginal prolapse: 1, dislocation of the urethra (urethrocele); 2, cystocele; 3, descent of the uterus and cervix; 4, enterocele (hernia of the pouch of Douglas); 5, rectocele; 6, deficiency of the perineum.

- Urethra and bladder: a urethrocystocele
- The cervix and uterus:
  - First degree – indicating some descent within the vagina but not reaching the vulva
  - Second degree – the cervix descends to the introitus
  - Third degree – the cervix and possibly the uterus descends such that the uterus lies outside the introitus (procidentia)
- Small bowel and omentum: enterocele
- Rectum: rectocele.

AETIOLOGY

Commonly childbirth, obesity and the menopause are major factors. It is probable that prolonged and difficult labour, forceps delivery and large babies are all important. Congenital weakness of the pelvic floor as in spina bifida causes a very small proportion of prolapse.

CLINICAL SYMPTOMS

Cystocele and urethrocele

The most common symptoms are of a dragging feeling in the pelvis or the feeling of a lump in the vagina. The patient will often say that she feels as if she is sitting on a plum or similar object. There may be associated urinary symptoms such as stress incontinence and urgency or frequency, particularly since the patient will wish to keep her bladder empty to avoid the stress incontinence.

Uterine prolapse

The patient is aware of a lump below, associated with low central backache. When the cervix protrudes through the introitus it may become traumatized by rubbing on underwear, leading to bleeding. Hesitancy or an inability to start the stream of urine may be a problem with second- and third-degree prolapse, and necessitate pushing the uterus back up the vagina to start the flow of urine.

Enterocele

This occurs more often after hysterectomy, and involves prolapse of the vault. Symptoms may be of a lump in the vagina or backache.

Rectocele

This leads to backache and a lump in the vagina. Often emptying of the bowel is difficult, and requires reducing the lump in the vagina digitally before bowel action is complete.

Treatment

Medical

Prolapse has been managed by the insertion of a ring pessary for many years (Fig. 25.2). With the introduction of much safer surgery and anaesthesia, particularly regional block, the necessity for long-term pessary use has reduced. The main indications now are:

- During pregnancy
- For the patient who has not completed her family
- For those medically unfit or refusing surgery
- For the relief of symptoms whilst awaiting surgery.

The modern pessary is made of inert plastic and is usually changed every 4 months.

For the very debilitated who have an extremely lax pelvic floor and perineum, it may be necess-

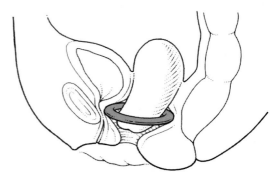

Figure 25.2 A ring pessary in position, tenting out the vaginal walls.

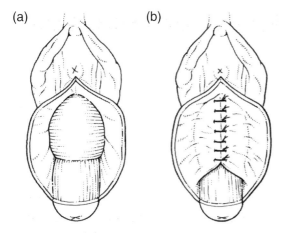

(a)   (b)

Figure 25.3   Essential steps in an anterior colporrhaphy.

ary to insert a shelf pessary, preferably of the solid plastic type.

Surgical

Cystourethrocele. This is treated by anterior colporrhaphy or repair, which involves a vertical anterior vaginal wall incision followed by dissection away of the skin from the underlying urethra and bladder (Fig. 25.3). Supporting stitches are placed on either side of the urethra, and the bladder is plicated. Redundant vaginal skin is removed, and the vagina then resutured.

Uterine prolapse. The best procedure for this condition is vaginal hysterectomy. In the past a Manchester repair was performed, where the cervix was amputated and the supporting ligaments resutured to the uterus. There is little place for this procedure today.

Enterocele or vault repair. This is the most difficult form of prolapse to repair. In the very elderly, obliteration of the upper part of the vagina may be all that is necessary, but in younger women various forms of fixation of the vagina to the sacrospinus ligaments or sling procedures may be necessary.

Rectocele. Gynaecologists approach this problem via the vagina, and the repair is very similar in principle to an anterior colporrhaphy. Levator ani muscles on either side of the rectum are brought together in the midline; the redundant skin is then excised and closed. Colorectal surgeons are taking an increasing interest in rectocele with its problems at defaecation, and they approach a rectocele through the perineal body. Anal sphincter repair can be carried out at the same time if there is an element of faecal incontinence. However, detailed investigations need to be carried out before such a procedure, and this will usually include endo-anal ultrasound studies and a defaecating proctogram. Such procedures are usually performed at a tertiary referral centre.

RECOMMENDED READING

Dorr C 1994 Relaxation of pelvic supports. In: de Chesney A, Pernoll M (eds) Current obstetrical and gynaecological diagnosis and treatment. Prentice Hall, London, pp 809–830

Hogston P 1995 Vaginal vault prolapse. Contemporary Reviews in Obstetrics and Gynaecology 7: 113–117

Mant J, Painter R, Vessey M 1997 Epidemiology of genital prolapse. British Journal of Obstetrics and Gynaecology 104: 579–585

Olsen A, Smith V, Bergstom J et al 1997 Epidemiology and surgically managed pelvic organ prolapse. Obstetrics and Gynecology 89: 501–506

Psychosexual problems

Problems of sexual dysfunction are often difficult to elicit from a patient but may become apparent when discussing other gynaecological symptoms. More often the patient will come to see the general practitioner for a totally different reason, and may only come round to the problem when she feels at ease and able to discuss it. Only a brief account of the diagnosis and management can be given here, and the reader is recommended to study more specialized books.

The incidence of sexual dysfunction varies according to the source of information, but Masters and Johnson, the pioneers of the study of sexual physiology, have estimated that approximately 50% of sexually active US couples had some problems at some time. Lack of orgasm in the female is noted in as many as 10% of women by Kinsey.

Normal sexual response has five elements, namely:

- Interest
- Arousal
- Plateau
- Orgasm
- Resolution.

Abnormalities in any of these five areas lead to dysfunction.

FEMALE SEXUAL DYSFUNCTION

Lack of interest varies according to the menstrual cycle or at other times in a woman's life, particularly during pregnancy. Lack of arousal, sometimes known as frigidity, means that the female has no particular desire for sex but if stimulated can become aroused and even orgasmic. Lack of arousability means that the patient neither desires sex nor can be aroused.

Orgasmic dysfunction can be either primary or secondary:

Primary orgasmic dysfunction implies that the woman has never achieved an orgasm. This is more often found in the obsessional, perfectionist type of woman who finds it hard to let go. Sometimes there may be guilt feelings or a sense of inadequacy.

Secondary orgasmic dysfunction occurs in women who have an initial successful sexual relationship but later fail to achieve orgasms, perhaps because their life takes on a rather boring repetitive fashion and there is little excitement.

Dyspareunia

Pain during intercourse will usually lead to an inhibition of sexual arousal. In turn this will cause lack of lubrication which will intensify the pain, thus creating a vicious circle. Dyspareunia may be superficial or deep.

The causes of superficial dyspareunia are usually due to past trauma, poor episiotomy suturing, or infection with thrush.

Deep dyspareunia is usually the result of pelvic disease, particularly endometriosis and pelvic inflammatory disease. Retroversion of the uterus with entrapment of the ovaries between the fundus of the uterus and the upper part of the vagina can lead to the condition. Pelvic congestion and even irritable bowel syndrome may cause deep dyspareunia.

Vaginismus

When the levator ani muscle goes into spasm, it seriously reduces the size of the introitus. This may be the result of dyspareunia. Vaginismus very seldom has a physical cause but often the patient will say that 'she is too small' or 'he is too big.' Treatment involves banning attempts at intercourse until the condition is cured. The patient is encouraged to examine herself with two fingers, preferably in private, perhaps while having a warm bath. The fingers are inserted into the vagina, and she is then instructed to squeeze them so that she is able to identify the muscle. By pushing down she can feel the muscles relax, and she must continue to practice this so that she can do it at will. When she feels ready to have intercourse she should adopt the superior position so that she is in control of the situation, and gently insert her partner's penis into the well-lubricated vagina. Should it cause pain, then she must not proceed until she feels absolutely comfortable. This process may take some considerable time, and the couple must be patient, but it is usually successful.

MALE SEXUAL DYSFUNCTION

The male problem may be either primary or secondary, or concern premature or retarded ejaculation.

Primary dysfunction

This is an inability to develop or to maintain an erection. It is often due to extreme anxiety about sex, engendered either by major psychological problems or by some unfortunate experience in the past, such as being caught during a sexual act at a most inappropriate moment.

Secondary dysfunction

There are both physiological and psychological reasons for this (Table 26.1).

Table 26.1 Some causes of male secondary sexual dysfunction

Physiological causes	Psychological causes
Endocrine	Anger
Neurological	Resentment
Chronic illness	Anxiety
Drugs	Guilt
Alcohol	Poor self-image
Fatigue	
Stress	
Pelvic pathology	
Prolonged continence	

Most men will have suffered this to some extent, perhaps the best known reason being excess of alcohol. Fatigue and stress at work are important factors, as are some antihypertensive drugs. Failure of satisfactory intercourse may cause disharmony between the couple, partly because the woman may suspect that either she is no longer sexually attractive or that her partner is having an affair with someone else. Problems such as these need to be sorted out at an early stage.

Premature ejaculation

Premature ejaculation may be the result of over-enthusiasm, but is often the result of anxiety, and careful counselling is required.

Retarded ejaculation

This is a condition in which the man is unable to ejaculate into the vagina during intercourse but is able to masturbate satisfactorily. This may be due to the result of drugs such as anti-depressants or β blockers, but it more often has a deep psychological cause.

HISTORY TAKING OF EITHER PARTNER

This must be approached with care, and if the doctor does not feel confident or competent then he should allow others to do it. Before attempting any form of counselling the following points should be borne in mind:

- The doctor should be relaxed and non-judgmental
- He should be able to discuss problems in a language with which the patient is comfortable and which can easily be understood
- The doctor should have knowledge of a range of sexual practices
- The doctor must be comfortable with his own sexuality.

An appointment time of at least 30 min must be given for the initial consultation. Enquiries must be made about family history and of the patient's relationship with his or her parents. A sexual history will include the date of first masturbation or menstruation, and the attitudes of the parents and the partner to sex. In the female, perhaps the most difficult area to approach is sexual assault as a child or teenager. Such abuse is now estimated to have occurred in 10% of adult women, and many, if not the vast majority, have never reported this. A contraceptive history is important, because a fear of pregnancy may be a major element in the sexual dysfunction, and assessment of the partnership is of great importance but may be difficult initially.

EXAMINATION

Physical examination of patients should be undertaken with their full permission. It may be necessary to point out the normality of their anatomy and, in the case of a female, a mirror may usefully be employed. Physical examination will also confirm that there is no physical cause for the underlying problem.

THERAPY

This is a complex area which requires considerable training. The basis of therapy is:

- *Sexual education of both partners.*
- *Discussion of sexual practice.* This is based on the premise that many patients feel that their sexual practices are wrong and that they feel guilty about it. The doctor must explain, if he believes it to be the case, that the sexual practice is normal and that no guilt should be attached to it.
- *A reduction of anxiety.* This may be difficult, depending upon the underlying cause of the anxiety. For instance, the sharing of a house with parents may only be remedied by the couple moving away.
- *Increase in communication.* This is of considerable importance, and refers essentially to communication between the two partners.

A number of therapies are based on these four points, the most important being behavioural techniques. Of these, sensate focusing is of great use, and is a gradual relearning of sexual behaviour. It is a recapitulation of the courting process. Couples are given assignments to carry out in privacy, and having achieved one target they will move on to a further one.

SEXUAL PROBLEMS OF DISABLED PEOPLE

The physical feelings and emotions of disabled individuals are precisely the same as the rest of the population. However, their ability to perform sexual acts may be severely limited, and it is only in recent years that these problems have been given the recognition they deserve. Only a number of specific conditions will be discussed here.

Spinal cord injuries

In the man this may lead to difficulties with erection, emission or loss of sensation. Where problems of fertility arise, samples of seminal fluid may be obtained by electrical stimulation of the male. In women they may be able to participate in a passive manner or else obtain pleasure from orogenital sex or caressing of the breasts. Counselling is aimed at bowel and bladder control, the use of catheters, care of the skin, positioning of the couple during intercourse and, of course, contraception.

Cerebral palsy

Individuals with cerebral palsy tend to be protected and brought up as if sexless, especially if female. Because of spastic movements, adductor spasm or facial grimacing, these patients may have problems in finding a sexual partner. Patients with cerebral palsy need to be treated with compassion. Society has not yet addressed the problem of providing sexual gratification for these people.

Diabetes with associated neuropathy

Affected males may have retrograde ejaculation

although no diminution in sexual pleasure. This may lead to fertility problems. Unless there is neuropathic dysfunction these patients usually perform normally.

Surgery

Gynaecological operations may be considered as mutilating. Hysterectomy itself means to some the loss of womanhood, and these areas should be explored prior to surgery. Repair operations on the vagina may lead to considerable narrowing, and sexual function must be considered prior to surgery. Some tightening of the vagina may be expected following surgery, but regular intercourse will help the vagina to stretch to accommodate the penis.

Colostomy and ileostomy

Major bowel surgery, particularly rectal surgery, may lead to lack of orgasmic response. The patient may be embarrassed about the odour from a colostomy bag and worry of spilling of contents or fear of hurting the stoma. Modern appliances and sympathetic professionals will ensure cleanliness with regular emptying of appliances and, more particularly, the creation of confidence in the patient.

Mastectomy

Radical mastectomy is less often performed nowadays, for it is perceived to be mutilative and other treatments give as good results. Most surgeons aim at lumpectomy and, if necessary, the insertion of a prosthesis at the time. Where there is a total removal of the breast, the patient must be carefully counselled along with her partner. He must offer continued support and a caring attitude, and an early return to sexual intercourse is recommended.

Cardiovascular problems

Individuals who have had a myocardial infarction, or who have angina, may be particularly worried about a recurrence of an attack during intercourse. Similar concerns can affect the partner, and both should be counselled carefully that intercourse is unlikely to cause any harm.

Blindness

There are particular problems here as there is an obvious taboo on learning through touching. Blind people are thus at a disadvantage as their ability to make comparisons between their own body and others is lessened, and they can have a poor self-image. There may be a fear of being watched or appearing in the nude.

Mental retardation

The sexuality of this group of people is not reduced but the fear lies amongst the general population that they will be unable to cope with contraception. This fear is totally unfounded, and compulsory sterilization is unwarranted. Efficient reversible contraception is needed, and the use of hormone-releasing intrauterine systems, which not only provide excellent contraception but reduce menstruation, are of particular use. Depo-progestogen preparations are also important.

RECOMMENDED READING

James K, Penketh R 1996 Psychosexual aspects of hysterectomy. Contemporary Reviews in Obstetrics and Gynaecology 8: 39–43

Kolodny A, Masters W, Johnson V 1979 Textbook of sexual medicine. Little, Brown, Boston

Paediatric gynaecology

DEVELOPMENTAL ANOMALIES

To understand the congenital abnormalities that occur in the female genital tract, the reader will have to recall some basic embryology. In the fifth week of embryonic life the nephrogenic cord develops, from which the mesonephron is formed, and the paramesonephric duct develops an ingrowth of the coelom (Fig. 27.1) antero-lateral to this duct. The paramesonephric duct later forms the müllerian system. In the female, the two mesonephric ducts move cordally until they reach the urogenital sinus. The lower part

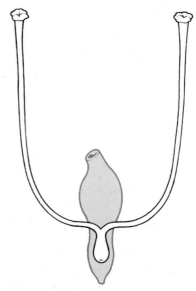

Figure 27.1 The paramesonephric ducts (or müllerian system) in a 7 week embryo. The lower ends have fused to form the upper one-third of the vagina, the cervix and the body of the uterus, in front of the hind-gut.

of this müllerian system fuses to form the upper two-thirds of the vagina, the cervix and the uterus, whilst the upper part of the müllerian system remains separate, forming the fallopian tubes. The division between the urogenital sinus and the müllerian system usually breaks down, but if it fails to do so it forms a transverse membrane across the vagina above the hymen, and this obstructs menstruation.

The vulva and vagina

Clitoral hypertrophy may result following the ingestion of androgens by the mother during pregnancy. This is now a rare cause as the androgenic progestogens used for the treatment of threatened abortion are no longer used. Congenital adrenal hyperplasia can cause masculinization and clitoral hypertrophy.

Labial fusion is a common problem in young girls, usually as a result of mild infection in the vulval area, possibly due to faecal contamination. The treatment consists of gentle digital division of the adhesion and the application of sparing amounts of a local oestrogen cream (preferably oestriol). The condition may recur. Congenital labial fusion is a rare complication, as is labial hypertrophy.

A number of congenital abnormalities of the vagina can occur as the result of failure in development of the müllerian system. These may include duplication of the vagina, agenesis, transverse vaginal septa and wolffian duct remnants. The so-called imperforate hymen is a misnomer, for the obstruction is an occluding membrane of the vagina, just above the hymen. It marks the junction between the müllerian system and the urogenital sinus (Fig. 27.2).

The classical presentation of this condition is of a young girl, about 15 years old, with normal secondary sexual development but admitted to hospital with a lower abdominal mass and acute urinary retention. There is always a history of primary amenorrhoea and, occasionally, cyclical lower abdominal discomfort. When examined, a mass in the lower abdomen is dull to percussion, smooth and cystic. It is the bladder. Examination of the introitus will reveal a

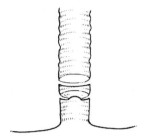

Figure 27.2   An occluding membrane not absorbed in fetal life can lead to haematocolpos later.

bulging membrane. A simple cruciate incision into this under anaesthesia will relieve the large collection of altered blood in the vagina (haematocolpos). The condition is often associated with endometriosis, perhaps because of retrograde menstruation, and laparoscopy may be necessary at a later date.

The uterus

Failure of fusion of the lower part of the müllerian system can lead to the anomalies seen in Figure 27.3. At the most extreme there is a double vagina and a double uterus, at the mildest a subarcuate uterus where the upper part of the uterus indents the cavity.

Renal system abnormalities are commonly found in association with uterine anomalies, and therefore intravenous urography or a renal ultrasound examination is an essential part of the investigations of those found with congenital anomalies of the reproductive tract.

If there is no obstruction in the vagina, or absence of the cervix at puberty, normal menstruation will occur. In pregnancy, an increased incidence of miscarriage, unstable lie, premature labour and fetal growth retardation are associated with irregular shapes of the uterine cavity.

Ambiguous genitalia

Androgen insensitivity (formerly known as testicular feminization) is a condition where the girl has the male karyotype 46XY but a female phenotype. The external genitalia are normally formed, but there is a short blind vagina and no

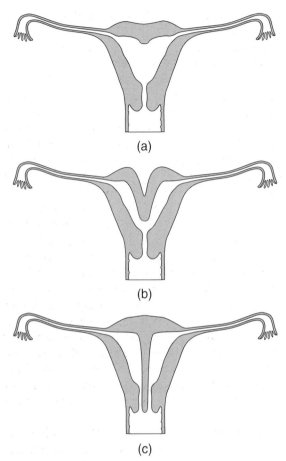

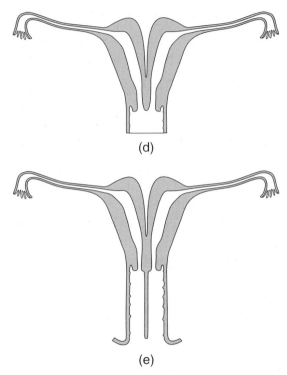

Figure 27.3 Uterine abnormalities following indifferent fusion of the paramesonephric ducts. **a** Arcuate uterus. **b** Bicornuate uterus. **c** Septate uterus. **d** Double uterus and cervix but no vaginal septum. **e** Double uterus and double vagina.

uterus. The testicles are undescended, and are either intra-abdominal or lying in the inguinal canal. Because the end organs in the skin are insensitive to androgens, these patients fail to grow any secondary sexual hair. There is normal breast development. Children are therefore brought up as females although they are unable to reproduce.

Other less common syndromes of ambiguous genitalia are listed in Table 27.1

The investigations for these abnormalities include:

- Karyotype
- Electrolytes
- Ultrasound check for uterus
- Steroid measurements, e.g. 17-hydroxyprogesterone
- Response to human chorionic gonadotrophin.

Table 27.1 Ambiguous genitalia at birth

Abnormality	Cause
Masculinized female	Congenital adrenal hyperplasia, particularly 21-hydroxylase deficiency Iatrogenic (danazol, etc.) Androgen-secreting tumour
Undermasculinized male	Partial androgen insensitivity Gonadal dysgenesis 5x-reductase deficiency Testicular failure
Hermaphrodite	Ovotestis

VAGINAL DISCHARGE

The most common cause of this is an infestation of threadworm from the alimentary tract via the anus. Diagnosis can be made by the Sellotape test in which a piece of clear adhesive tape is placed across the anus and then removed and examined under a microscope for ova. Suitable therapy with piperazine will remove the infestation, both from the anus and the vagina.

Occasionally children insert foreign objects into the vagina, and this can give rise to persistent discharge. Examination under anaesthesia may then be necessary, when a fine hysteroscope or laparoscope can be passed into the vagina without disrupting the hymen and the foreign object removed. An auroscope is sometimes helpful in locating the foreign body, and ear, nose and throat forceps can be used to remove it.

Other problems affecting children include herpes infection, condylomata acuminata (warts) or trauma. The last may be as a result of accident or sexual assault. In cases where there is trauma to the hymen or fourchette, the latter must be suspected.

SEXUAL INTERFERENCE

The general practitioner may, very occasionally, be asked to examine a prepubertal child where a sexual assault is suspected or where he believes that some form of abuse may have occurred. Some of the more relevant points are considered, but it must be stressed that the interpretation of physical findings is a matter for a doctor with experience in the field.

A substantial proportion of sexually abused children show no abnormal physical findings, and the single most important feature in the diagnosis of abuse is a clear statement by the child.

The recommended position for examining female genitalia in children is in the supine frog-legged position, so that the ankles are together and the knees flexed. Very gentle labial separation and gentle labial traction is used to display the hymeneal orifice. The anus can be examined in the left lateral position, with the hips and knees well flexed.

Where penetrative abuse is suspected, measurement of the hymeneal orifice has previously been considered to be of importance. However, even in cases where the perpetrator has admitted penetration, the genitalia may appear normal. At puberty the transverse hymeneal diameter is about 1 cm, and diameters greater than 1.5 cm, particularly in association with other evidence of trauma, is highly suggestive of abuse, but it cannot be used as the sole basis for diagnosis. Lacerations of the hymen, particularly posteriorly, are associated with penile penetration. Anterior changes have been associated with digital penetration, but this has since been shown to be normal in many children. Where there is definite evidence of perineal scarring, penile penetration should be suspected. Other signs seen within 72 h of abuse include bruising, abrasions and tears in the hymen, which may extend to the posterior vaginal wall. In chronic abuse there are scars or old transections of the hymen and attenuation or rubbing away of the hymen. The opening is usually greater than 1.5 cm.

Other signs which occur in abused children, but can also be seen in non-abused children and are therefore non-specific, include inflammation, superficial friability of the posterior fourchette, fusion of the labia minora, vaginal discharge, anal fissure and perianal venous distension. Poor hygiene and scratching are contributory factors.

Some children subjected to anal abuse will show dilatation of the anal canal. However, reflex anal dilatation is not a strong sign, and cannot, by itself, be regarded as a sign of abuse. It may, however, help to support a child's story of abuse.

In summary, physical findings including normality are consistent with abuse, and it is therefore important to document carefully even minor anogenital signs as well as negative findings.

RECOMMENDED READING

Royal College of Physicians 1997 Physical signs of sexual abuse in children, 2nd edn. RCP, London

Sanfilippe J 1999 Pediatric and adolescent gynaecology. Lippincott, Philadelphia

Dysmenorrhoea

Dysmenorrhoea, or painful menstruation, is differentiated into primary and secondary conditions. Primary dysmenorrhoea is painful menstrual cramps occurring in the absence of pelvic pathology; it is often referred to as spasmodic dysmenorrhoea. It is a uterine problem. Secondary dysmenorrhoea is pain arising from structures around the uterus, and is referred to as congestive dysmenorrhoea. The most common pathologies associated with the condition are endometriosis and pelvic inflammatory disease.

The patient typically complains of lower abdominal pain, backache and pain radiating down the front of the thighs. It is usually bilateral, but can occur on one side. Unilateral pain is more often due to caecal or colonic spasm, although one-sided endometriosis or spasm in one horn of a deformed uterus may be a cause.

At least 75% of women have painful periods at some time in their reproductive life. This is probably an underestimate, as many never present to a doctor and will treat themselves with over-the-counter medication.

PRIMARY DYSMENORRHOEA

Primary dysmenorrhoea is mostly a complaint of women in their teens and early twenties, the pain coinciding with the onset of ovulatory cycles. Up to 15% of females are incapacitated every month, leading to a significant amount of time off school and work. Dysmenorrhoea may result from a girl having a lack of information,

Table 28.1 Some causes of primary dysmenorrhoea

Primary	Secondary
Ischaemia of the myometrium	Endometriosis
Increased prostaglandin	Adenomyosis
secretion	Chronic pelvic inflammation
Increased leukotrienes	Other adhesions tethering
Increased vasopression	ovaries
Increased endothelins	Ovary trapped by retroversion
Increased tumour	
necrosis factor	
Increased interleukins	
Passage of clots because of	
adolescent menorrhagia	

and is more commonly seen in daughters whose mothers suffered in their youth. It is true that there is usually an improvement with time and after childbirth, although nothing could be more disheartening for a young sufferer than to be told that she will grow out of it or that 'It will get better after you've had a baby.'

The pain, which is cramping in nature, starts on the first day of menstruation, and is often accompanied by faintness, headaches and alimentary symptoms. It usually passes off on the second day of the period (Table 28.1).

Cause

Hypotheses that the cervix is too narrow, or that the uterus is underdeveloped, are false; no evidence has ever been produced to substantiate these views. A hormonal cause is probable. Spasmodic dysmenorrhoea is very uncommon in anovulatory cycles, hence the absence of the problem in the first few cycles after the menarche.

There is strong evidence that the pain is associated with increased uterine activity, resulting in increased uterine tone and excessive spasmodic contractions. This combination is capable of inhibiting uterine blood flow, causing ischaemia. Simultaneous recordings of intrauterine pressure and uterine blood flow have shown that the pain is at its maximum when the flow is at its minimum.

Paradoxically, high pressure in the uterus has been seen without excessive pain, and pain can be produced by autologous transfusion of plasma from a dysmenorrhoeic woman. This suggests that there are other mechanisms of pain production independent of uterine spasm.

There is now strong evidence to suggest that prostaglandins are associated with the condition. They have been isolated in high concentrations in menstrual washings of dysmenorrhoeic women. Furthermore, *in vitro* synthesis of PGF_2 from arachidonic acid is significantly greater in the endometrium of sufferers.

Other substances have also been implicated, including leukotrienes, vasopressin, endothelins, tumour necrosis factor and interleukins. The part they play is not yet clearly known, although vasopressin has been shown to produce a decrease in uterine blood flow and cause dysmenorrhoea-like pain.

At present, vasopressin antagonists are not suitable for the clinical treatment of the condition because of their short half-life and their route of administration.

In the older woman with heavy periods, the passage of large clots is sometimes associated with pain. The pain can be particularly severe in the presence of intrauterine fibroid polyps, and can be seen associated with intrauterine contraceptive device users, particularly in the nulliparous.

Management and treatment

Management should commence with a detailed explanation of the physiology of the condition and its implications. There is some evidence that patients suffering with primary dysmenorrhoea later develop endometriosis. This may be due to increased retrograde menstruation.

The expectation of pain may be fostered by an overanxious mother and by the curtailment of activities during menstruation. General advice, reassurance and relief of pain with simple analgesics may be all that is needed.

An oral contraceptive will provide relief in up to half for those who will accept it; and this depends upon the age of the girl and parental attitude. Anovulatory cycles are associated with a decrease in $PGF_{2\alpha}$ synthesis by the endometrium, and this is the presumed mechanism by which the contraceptive pill works.

Non-steroidal anti-inflammatory drugs

A further 30–40% of sufferers will be helped by non-steroidal anti-inflammatory drugs (NSAIDs) given at the time of bleeding. These have become one of the main therapeutic agents for the treatment of primary dysmenorrhoea, and have been shown to be highly efficacious in double-blind controlled trials.

Most agents have a strong placebo effect in the first two or three cycles but the effect usually wears off. This is not the case with NSAIDs: they are easy to take and are relatively free of side-effects. Started at the onset of the pain (or when it is possible to judge, 1–2 days before the onset of menses) they provide an easy and effective regimen when used with oral contraception.

Compliance may be a problem in young patients, and long-acting agents such as ketoprofen or diclofenac may be particularly useful. However, ibuprofen and mefenamic acid remain the most popular although, as with all NSAIDs, alimentary irritation may be a problem. Care should be exercised when prescribing to asthmatics because of the danger of inducing bronchospasm.

Antispasmodics such as alverine citrate and anticholinergics such as hyoscine butylbromide have a limited place, and may be tried in conjunction with oral contraception or where other treatments have failed.

Progestogens have been used for many menstrual disorders including dysmenorrhoea although their effect is variable; they may induce premenstrual-type symptoms and generally have little to commend them unless there are strong contraindications to oral contraception. The latter may be tricycled, i.e. three courses of a monophasic preparation given continuously, although breakthrough bleeding is occasionally a problem. Anti-emetics may be needed for those who have severe associated symptoms of nausea and vomiting.

A theoretical link between primary dysmenorrhoea and migraine (arterial spasm, nausea and headaches) has led workers to use substances such as clonidine, although this has no greater effect than placebo. Selective β_2 agonists such as terbutaline and calcium antagonists may be useful as part of the therapy.

The levonorgestrel-containing intrauterine system is associated with reduction in blood flow and pain. However, among nulliparous patients it should only be considered in those needing contraception who are in a long-term monogamous relationship. Careful counselling is required. Local anaesthesia, such as a para-cervical block, may be necessary for fitting.

In the most extreme cases of primary dysmenorrhoea, amenorrhoea can be induced with gonadotrophin-releasing hormone agonists. However, no more that 6 months of treatment should be given because of potential bone loss, unless a continuous combined form of hormone replacement therapy is added. Such therapy is very effective but also very expensive.

Alternative remedies

Alternative measures such as hypnotherapy, aromatherapy, acupuncture and behavioural modification therapies may have a part to play. However, a sympathetic and understanding doctor is often the best adjunct to simple analgesic therapy with NSAIDs.

SECONDARY DYSMENORRHOEA

This is pain associated with pelvic pathology around the uterus. The pain is typically dull, commences before the onset of bleeding and may persist through the period and sometimes remain after the period has finished. It is often associated with heavy periods and deep dyspareunia. Commonly there is low central backache, and the pain may also radiate down the inner aspect of the thighs to the knees.

Causes

Chronic pelvic inflammatory disease and endometriosis are the two most common causes of the condition. Clinical examination of the pelvis will often reveal marked adnexal tenderness, the classic nodules of endometriosis in the pouch of Douglas, or a fixed uterus. A tender bulky uterus is typical of adenomyosis (endometriosis involving the myometrium). Other causes of menorrhagia may also lead to secondary dysmenorrhoea.

Treatment

Sufferers of secondary dysmenorrhoea are usually older women. Because of the aetiology of the condition many will be childless, and conservation of the reproductive organs is of paramount importance to them. Treatment of the condition is dependent upon the cause, and laparoscopy is often an essential part of the diagnostic procedure. Apart from simple analgesics and NSAIDs, the treatment is dependent upon the cause.

29

Fertility

At least 90% of couples under the age of 35 years will achieve a pregnancy within 1 year if they are having regular, frequent and contraception-free intercourse. The actual chance of becoming pregnant in any one cycle is about 15%, but it is cumulative over 6 months, after which it remains relatively static until 12 months. It is therefore reasonable not to investigate a couple until 1 year of time has passed. This is a generalization, and the needs of each couple must be taken into account. For instance, a newly married couple, both of whom are over the age of 35 years, may feel there is a greater sense of urgency than a couple who are in their early twenties.

Investigations should be simple, useful and non-invasive wherever possible. To perform a whole series of complicated and expensive hormonal assays is usually unhelpful. The essence of investigations is to show that each of the couple is producing gametes (sperm or eggs) and that they are able to deliver them to the right anatomical place. For a man it is relatively simple because he can produce a specimen by masturbation and present it for analysis. Unfortunately, it is obviously impossible for a woman to produce an egg on demand and deliver it to her uterus. Therefore, for the female, tests are aimed at firstly establishing that she can produce an egg and secondly that her anatomy is functioning normally.

Treatment for infertility has advanced enormously since the introduction of assisted reproductive techniques, and whilst a few years ago most treatments were empirical, now a proper scientific approach can be made and help given in most cases.

HISTORY AND EXAMINATION

Although it has been traditional for the gynaecologist to investigate and treat infertility, it is important to remember that it is a couple who are being investigated and, wherever possible, both should attend at least the first appointment.

The male

Points of particular importance in the past history of a male are previous surgery, trauma to the testicles and infections of the testes. A widespread myth has built up concerning the effect of mumps in postpubertal men. However, the infection affects the testes in less than 50% of cases and, even when there is bilateral orchitis, a major effect on the sperm is unusual. Of much more importance is a history of smoking, drinking or drug intake. Smoking more than 20 cigarettes a day can severely affect sperm motility. Although moderate amounts of alcohol seem to have little effect, excessive drinking may cause liver damage, which in turn can severely reduce the sperm count. Most drugs have little effect on sperm concentration except salazopyrin, which can severely reduce the count. However, this is reversible on stopping the drug. Anabolic steroids may have a profound effect on both sperm concentration and testicular volume, and long-term use may permanently damage sperm production. Certain antihypertensive drugs can lead to erectile problems. The penis and scrotal contents should be assessed, but examination is usually normal. Excessive enlargement or diminution of testicular size may be quantified with an external aid.

The female

A detailed menstrual history is required which may give some indication if ovulation is taking place. Midcycle pain suggestive of ovulation may be helpful. A history of pelvic infection should be sought and, of course, a history of previous pregnancies and any complications. A detailed abdominal and pelvic examination should be carried out, with particular emphasis on the pelvic findings of adnexal masses or fixed retroversion of the uterus, suggestive of pelvic inflammatory disease or endometriosis.

INVESTIGATIONS

The male

Semen analysis

A sample should be collected by masturbation into a clean plastic pot. It is essential that samples are not collected in a condom as these contain spermicides. Prior to production of the specimen there should be a period of abstinence of between 1 and 3 days. The specimen should be delivered to the laboratory within an hour, and it should be examined microscopically ideally within 2 h of production. A normal semen analysis is shown in Table 29.1. With higher concentrations, lower motility and morphology scores are acceptable.

In the past much emphasis has been placed on the concentration of sperm present, but it now appears that motility and particularly progression are more important. Concentrations below 20 million/ml are still associated with relative fertility, albeit with a reduced chance.

Oligozoospermia

Where sperm concentrations are below 5 million/ml the chances of conception by

Table 29.1 Semen analysis – normal values

Test	Value
Volume	2–5 ml
Liquefaction	<30 min
Concentration	>20 million/ml
Motility	>50% at 4 h
Progression[a]	3–4
Morphology	>60% normal forms
Sperm clumping	None

[a]Progression is a subjective score of forward movement of the sperm. A score of 4 represents rapid forward movement, and a score of 1 a shaking movement with no progression

normal intercourse become much reduced. Causes are seldom found; low concentrations are usually associated with poor motility and progression scores and a high percentage of abnormal forms. This suggests a basic defect in sperm production rather than a drug effect or some other external cause.

Azoospermia

If two semen analyses show a total absence of sperm, a follicle-stimulating hormone (FSH) estimation should be carried out. If raised it confirms testicular failure, and there is no remedy. If the FSH level is normal, there is a suggestion that there may be some obstructive lesion, and further investigation by an andrologist is warranted.

The female

A woman with a regular menstrual cycle (anything between 28 and 42 days) is probably ovulating. This can be confirmed by measuring the levels of serum progesterone, a sample being taken at the *midluteal* phase, 7 days prior to menstruation. Many women have a 28 day cycle, so their midluteal phase is on day 21. Hence, it has become common practice to measure progesterone on day 21, but this becomes a meaningless reading in women who have longer cycles. As the luteal phase is a fairly constant 14 days, it is very important to gain a reasonable idea of the length of the patient's cycle and work back 7 days to arrive at the correct day to take the blood. In cases where the cycle is irregular, it may be necessary to start on day 21 and take blood every third day. Levels of over 30 nmol/l indicate ovulation.

If ovulation is confirmed, there is no sense in performing other endocrinological investigations. However, if the progesterone assay is below this level, then blood should be taken to measure thyroxine, FSH, luteinizing hormone (LH) and prolactin levels. Ideally these should be done in the *midfollicular* phase. High prolactin levels (> 1000 i.u.) indicate adenomata of the pituitary gland. CAT scans or magnetic resonance imaging can show tumours over 1 cm in diameter. If they are not seen, microadenomata are diagnosed.

Traditionally, basal body temperature recording has been used to confirm ovulation, taking the temperature either orally or rectally upon wakening. It is then recorded on a chart, and a preovulatory dip in temperature followed by a rise of approximately 0.5°C will confirm ovulation. This rise is maintained throughout the luteal phase. Unfortunately, temperature charts are notoriously unreliable, and they may concentrate the patient's mind on her problem, causing unnecessary stress. As a result they have been abandoned by most people for they serve little purpose.

Hormone assays

Abnormalities of thyroxine levels need to be treated accordingly with pharmacological agents or surgery as appropriate. The FSH and LH levels are of considerable importance if ovulation has been shown to be defective. A rise in the FSH level is indicative of ovarian failure, and is mostly seen in women over the age of 40 years with oligo- or amenorrhoea. A rise in the level of LH suggests either that the blood has been taken too close to the midcycle surge of LH or, if taken at the correct time, there may be polycystic ovarian disease. Biochemical evidence of this is associated with an LH level three times that of the FSH concentration, or levels of LH over 12 IU/l. In these circumstances, transvaginal ultrasound scanning of the ovaries should be undertaken to confirm the diagnosis.

Moderate rises in prolactin levels are of little concern. Elevated levels can be found after breast and pelvic examination, and the test should be repeated. If there are persistent levels of over 1000 IU/l, then further investigation is warranted. This should include a computerized tomography scan of the pituitary fossa and an estimation of the visual fields to exclude a micro- or macroadenoma of the anterior pituitary. The condition of hyperprolactinaemia is usually associated with inappropriate galactorrhoea and oligo- or amenorrhoea.

The postcoital test

This test of sperm/mucus compatibility is carried out at any time in the 4 days prior to ovulation. The mucus should have the consistency of raw egg white, being slippery, stretchy and plentiful. It is the ideal medium for sperm. The stretchability of the mucus is known as *spinnbarkeit*, and usually a string of about 10 cm can be obtained at the optimum time of the cycle.

The couple are asked to have unguarded intercourse 8–12 h before the visit. The test itself involves aspirating a small quantity of cervical mucus into a fine plastic tube. The mucus is then placed on a slide and examined microscopically. A positive test implies that there are more than five sperms per high power field which are motile progressively. The presence of non-motile sperm in the mucus when the partner has a normal sperm count may suggest the presence of sperm antibodies.

Tubal patency tests

Laparoscopy. At endoscopic examination of the pelvic organs, the uterus, tubes and ovaries can be inspected thoroughly. Blue dye is introduced through the cervix, and its passage along the tubes can be observed and spillage noted. As well as assessing tubal patency, the presence of a follicle or corpus luteum on the ovary is useful information. At the same time the pelvis can be examined for evidence of past pelvic inflammatory disease or endometriosis. Abnormalities of the uterus such as the presence of fibroids can usually be seen, but distortion of the cavity cannot be detected unless hysteroscopy is performed at the same time. The procedure has the disadvantage that it is an invasive technique requiring general anaesthesia.

Hysterosalpingography. This investigation can be carried out using radiography or ultrasound. In the former a radiopaque dye is injected into the uterus by means of a cervical cannula, and fluoroscopic screening is performed. This shows the uterine cavity and the fallopian tubes, and spillage of dye may be seen (Fig. 29.1). Unfortunately, the procedure can be painful and may

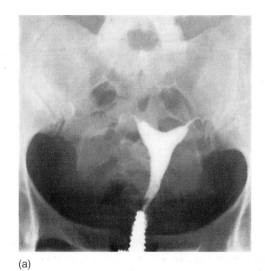

(a)

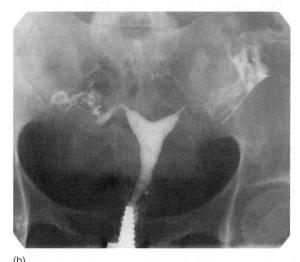

(b)

Figure 29.1 Radiographic hysterosalpingogram. **a** The uterine cavity and intramural parts of the tubes have filled. **b** The dye passes easily along each tube and spills readily on the left. Once the pressure is lowered by spill on the side it does not always do so on the other.

lead to false-negative results, usually through tubal spasm. It gives little idea of pelvic disease unless there is tubal occlusion, and the ovaries cannot be seen. Selective salpingography measuring tubal pressures is of use.

Tubal visualization by ultrasound is a new technique when a fluid medium that reflects ultrasound is injected into the uterine cavity and hence the tubes. The cannula used is extremely fine, and the procedure is considerably less painful than conventional radiographic procedures. The technique is simple to perform; it shows tubal filling and spill while at the same time the ovaries can be inspected for evidence of activity. Otherwise it has similar disadvantages to the radiographic technique. Imaging techniques have the advantage of delineating the uterine cavity.

TREATMENT

The male

The testicles lie outside the body cavity as they perform most efficiently at a temperature below that of the core temperature. Working in very hot environments and the wearing of very tight clothing, which may return the testicles to an intra-abdominal position, or sitting on the testicles for prolonged periods of time such as in long-distance lorry driving, have all been associated with low counts. In addition, varicosities of the testicular veins have been implicated. From this a number of treatments have evolved which aim to reduce the temperature of the testicles. The wearing of loose underwear, taking cold baths or showers, or the ligation of varicosities have all been tried. None have been shown to be very effective. Many drugs have been used, including mesterolone and other androgen-like substances, vitamin E and zinc supplements. The multiplicity of remedies strongly suggests that there is no truly effective therapy.

Isolation of highly motile sperms is now possible using a wash and swim-up technique. This involves mixing semen with a culture medium, centrifuging the sample for 5 min, removing the supernatant and replacing it with further culture medium. The sample is then incubated at body temperature for an hour, and the highly motile sperm will swim up from the plug at the bottom of the tube into the culture medium. This is then drawn off, and the sperm can be utilized by a number of techniques which will be detailed later.

The major advance in the treatment of male infertility has been intracytoplasmic sperm injection (ICSI). This now affords the possibility of a man fathering his genetic child even with extremely low sperm concentrations, and will be dealt with in the section on *assisted conception* later in this chapter.

The female

Hormonal problems

In cases where the progesterone level in the midluteal phase is below the optimal level and other hormonal assays (e.g. FSH, LH and T_4) are normal, treatment is usually instituted using clomiphene citrate. The initial dose is 50 mg, and is given from days 2 to 6 of the menstrual cycle inclusive. The effect of this is to increase FSH levels and thereby promote follicular development. The cycle should return to approximately 28–30 days, and a midluteal serum progesterone level should be measured to ensure that the dose given is sufficient. If progesterone levels indicate non-ovulation then the clomiphene dosage can be increased incrementally in steps of 50 mg to a maximum of 200 mg for 5 days. If pregnancy has not occurred following six ovulatory cycles, then this form of treatment should be abandoned. Tamoxifen, initially at a dose of 10 mg twice a day from days 2 to 6 inclusive, can be used instead of clomiphene but has no distinct advantages over it. The dose may be doubled if necessary.

In cases where ovulation does not occur with either of these drugs, the patient will need to be referred to a more specialized unit where treatment with human menopausal gonadotrophins can be used. This requires careful monitoring with at least a facility for ovarian follicular tracking by ultrasound scanning.

Hyperprolactinaemia

Hyperprolactinaemia, when significant, is usually treated using bromocriptine. The drug can lead to marked nausea or vomiting unless it is started at a low dose (e.g. 1.25 mg/day) and then gradually increased as tolerance develops. A maximum dose of 2.5 mg three times a day is usual. The drug is given on a daily basis as long-term medication, and can be continued through-out pregnancy. Careful surveillance of the patient with repeated measurement of prolactin levels and regular checks of her visual fields are necessary.

Polycystic ovarian disease

In mild cases, where there is elevation of LH levels and ultrasound evidence of the disease, the patient may respond to clomiphene or tamoxifen as detailed previously. In more severe cases, especially associated with gross weight gain, it is advisable for the patient to make every effort to lose weight so that her body mass index does not exceed 26 (weight in kilograms divided by the square of the height in metres). These patients may fail to respond to high doses of clomiphene and will then require pituitary downregulation with a gonadotrophin-releasing hormone analogue followed by purified FSH injections. Alternatively, ovarian drilling at laparoscopy may lead to a return of ovarian function.

Cervical factors

Many cases of cervical mucus hostility are due to anovulatory cycles, and a resumption of ovulation leads to good mucus. However, where there is a persistence of hostile mucus, intra-uterine insemination of prepared sperm (see later) is of benefit.

Tubal factors

Tubal occlusion needs careful assessment by laparoscopy and salpingography. Tubal surgery can be offered where there is a reasonable chance of success, i.e. flimsy peritubal adhesions or simple fimbrial occlusion without hydrosalpinx. Salpingostomy is a relatively easy operation, but there should be a reasonable length of residual tube and relatively free fimbria. Although tubal patency may be demonstrated, there is an increased incidence of ectopic pregnancy. In all cases of tubal occlusion, careful consideration should be given to in vitro fertilization (IVF),

which may offer the patient a much greater chance of a successful pregnancy.

ASSISTED CONCEPTION

There are many assisted reproductive techniques available, all of which involve sperm preparation (wash and swim up or similar techniques) and superovulation with gonadotrophins, monitored by ultrasound scanning. These techniques are known by a variety of acronyms and initials, but only the three most commonly used will be considered here.

In vitro fertilization (IVF)

This was pioneered by Steptoe and Edwards. The technique involves initial stimulation of the ovaries with intramuscular gonadotrophins, aiming at a large number of follicles. When a reasonable amount of these exceed 16 mm in diameter, a dose of human chorionic gonado-trophin (LH) is given. Approximately 34 h after this, the oocytes are retrieved using a trans-vaginal approach. An ultrasound transducer is placed into the vagina, alongside of which lies a guarded needle. This is passed through the posterior fornix of the vagina into the pouch of Douglas and then, by ultrasound guidance, into the follicles. The aspirated oocytes are placed in culture medium, and a measured amount of sperm introduced (approximately 500 000 per egg). The eggs and sperm are incubated at body temperature for a varying amount of time. Fertilization can usually be confirmed within 24 h, but sometimes requires 48 h. Three zygotes (pre-embryos) are selected and are returned via a cannula to the uterine cavity. It is usual for the remaining zygotes to be frozen for future use. The luteal phase of the cycle is often supported by the use of progesterone, which may be given vaginally or intramuscularly.

Success rates for fertilization after IVF may be 90% or more. Pregnancy is only diagnosed when a fetal heart can be identified by ultrasound scanning; success rates of 30% at this stage are reported from many larger units, but the overall live birth rate is no more than 15% taken over

Table 29.2   Advantages and disadvantages of IVF

Advantages	Disadvantages
It is the only form of assisted conception which confirms fertilization	Complexity of the procedure Ovarian hyperstimulation syndrome (OHSS)
Tubal patency is not required	Multiple pregnancy Emotional stress Cost

Table 29.3   Advantages and disadvantages of GIFT

Advantages	Disadvantages
The transfer of egg and sperm to the fallopian tube provides a natural environment for fertilization	Fertilization cannot be confirmed if the procedure is unsuccessful The risk of ectopic pregnancy is increased General anaesthesia is required Patent tubes are necessary OHSS Multiple pregnancy Emotional stress Cost

all. It is therefore important that the patient should understand that when she embarks upon this highly technical and expensive treatment her chance of success in any one cycle is no more than 1 in 6. The advantages and disadvantages of IVF are given in Table 29.2.

Intracytoplasmic sperm injection (ICSI)

ICSI involves manipulating an individual sperm and injecting it into an oocyte (Fig. 29.2). This is a highly technical procedure, but fertilization rates are high. Once fertilization has occurred, the procedure is as for IVF.

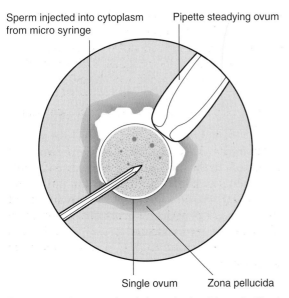

Sperm injected into cytoplasm from micro syringe
Pipette steadying ovum
Single ovum   Zona pellucida

Figure 29.2   Intracytoplasmic insemination. The unfertilized oocyte is steadied by a blunt probe while a single sperm from the male is injected into the cytoplasm.

Gamete intrafallopian transfer (GIFT)

This procedure involves a similar ovarian stimulation as described previously, but oocyte retrieval is by laparoscopy under general anaesthesia. Once the oocytes are retrieved, they are examined microscopically, and the three best are mixed with prepared sperm. They are reintroduced to the fimbrial lumen of one of the fallopian tubes through a cannula under laparoscopic guidance. Success rates are similar to IVF. The advantages and disadvantages of GIFT are listed in Table 29.3.

Intrauterine insemination (IUI)

This procedure can be carried out at a district general hospital with a good laboratory and with good ultrasound facilities. It involves similar follicular development, although in this case the aim is to achieve three mature follicles. Rupture of the follicles is ensured by the injection of human chorionic gonadotrophin, and prepared sperm are placed high in the uterine cavity by the introduction of a fine cannula through the internal os. The procedure is a simple outpatient one requiring unsophisticated equipment. In some units, three treatment cycles achieve similar success rates to those of IVF or GIFT. The advantages and disadvantages of IUI are given in Table 29.4.

All forms of assisted conception require an enormous emotional outlay for the couple

Table 29.4 Advantages and disadvantages of IUI

Advantages	Disadvantages
Less invasive	Fertilization is not confirmed
Less emotional commitment	Patent tubes must be present
Less expensive	It is not as successful as IVF
Less time-consuming	and GIFT
	OHSS
	Multiple pregnancies

involved. The NHS can seldom afford to offer either IVF or GIFT, and this is largely found within the private sector. IUI, however, is offered in many hospitals although there is increasing limitation of budgets for such treatments.

DONOR INSEMINATION

With the introduction of ICSI this is likely to become a much reduced need. However, there are a small number of men with problems such as chromosomal abnormalities, e.g. Klinefelter's syndrome (47XXY), rhesus incompatibility or who have total testicular failure whose partners may only be able to reproduce successfully by means of donor insemination.

At present specimens of seminal fluid are obtained from volunteers. The Human Fertilisation and Embryology Authority does not allow them to be paid a fee for this service, but travel expenses, up to £15, are permitted. The medical and genetic history of the donors are carefully screened, and they must produce a sample of sperm which meets the required standards of normal fertility. Specimens are checked bacteriologically, and the donors need blood tests for human immunodeficiency virus (HIV) and hepatitis B. Specimens are then stored by freezing for 6 months and, once again, the donors are checked for HIV infection. Provided both tests are negative, the specimens are then released. Recipients are able to choose donors in terms of skin and eye colour, height and blood group and other racial characteristics, although it is not easy to persuade donors from some ethnic minority groups to volunteer. Success rates using donor sperm depend upon the age of the recipient, but are approximately 50% after six cycles of therapy. The anonymity of the donor is always maintained, and the donor has no legal rights whatsoever over his donated sperm. However, his progeny, if told about their genetic origin, may be entitled to seek the identity of the donor, and records will have to be kept for many years.

THE HUMAN FERTILISATION AND EMBRYOLOGY AUTHORITY

This regulatory body was set up by an Act of Parliament to govern assisted conception and similar techniques including donor sperm insemination. Its task is to regulate any research or treatment which involves:

- The creation and use of human embryos outside the body
- The storage or donation of human eggs and sperm.

Its code of practice underlines:

- The respect which is due to human life at all stages of its development
- The right of infertile people to the proper consideration of their request for treatment
- A concern for the welfare of the child
- A recognition of the benefits from the responsible pursuit of medical and scientific knowledge.

All units licensed by the authority are inspected annually, and there is considerable emphasis on good record keeping and confidentiality. Unfortunately, as a consequence of this, direct communication between the unit and the patient's family doctor is not possible, and can only be done through the patient and with her consent.

RECOMMENDED READING

Ayede G, Balen F, Balen A 1996 The usefulness of ultrasound in infertility management. Contemporary Reviews in Obstetrics and Gynaecology 8: 32–38

Nugent D, Rutherford A 1997 Micromanipulation for male infertility. Contemporary Reviews in Obstetrics and Gynaecology 9: 67–73

Yovich J, Grudzinkos G 1990 The management of infertility. Heinemann, Oxford

30

Family planning

INTRODUCTION

Family planning is one of the success stories of the last 50 years. Now over half of the couples in developing countries are using contraception, and in most such countries the family size has dropped. During the same time the health of women and children has improved. However, the global population continues to increase. The need for services continues to grow – the number of women of child-bearing age in the developing world will rise from 1 000 000 000 000 in 1990 to 1 500 000 000 000 in 2010. Although oral contraception remains the most popular form of family planning in the UK, breast feeding, a most unreliable method, still prevents more pregnancies in the underdeveloped countries than anything else.

The efficiency of any contraceptive is measured as the pearl index (Table 30.1). This represents the number of pregnancies that occur with a particular form of contraception per 100 woman years of use (equivalent to the number of pregnancies in 100 women using a method for 1 year).

People use different methods at different times in their lives as their medical, emotional or relationship needs alter. The choice of a contraceptive is dependent upon its effectiveness, its suitability for that person or partnership, the risks and benefits of its use, how it is used and how it works. The most efficient contraceptive is that which is anatomically, physiologically and psychologically best suited to that partnership.

Table 30.1 The pearl index. Failure rates of various forms of contraception expressed as failures occurring in 100 women per year of use. Rates alter according to the age of the woman

Method	Failure rate per 100 woman years
Abstinence	0
Withdrawal – coitus interruptus	4–19
Rhythm method	9–20
Condom	3–12
Diaphragm	4–12
Spermicides	6–21
Sponges	9–36
Intrauterine contraceptive device	1–4
Intrauterine contraceptive device (levonorgestrel)	0.05
Depo-progestogen	0.3
Progestogen-only pill	0.5–3
Combined oral contraceptive pill	0.03
Sterilization	0.02

HORMONAL CONTRACEPTION

The hormonal contraceptives available today are either combinations of synthetic oestrogens with a progestogen or progestogen on its own. The combined oestrogen/progestogen preparation (the combined oral contraceptive, COC, or the pill) was first introduced in the mid-1960s, and over the last 30 years there has been a gradual reduction in the oestrogen content and also a change in the progestogens.

The combined oral contraceptive pill

Most COCs contain ethinyloestradiol as the oestrogen component, whereas there are a number of progestogens, which are broadly divided into two categories:

- Second-generation progestogens – norethisterone and levonorgestrel
- Third-generation progestogens – desogestrel, gestodene and norgestimate.

Mode of action

The pill inhibits ovulation by its suppressive effect on the anterior pituitary, and follicle-stimulating hormone (FSH) and luteinizing hormone (LH) secretion in particular. It also has a direct effect on the endometrium, making implantation difficult, and the progestogens alter cervical mucus, affording further contraceptive protection.

Metabolic effects

The oestrogen content has a direct effect on platelet aggregation and increases the incidence of deep-vein thrombosis. The second-generation progestogens have a depressive effect on high-density lipoproteins (HDLs), and this increases the risk of atherosclerosis and ischaemic heart disease. The third-generation progestogens do not have this effect, and appear to have very little androgenic activity. They are considered to be relatively oestrogen-dominant, and may increase the risk of venous thromboembolic phenomenon compared with the second-generation progestogens.

Taking the oral contraceptive

The majority of oral contraceptives contain 21 days of active ingredients followed by a pill-free week. Some preparations include seven blank pills to be taken during the active pill-free week to aid patient compliance. For new users, the oral contraceptive should be started on the first day of the period, and contraception will be effective from the start. The first cycle will be of 23 days, but thereafter a 28 day cycle will be maintained. Detailed instructions for taking the contraceptive are given with each packet of the pill, and users should be instructed to read these carefully before commencing the preparation.

Drug interactions

A number of enzyme-inducing drugs of clinical importance will interfere with the metabolism of the oral contraceptive. These are all the antiepileptics (except for sodium valproate), rifampicin, griseofulvin and spironolactone. Patients who are taking these drugs in the long term should be advised that they must take a higher dose oral contraceptive to provide effective contraception.

Broad-spectrum antibiotics, in particular those derived from penicillin and tetracycline, may reduce the level of gut flora and therefore prevent the full absorption of ethinyloestradiol. Therefore, patients taking short courses of antibiotics should be advised to use alternative contraception as well as the oral contraceptive during the treatment and for 7 days afterwards.

Which oral contraceptive?

The present recommendations are that the patient should take a low-dose oral contraceptive (i.e. 35 µg or less of ethinyloestradiol) containing a second-generation progestogen. Because of the lower incidence of venous thromboembolism, women wishing to take oral contraceptives containing third-generation progestogens (gestodene, desogestrel) must be advised that there is a slightly higher risk of venous thromboembolism although that risk remains half of the risk posed by pregnancy. Because of the lipid-friendly profile of third-generation progestogens, those over the age of 35 years are best started or changed to these oral contraceptives.

There is no time limit to taking the pill. However, for women who have taken it continuously for 10 years and are over the age of 30 years when they cease, there is a small delay in the return of fertility; by 18 months fertility rates are precisely the same as those who have formerly used barrier methods of contraception. Amenorrhoea following cessation of the oral contraceptive (previously and incorrectly known as post-pill amenorrhoea) merely indicates a disturbance of the pituitary–ovarian axis that has been masked by the use of the oral contraceptive and which should be investigated. There is no real association between amenorrhoea and taking the oral contraceptive.

The combined pill and cancer

There is strong evidence that taking the pill has a protective effect on the endometrium and the ovary, reducing the incidence of cancer in either by about 40%.

Data relating to cervical cancer is complex. The pill may be a co-factor in cervical cancer, but this possibly reflects the interaction of direct contact of seminal fluid and infection with the cervix rather than a direct effect of the pill.

There is a small increase in the risk of breast cancer for women who commence the pill under the age of 25 years, but there appears to be no increase in risk for women taking the pill between the ages of 25 and 45 years. New pills with lower doses of oestrogen and third-generation progestogens may diminish this risk still further.

The progestogen-only pill

The progestogen-only pill (POP) accounts for only a small percentage of the hormonal contraceptive market. It works primarily by causing the cervical mucus to become thick, viscous and hostile to sperm. At the same time there is a direct effect on the endometrium, which makes it inhospitable to nidation. Tubal motility is also altered. In younger women there may be a direct effect on the pituitary, with at least 10% developing amenorrhoea. This implies that ovulation is inhibited. Unfortunately, interference with FSH and LH secretion may lead to the development of functional cysts of the ovaries.

Efficacy

Like all modes of contraception, the efficacy of the POP is dependent upon the age of the woman taking it. In those under the age of 35 years the pearl index is around 2, but this reduces to 0.5 by the age of 40 years. In view of this, the preparation is most suited to women over the age of 35 years in whom there are contraindications to the use of the COC pill. This would particularly apply to those who smoke, are hypertensive, obese or have migrainous headaches. It is also suitable for those women who are lactating as it does not inhibit milk secretion (unlike the COC). Because of the contraceptive effect of lactation, the use of the POP during this time makes its efficiency close to 100%.

Side-effects

The main problem with the POP is unscheduled bleeding. About 40% of users will regain a normal menstrual pattern, but the remainder will have irregular bleeding or amenorrhoea. Those who develop amenorrhoea are the most worried because of the fear that they may have become pregnant, but are probably the safest as the pill has led to anovulation and therefore a higher efficiency rate.

Taking the POP

The pill must be taken every day and within 3 hours of the same time each day. As metabolism of the pill takes about 4 h from ingestion, this is probably best taken at a time which does not coincide with the usual time for intercourse.

Injectable progestogens

The most widely used is depot medroxy-progesterone acetate (DMPA). This is given every 12 weeks, and it is estimated that over 4 million women around the world use this method of contraception. There has been well-publicized adverse criticism of DMPA over the years, but much of this is unfounded. The injection of DMPA (150 mg) is given within the first 5 days of the cycle into a deep intramuscular site, usually the gluteal muscles. In postpartum mothers it should be given approximately 5 weeks after birth.

Advantages

The injectable progestogens are highly effective for they inhibit ovulation and are virtually 100% effective. They do not require any day-to-day motivation by the user, and the method is not related to intercourse. It is particularly suitable for the woman who shows poor compliance with oral contraception. There is a reduced incidence of pelvic inflammatory disease because of the direct effect on the cervical mucus. It is the contraceptive choice for women with sickle cell disease, and as there are no oestrogen related side-effects it is suitable for those in whom the COC is contraindicated.

Disadvantages

The most obvious of these is that once the injection has been administered, it cannot be removed, and therefore its effects are likely to last for a minimum of 3 months and possibly considerably longer. Patients must be advised of this. There may be disruption of the menstrual cycle, and on average this will last for about 6 months after the last injection, although it may be as prolonged as 2 years. Similarly, return of fertility may be disrupted for as long as this, although the mean time is approximately 5 months. Headaches, weight gain and depression are common problems associated with progestogens, and may occur with DMPA.

Depot progestogens remain an extremely useful form of contraception, particularly amongst the non-compliant and for those who have finished having children. However, careful counselling about the side-effects of the preparation must be given prior to administration of the drug.

Postcoital contraception (emergency contraception)

If a woman had the first act of unprotected intercourse within 72 h of seeking advice, then hormonal contraception can be given. This consists of taking two oral contraceptive tablets, each containing 50 µg of ethinyloestradiol and 250 µg of levonorgestrel. This dose is then repeated 12 h later. Nausea is a common side-effect, and occasionally vomiting may occur. If this happens within 3 h of taking a dose, it should be repeated. The efficiency of the method is dependent on what time of the cycle intercourse occurred. If at midcycle, then the failure rate is approximately 4%; at other times about 2%. There is an extremely small risk of teratogenicity should pregnancy go on; women should be warned about this.

Women must be advised that they should return to the clinic within 3 weeks, and that there will be no delay in the return of their period if the method has worked satisfactorily. It is essential that good contraception is initiated at this visit.

If the first act of unprotected intercourse was 5 days ago or less, the alternative form of postcoital contraception is the introduction of an intrauterine contraceptive device of an (IUCD). The usual contraindications apply, and nulliparity remains a strong relative contraindication.

THE INTRAUTERINE CONTRACEPTIVE DEVICE

The IUCD is a foreign body placed in the uterus; it is highly effective in protecting against pregnancy but has a number of undesirable side-effects.

The initial concept of placing a foreign object within the uterus to prevent pregnancy is said to have derived from the habit of camel owners placing stones in the uterus of their animals to prevent pregnancy during long journeys. The initial human devices were of silver or gold. In 1960, second-generation IUCDs were launched: silastic devices in many flexible shapes containing radiopaque barium sulphate.

The most widely used in the UK were the Lippe's loop and the Saf T coil. Each has an attached thread that protrudes through the cervix and lies in the vagina. Not only does it allow the patient to check that the device is still present but is a simple means of removal of the IUCD by traction on the threads.

In the 1970s, devices consisting of a silastic frame, bearing copper, were introduced. These are considerably smaller in size than the inert devices, have a greater efficiency and are easier to insert. However, unlike the inert devices they have a limited life, of 3–5 years, but the modern T-shaped device will last up to 8 years (Fig. 30.1).

The most important problem with IUCDs is the possible increased incidence of pelvic inflammatory disease and subsequent tubal damage. This has led to many law suits in the USA, with judgements being given both for and against the devices. Because of the enormous

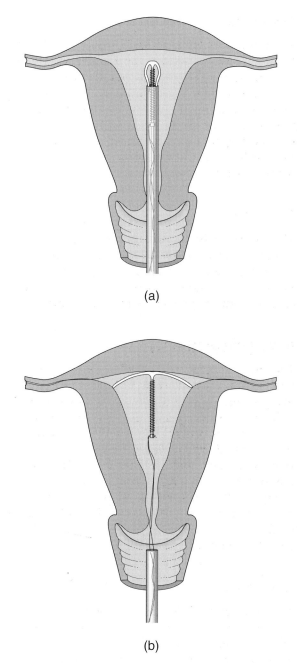

(a)

(b)

Figure 30.1 Insertion of the copper T IUCD. **a** The limbs of the coil are bent down whilst in the tube and the device passed through to the cervix. **b** Withdrawal of the outer tube allows the limbs to open out at the fundal end of the uterus.

sums of money involved in defending these cases, the manufacture and distribution of IUCDs has declined dramatically in the USA.

Mechanism of action

A World Health Organization scientific group reported that although raised β-human chorionic gonadotrophin levels can be identified in the late luteal phase of some IUCD users, it is unlikely that prevention of implantation of a fertilized ovum is the main method of action. There is a foreign body reaction in the endometrium with an increase in white cells, particularly macrophages, not associated with bacterial infection. Sperm migration into the fallopian tubes is considerably reduced, and transport and development of ova are impeded. It is probable that IUCDs exert their effect beyond the uterus. The uterine and tubal fluids are altered in the presence of a device, and so impairs the viability of gametes, reducing their chances of union. This effect is probably potentiated by copper ions. The IUCD remains contraindicated for those who have an ethical or moral objection to a process that could possibly interfere with implantation of a fertilized ovum.

Effectiveness

A number of factors influence the effectiveness of IUCDs, the most important of which is the skill of the doctor inserting the device. The other two factors are the age of the patient – fertility decreases with increasing age, especially over 35 years – and the length of time the IUCD is in place – the first year of use is associated with the highest failure rates. The failure rate for copper-bearing devices ranges from 0.3 to 3.0 per 100 woman years.

Advantages and disadvantages

The advantages of the IUCD are:

- It is highly effective
- It is not related to intercourse
- The effect is reversible
- Little patient compliance is required
- It is relatively cheap
- It has no known systemic effects
- It has no effect on lactation as hormonal methods may.

The main disadvantages are:

- The insertion must be by a trained doctor or nurse, and so is labour-intensive and expensive.
- There is an increased risk of miscarriage if pregnancy does occur and possibly of infection. In a woman who wishes to continue with her pregnancy the device should be removed in the first trimester if the threads are visible.
- About 1 in 20 IUCD-related pregnancies are ectopic compared with 1 in 200 when there is no IUCD present. This is because the devices are not as effective in preventing tubal pregnancies, and tubal inflammation may be a factor. However, because the overall pregnancy rate among IUCD is very low, the incidence of ectopic pregnancy is extremely small (approximately 0.05 per 100 woman years).
- Expulsion may occur, especially in the first few months. This is related to the efficiency of the insertion, the age of the patient and her parity.
- Pain is quite common both during and after insertion. Infiltration of the cervix with a local anaesthetic may be helpful, as is the use of non-steroidal anti-inflammatory drugs. Severe persistent pain is an indication for removal of the device.
- Perforation of the uterus may occur at the time of insertion. The incidence is usually less than 1 in every 1000 insertions but is influenced mainly by the experience of the inserter.
- Bleeding may increase in amount and duration, but not frequency. Some irregular bleeding is common in the first days after insertion.
- Pelvic infection – the risk of a sexually transmitted disease is increased in women who are not in stable relationships and therefore is much more common in single nulliparous women. For this reason nulliparity is considered to be a relative contraindication. There is no increased risk of tubal infertility amongst IUCD users in stable, monogamous sexual relationships.

Contraindications to use

- Undiagnosed irregular genital tract bleeding.
- Suspicion of pregnancy (except when used as a postcoital contraceptive).
- Pelvic infection – past or present.
- Previous ectopic pregnancy, tubal disease or tubal surgery.
- Distorted or congenitally abnormal uterine cavity.

Removal and replacement of devices

All inert devices can stay in until menstruation ceases unless problems supervene. The majority of copper-bearing devices can be left in place for up to 8 years in women under the age of 40 years. For those over 40 years of age at the time of insertion, they may be left in place until 1 year after the final menstrual period. Devices can be removed at any time during the cycle, but replacement is best carried out towards the end of menses as the cervical os is slightly dilated and it is a time when the patient cannot be pregnant.

The hormonal intrauterine system

A plastic T-shaped device with progesterone in a rate-limiting membrane attached to the main stem of the device has been available for many years. However, it was bulky and had an effective life span of only 1 year. More recently, a levonorgestrel-containing device has been introduced. This releases 20 µg of the hormone daily, and has a life span of 5 years. It has the enormous advantage of an extremely low pregnancy rate, equivalent to that of steriliz-ation, a marked reduction in menstrual flow and a protective effect against pelvic infection. Its major problems are associated with initial irregular menstrual loss and a slightly more difficult insertion because of its increased diameter.

New devices

A frameless device consisting of copper bands mounted on a nylon thread has been devised. It

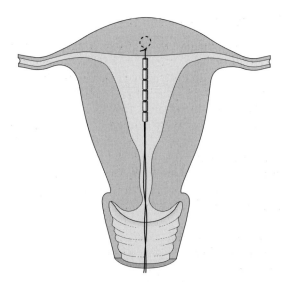

Figure 30.2   A stemless copper-releasing IUCD. It is fitted as an outpatient procedure transcervically like the other IUCDs. It is frameless, and a special inserter allows it to be secured into the myometrium.

is held by a fixation device into the myometrium at the uterine fundus and can remain in place for many years (Fig. 30.2). Initial clinical trials have shown it to be highly acceptable, easy to insert and to have a lower rate of heavier periods.

DIAPHRAGMS

Diaphragms are dome-shaped rubber devices with a spring on the outer rim. When placed correctly in the vagina, they occlude the cervix and act as a carrier for spermicide. The arcing diaphragm has a firm double metal spring in the rim (Fig. 30.3). When compressed it forms an arc, directing the posterior part of the diaphragm downwards into the posterior fornix. It is particularly suitable for women with a retroverted uterus, and it is now used by 2% of women seeking contraceptive advice.

Effectiveness

This is dependent upon the motivation of those using it. Higher failure rates can be expected among the younger age group and in the first year of use. Increasing use of the method and

(a)

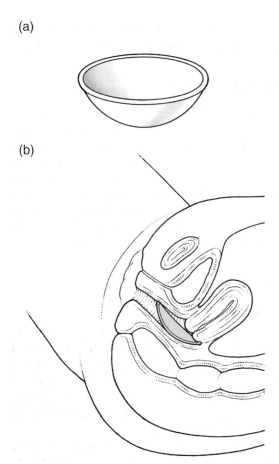

(b)

Figure 30.3 **a** A vaginal contraceptive diaphragm. **b** The diaphragm correctly lodged in the vagina covering the cervix and much of the anterior vaginal wall.

increasing age both reduce failure rates, which range from 1 to 6 per 100 woman years.

Advantages and disadvantages

The main advantages are:

- It is effective
- It has no serious health hazards
- It has some protective effect against pelvic infection
- It may be associated with a reduction in the incidence of cervical neoplasia.

The disadvantages are:

- It does require a high degree of personal motivation to use

- Trained personnel are needed to teach its use
- It is coitally related
- Some women find it messy to use
- There is a slightly higher rate of urinary tract infections
- A small number of women are allergic to the latex rubber used in its construction

Fitting and removal

The initial fitting must be carried out by trained nurses or doctors. Patients should be advised to recheck the size after childbirth or if there is a marked change in their weight. It is wise to use spermicidal cream both on the inner aspect of the diaphragm and around the rim. Users must leave the device in place for a minimum of 6 h after each act of intercourse.

Other vaginal occlusive devices

The cervical cap, the vault cap and the Vimule are all designed to fit over the cervix, and are held in place by suction. They have the advantages of the diaphragm but require more detailed fitting and teaching. They are rarely used now except by professional sex workers.

THE VAGINAL CONTRACEPTIVE SPONGE

This is a soft, white, circular sponge 5.5 cm in diameter impregnated with nonoxynol-9, with a polyester loop to facilitate removal. It must be fitted high in the vagina to cover the cervix, and can be worn for up to 30 h. The sponge requires no training to fit, and is available without prescription. In young people the failure rates have been unacceptably high, but the sponge can be recommended in women in their forties whose fertility is lower. If intercourse is less frequent, the method may have some attraction.

CONDOMS

Most modern condoms are made of fine latex rubber and consist of a circular cylinder with a closed plain or teat shape at one end and an integral rim at the other. They come in a great variety of shapes, textures, flavours and colours but, despite popular opinion, are usually of one size only.

Their effectiveness is dependent upon the experience of the user. Failures occur because of mishandling before use, failing to expel the air from the teat, genital contact before and after use and, very rarely, due to breakage. In the UK they are manufactured to a very high standard and provide an effective means of contraception, failure rates depending upon the age of the female and user experience. The pearl index ranges from 0.4 to over 10 per 100 woman years, but on average is about 4 per 100 woman years.

An estimated 40 million couples use the method throughout the world and, in Japan, 70 per cent of couples use them. In the UK only 13% rely on the condom alone; but the well-publicized risk of HIV infection is increasing this figure considerably, especially among younger unmarried couples.

Advantages and disadvantages

The advantages are:

- Ready availability, e.g. from vending machines
- No need for medical help to use
- Lack of medical complications
- Protection from sexually transmitted disease
- Protection from cervical neoplasia.

The disadvantages are:

- Coitally related
- May lead to loss of sensation
- Very occasional erectile impotence
- Allergy in one of the partners to latex.

SPERMICIDES

These are chemical agents that destroy sperm. Nonoxynol-9 is the commonest used in the UK. It is a surface-active agent disrupting the lipoprotein cell membrane of the sperm. Bactericides may also be used in combination.

Spermicides are available as foams, pessaries, creams, jellies and as a film. They are generally used as an adjunct to other forms of contraception such as barrier methods or the IUCD.

STERILIZATION

Sterilization of the male or female has become one of the most popular forms of contraception, particularly within the Western world. It has been open to abuse in certain third-world countries where major compulsory sterilization programmes have been carried out. It has now become a simple reliable procedure both for the male and, especially, the female, with the introduction of laparoscopy for the latter.

Female sterilization

Laparoscopy

This was first introduced in the late 1960s and has been in extensive use since the mid-1970s. It is popular, for the incision is less than 1 cm at the lower border of the umbilicus, and the operation is usually done as a day case. It needs, however, a general anaesthetic. The following methods have been used.

Unipolar diathermy. This coagulates approximately 3 cm of each tube, and is not used widely any longer. There is an unacceptable morbidity rate due to bowel and abdominal burns, and reversibility is considered to be almost impossible.

Bipolar diathermy. This allows a much smaller segment of tube to be destroyed, but is not widely used because of the risks of damage to bowel.

Falope ring. This is a silicone rubber ring containing barium sulphate. Viewed through a laparoscope, the applicator draws up a loop of tube (usually in excess of 2 cm), and the ring is then forced off, occluding the piece of tube. The loop of tube becomes necrotic, and the proximal and distal remaining portions of the tube fall away. The principle of the procedure is precisely the same as that used for castrating male sheep (but probably far less painful!).

Hulka Clemens clip. This was widely used throughout the 1970s, and is made of plastic

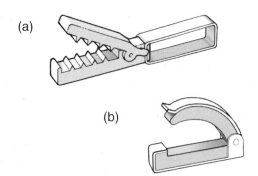

Figure 30.4 Clips used for laparoscopic occlusion of the fallopian tube. **a** Hulka Clemens clip. **b** Filshie clip.

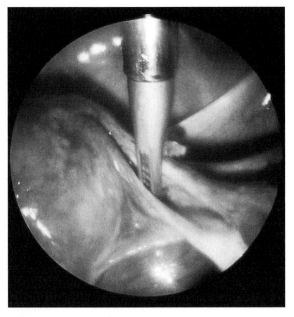

Figure 30.5 Laparoscopic application of the Hulka Clemens clip.

with teeth that interlock when the clip is closed (Figs 30.4 and 30.5). It is locked in place with a gold-plated stainless steel spring. It destroys approximately 3–4 mm of tube.

Filshie clip. This was introduced in 1975, and is now the main occluding clip used within the UK. It destroys approximately 4 mm of tube, ensures complete occlusion and complete tubal ischaemia due to the constant pressure of the silicone rubber insert (Fig. 30.4). It is not uncommon for the clip to migrate away from the site of application some weeks after the procedure. However, the two separated pieces of tube are by then occluded and separate. The failure rate for the procedure is reported to be as low as 1 per 1000 cases. A cheaper, all-plastic improved version of the clip is likely to be introduced shortly.

Other methods

Mini-laparotomy. This involves a small transverse suprapubic incision of about 3–5 cm in length. The tubes are mobilized and either cut and divided or a clip or ring is applied.

Culdotomy. An incision in the posterior fornix under anaesthesia allows access to the pouch of Douglas, and the fimbrial end of each tube can usually be brought down and removed. The procedure is easy if the uterus is mobile and there are no adhesions, but it has a higher complication rate than laparoscopy.

Transuterine tubal occlusion. A number of techniques have been developed, including diathermy, the introduction of chemical sclerosing agents, silicone splints and tubal plugs. Unfortunately the failure rate is unacceptably high, and there is a high ectopic pregnancy rate among these failures.

Sterilization at the time of caesarean section

This is still widely practised but should be avoided. The risk of failure is increased but, more importantly, the newborn child is most at risk in the first 6 weeks of life, and it is best to allow this time to elapse before admitting a patient for sterilization, when it can be carried out as a day case using a laparoscopic method. Sterilization at caesarean section should not be carried out when the request is made during labour and an emergency section is performed.

Morbidity

Laparoscopic techniques have been shown to be safe with low morbidity. However, surgical difficulties may be encountered because of the size of the patient and due to pelvic disease, particularly inflammatory disease or endometriosis. Bleeding problems are rare, but where diathermy is used, adjacent structures may be damaged.

Immediate postoperative pain is more common when using occlusive rings as opposed to clips. From long-term studies there is no evidence to support the view that women undergoing sterilization have an increase in menstrual problems compared with a matched group of women whose partners have undergone sterilization. In the UK one-third of all women over the age of 35 years are sterilized, and so it follows that one-third of women over 35 years of age presenting with gynaecological problems will also have been sterilized.

Preoperative counselling

Counselling is an essential part of the sterilization process. It is important that the procedure is explained carefully to the patient, and she is told that there is a small failure rate (usually given as 1 in 500). The patient must understand that sterilization is considered irreversible. She must continue to use contraception up to the time of the operation and, if she is taking the oral contraceptive pill, continue to do so until she has finished the current packet.

Ideally the operation should be in the first 10 days of the menstrual cycle. If not, a pregnancy test should be done, and the sterilization accompanied by a dilatation and curettage.

Every woman should be considered on an individual basis, and her own wishes taken into consideration. There should be no rules concerning the number of children, stability of the partnership or age when considering sterilization. However, approximately 10% of women under the age of 30 years who undergo sterilization request reversal at a later date. The most common reasons for this are change of partner, desire for another child, loss of sense of fertility and, occasionally, sexual problems.

Failure

Recanalization as a cause of true method failure is uncommon, and more likely is surgical error, where the wrong structure has been occluded such as the round ligament. Alternatively the occluding clip may not be correctly placed across the tube, which consequently is not fully blocked. Occasionally the patient may have been pregnant at the time of the sterilization, and the ovum already in the proximal part of the tube, travelling to the uterus.

The design of the Filshie clip makes it the least likely to be associated with method failure. The Falope ring can leave two pieces of viable tube in apposition either side of the ring, and it is possible for reanastomosis to occur at that site.

Reversibility

If sterilization is to be reversed by operation it is essential for there to be at least 4 cm of viable tube and normal fimbriae for there to be any chance of success. The greatest success is achieved when the least amount of tube has been previously destroyed, as with occlusive clips. In women under the age of 35 years, success rates of up to 80% have been reported for reanastomosis, depending on the skills of the surgeon and the selection of cases for surgery. It is important for the patient to understand that reversal of sterilization involves a laparotomy, a more prolonged stay in hospital and that there is an increased ectopic pregnancy rate. In most parts of the UK the procedure is no longer available under the National Health Service.

Male sterilization

Because of the accessibility of the vas deferens immediately below the scrotal skin, the procedure of vasectomy can be carried out as an outpatient procedure under local anaesthesia. Either a midline scrotal incision or bilateral incisions can be used, and the vas then occluded by ligation with division or diathermy.

The major problem associated with vasectomy is that it is not immediately effective. Clearance of the reproductive tract of viable sperm is dependent upon time and the rate of ejaculation. It is usual to ask for two semen samples a month apart at approximately 3 months after the operation to check this. Provided that both of these show a complete absence of sperm, then the vasectomy is considered successful. Prior to this, contraception by one or other of the partners must be continued. The failure rate for the procedure is similar to those encountered with female sterilization.

Morbidity

The most common problem associated with the procedure is haematoma formation, but occasionally infection is also encountered. Sperm granulomata may form at the site of ligation of the vas, leaving a painful lump. Long-term problem rates are low. Antisperm antibodies will develop in over 50% of patients after 5 years, and may affect the success of subsequent reversal procedures. Their influence on connective tissue disorders in later life is uncertain and being watched.

Counselling

As with females this is very important, and the patient is required to sign a consent form stating that he understands that the procedure is considered to be irreversible and that there is a small failure rate. Unfortunately, some men confuse virility and potency with fertility. They believe that procedures which render them infertile will similarly make them impotent. These fears need to be dispelled at an early stage; if the doctor feels that there may be psychological problems, then the procedure should not be undertaken.

In both male and female sterilization there is no longer a requirement for the partner's consent to the procedure, but mutual discussion is wise.

RECOMMENDED READING

Filshie M, Guillebaud J 1990 Contraception – science and practice. Butterworth, London
Guillebaud J 1997 Contraception today, 3rd edn. D Units, London
Hickey M, Fraser I 1995 Contraception in the future. Contemporary Reviews in Obstetrics and Gynaecology 7: 160–166

Kaunitz H 1997 Contraception and the adolescent patient. International Journal of Fertility 42: 30–38
Mansour D 1997 Effect of recent advice on the uses of oral contraception. Contemporary Reviews in Obstetrics and Gynaecology 7: 61–66

Medicolegal matters

31

Medicolegal matters

It is said that in politics 'When America sneezes, Europe catches a cold'. Certainly in the medicolegal avalanche of proceedings, the USA has led us on the steep slope down which we are sliding. More medicolegal work is being done now than ever before, with the obstetrical and gynaecological department responsible for more claims and damages than any other in hospital practice. Annually, £280 000 000 is spent in this area; this has to be taken from a stringent budget for health care. The anxiety produced among both junior and senior obstetricians is mounting with their exposure to threats of litigation, and is in some instances acting negatively in the performance of the management of women. For example, in a recent survey when senior obstetricians were asked their opinions about the reasons for the increase of caesarean section rates, over 40% gave the fear of litigation. Thus, defensive medicine creeps in, and this is not of necessity good for the patients we look after.

In the early 1990s the Department of Health introduced Crown Indemnity, so that all doctors working in National Health Service hospitals would be covered for fees of a legal nature and damages if these should be given by the courts. Although this was superficially helpful to the profession, it did shift the responsibility for deciding on the conduct of defending cases from trained doctors and the defence unions to administrators in the National Health Service and the health authority lawyers. This situation was worsened in April 1998 by the establishment of a special health authority, the NHS Litigation Agency, which deals with all medicolegal matters centrally, thus even further distancing decisions from the clinical workers.

This led to a downgrading of the level at which cases were defended and often to the reactions of obstetricians. It has now been accepted within the National Health Service that this goes on. Doctors should remember that they are not covered by Crown Indemnity if working in general practice or at any events outside the hospital even though these may be emergency actions, for example attendance at a road accident or unexpected home delivery. Neither does cover extend to the private sector. It is important that obstetricians and gynaecologists retain their membership of defence societies or unions at an appropriate level of any earnings in the private sector. Another good reason for keeping up membership of a defence union is the need for help should there be criminal proceedings against a doctor or disciplinary ones by the General Medical Council or the health authority. Here the unions will aid the insured.

The subject is a large one, and there are many good books about it (see the recommended reading list). An outline only will be given in this section to help those working in obstetrics and gynaecology to find their way through the thorny jungle where the predators are not just the patients but their lawyers also.

CAUSES OF LITIGATION

The commonest allegation in our field is that of intrapartum hypoxia which results in cerebral damage, accounting for about 30% of claims. Although we know that about 80% of hypoxic damage is due to antenatal events, still any sign of fetal distress in labour is often falsely associated by the courts with intrapartum cerebral damage. This leads to very expensive legal cases and, should the case be lost, to very heavy damages of over £3 000 000. To this one must always add another 50% for legal fees in these cases.

About 15% of claims are connected with perinatal death, and a further 15% to injuries, either to the mother or baby. No other set of problems rise above 5%.

In gynaecology about 25% of claims are linked

to failure of sterilization, and about another quarter to operative complications such as damage to a ureter, failed termination or perforation of the uterus.

It is the experience of those who are skilled in giving expert witness that in about half the cases submitted there is no sustainable case. Despite the expert witnesses statements of this to the plaintiff's side, only in 5% of cases is the action discontinued by the solicitors. When cases proceeded in as many as 90%, liability is admitted and settlement is reached out of court, thus saving the health authority the legal fees of continuing to defend the case. In the experience of Clements, a knowledgeable medical expert, only 4% of the many cases he advised had a case proceeded to trial (about 1% of the total anyway). The courts decided in favour of the plaintiff in half. Hence of all the cases started, it would seem that less than 1% go to court and only half of those are won by the plaintiff. Among those cases that do not go to court, a large number are settled in order to save the legal fees and the risk of damages.

There is obviously something wrong with the legal system of a country when this is the way in which cases are settled. A *no claim, no blame*

Box 31.1   Common antenatal causes of litigation

- Records
  - Poor completion
  - Poor filing (e.g. lost notes)
- History
  - Poor completion. Inaccurate recording (e.g. woman's age)
  - Gaps in shared care
- Fetal testing:
  - High-risk pregnancy not identified
  - Growth retardation not diagnosed
  - Congenital abnormalities not diagnosed
  - Diagnostic tests not done
  - Results of tests not scrutinized
  - Results of tests not recorded or reported correctly
- Patient's requests and birth plan:
  - Deviation from the woman's preferences. Pay particular attention if these are not in accordance with hospital protocol
  - Failure to discuss antenatally variation of hospital practice from the birth plan
  - Lack of awareness of those who would not wish monitoring

Box 31.2   Common causes of litigation in labour

- Records:
  - Not written clearly, or not dated, timed or signed
  - Partograms – not used properly and not all readings initialled
  - Not following protocols or guidelines
  - No retention of copies of old superseded protocols for future defence
- Monitoring of fetus:
  - Lack of understanding of cardiotocogram (CTG) at different levels of labour ward staff
  - No full handover between members of staff at end of periods of duty
  - Senior staff not kept well informed of early changes in fetal hypoxia
  - Unlabelled CTG (without name, date or time)
  - CTG records and partograms not kept properly
- Normal delivery:
  - Indiscreet remarks between staff members in a woman's hearing
  - Inadequacy of training of staff who do the delivery
  - Ignoring women's wishes about giving of oxytocic drugs for third stage labour
  - Absence of paediatrician if risk of hypoxia
  - Retained vaginal swabs when sewing up episiotomy or tears
- Forceps:
  - Lack of experience of staff who do various degrees of difficult deliveries
  - Not ensuring correct traction is used. If unsuccessful, record number of attempts
  - Not doing forceps in theatre if there is any doubt about vaginal delivery
  - Not being prepared to move to caesarean section
- Seniority of deliverer:
  - The consultant on duty is not kept informed of events
  - Consultants on duty not easily available, or did not do labour ward rounds
  - Senior staff not present for difficult operative deliveries
  - Senior and experienced anaesthetists not working on delivery suite
- Caesarean section:
  - Inexperienced person does an operation. Senior staff must perform difficult procedures (e.g. repeat placenta praevia)
  - Damage to bladder, ureter or bowel
  - Retained instruments and swabs

Box 31.3   Common postnatal causes of litigation

- The baby:
  - No early examination to reveal any obvious abnormalities
  - Paediatric care not available in the labour ward when necessary
  - Baby not tested appropriately with agreed screening tests
  - Results of any tests not discussed with the mother
- The mother:
  - Need for rubella immunization not checked for seronegative mothers
  - Anti-D immunoglobulin not given when required
  - Retained swabs in the vagina not checked for after a vaginal delivery

Box 31.4   Common gynaecological causes of litigation

- Consent form:
  - Informed consent not given to the doctor who should have explained and witnessed the signature on the consent form
  - Poor discussion about the potential removal of ovaries at total abdominal hysterectomy. If there is any possibility, get consent
  - Failure rates of sterilization not understood and not recorded in the notes
  - No discussion that if a laparoscopy operation is not possible, a laparotomy will be done under the same anaesthetic. No consent for this
- Operative injury:
  - Injury to ureter, bladder or rectum
  - Did not get help from relevant specialist in urinary or alimentary surgery if damage occurred at operation
  - Did not get early consultation from specialists if complications suspected after operation
  - Swabs and instruments not checked with the scrub nurse at operation (even though she says they are complete, it is still the surgeon's responsibility)

system would be better, where compensation would be offered to cover financial need produced by an independent enquiry. Further, damages could be awarded annually instead of as a lump sum. In obstetrical cases, the infant does not always survive the early years, yet damages are calculated on a life expectancy of reaching adulthood. Hence in the event of early demise, the damages are excessive but are not paid back. Another useful idea is the pre-court hearing, where the case can be settled in a less formal, speedier and less expensive way. Pilot studies are proceeding, but this is for the future. At the moment we are saddled with the adversarial system in the courts. The major features of obstetrical and gynaecological areas where negligence may arise are briefly considered in Boxes 31.1–31.4, the first three relating to obstetrics and the last to gynaecology.

Box 31.5 Ten important ways to avoid medicolegal problems in obstetrics and gynaecology

1. Be concerned
Ensure that you are available and prepared to talk to a woman or her family, particularly if anything has gone amiss
  Show your concern to the family for the problem and, whilst not of necessity admitting blame, be sorry with the woman for any problems that have happened

2. Understand the current legal position
Ensure you know what is happening in the current medicolegal world about the matters which concern your practice; for example, consent for sterilization of the mentally handicapped over 18 years or therapeutic abortion after 24 weeks of gestation

3. Know your own medicolegal advisers
If you are working in the National Health Service in hospital and covered by Crown Indemnity, ensure that you know who is the hospital manager dealing with medicolegal affairs and who are the legal advisers to your health authority. Be prepared to communicate with them swiftly if you think anything may proceed to legal action
  If you work outside the hospital or in the private sector, ensure that your medical defence organization subscription is at the right level, and report early any potential problems

4. Explain carefully
Discuss with the patient what is likely to happen in labour (particularly if it is likely not to be straightforward) or in an operative procedure in gynaecology. Make sure the woman understands what you have said, and go over with her the risks of any procedure. Enter into the medical records that you have done this, and sign it. The provision of printed leaflets or books is no substitute for telling people personally
  Before the operation begins, ensure that the consent forms are correctly filled in and signed by the patient and doctor

5. Keep good medical records
Medical records should be made by the doctor concerned at the time of the procedure, whether a consultation or treatment
  If involved with an operation, write the records in theatre. Always date (and, if relevant, time) records and sign them
  Remember that your records may be read years later, so make them clear. Avoid amusing, slang or derogatory remarks, for they sound awful out of context in the courts later
  Enter what you told the woman or her relatives if problems arise

6. Investigations
Do the appropriate investigations at the right time. In pregnancy, know the local protocols for fetal monitoring
  Explain these to the woman beforehand, particularly stressing what the test is looking for and what it is not. Make sure that she understands the potential management of any results
  Ensure that the results are seen by someone of appropriate seniority and that action is taken if indicated

7. Adequate medical staff
Ensure that sufficient medical staff are available to cover the service required, which in obstetrics is 24 h a day and no less
  Ensure sufficient and experienced enough staff are on duty
  Be especially cautious when locums are employed, and with newly joined junior staff at weekends
  If the workload of the timetable exceeds the practicality of covering all duties, ensure that the health authority knows about this in writing and work with them towards getting it altered
  Try to close split sites. Record all untoward incidences associated with staff on two sites

8. Appropriately skilled doctors
Ensure that an appropriately skilled obstetrician and anaesthetist perform procedures, particularly if these are elective ones
  If emergencies arise, ensure that the junior doctors inform senior cover immediately and that they act according to local practice. Make sure that there is full and readily available senior cover for junior staff

9. Working inside skills
Only perform procedures that are inside your comfortable practice and skills. If training is required, ensure that it is done properly and thoroughly before offering the procedure as a service one
  Know the effects and side-effects of all new drugs fully before using them (e.g. mifepristone)

10. Adequate equipment
Ensure that the health authority or private hospital has adequate equipment for the procedures being performed and the facilities for investigation needed for the care of women at all stages. If these are missing or not working efficiently, consider postponing the work and ensuring that the employing authority knows of this

AVOIDANCE OF MEDICOLEGAL PROBLEMS

Avoidance of medicolegal problems is not defensive medicine but good medical practice. One must know one's subjects both in theory and in the techniques. The practising of surgical procedures on women by staff in training is laudable if done under supervision and with some knowledge. It is inexcusable without both of these.

Communication with the woman and her partner must be complete, and trust must be evolved. If things go wrong they should be admitted without admitting actual liability. Human sympathy should, of course, be expressed, again without allocating blame.

Careful records are the essence of preventing or limiting litigation. They should be well written, signed, dated and kept available for up to 25 years in obstetrical cases, and 7 years in gynaecology. New court rules came in the spring of 1999 for dealing with the process of litigation (the Woolf reforms). The time-scale for the management of claims will be governed by a judge rather than being plaintiff–defendant driven. There will be financial penalties for failure to meet time-scales. For example there will be 3 months only for Trust's claim managers to fully investigate their side of a claim.

Ten important ways to avoid medicolegal problems were published by the Royal College of Obstetricians and Gynaecologists in 1992. They have been reproduced here (Box 31.5) with permission of the college, and contain the essence of good obstetrical and gynaecological behaviour.

RECOMMENDED READING

Chamberlain G (ed) 1992 How to avoid medico-legal problems. RCOG, London

Clements R (ed) 1992 Safe practice in obstetrics and gynaecology. Churchill Livingstone, London

Gupta S, Bewley S 1998 Medico-legal issues in fertility regulation. British Journal of Obstetrics and Gynaecology 105: 818–826

Appendix

Example questions for the MCQ examination

Examples for the multiple choice question (MCQ) paper of the Diploma examination of the Royal College of Obstetricians and Gynaecologists (DRCOG) are given in this appendix to familiarize candidates with the format of the examination. It is suggested that the questions are not attempted until the relevant chapters have been read and digested.

Go through the instructions given in Chapter 1 of this book again, and only then attempt each question. Do a full page of questions at a time, and only then turn over to look at the answers.

Chapter 5. Antenatal care

External cephalic version

a. is a recognized cause of fetal tachycardia
b. is a recognized cause of transplacental haemorrhage
c. can be performed in the presence of a twin pregnancy
d. can lead to placental abruption
e. is never attempted after 38 weeks of gestation

Chapter 6. Fetal progress

Amniocentesis

a. is associated with a 1% abortion rate
b. is routinely carried out in the first trimester
c. is used for the detection of Down's syndrome
d. carries a risk of subsequent fetal orthopaedic deformity
e. is necessary prior to cordocentesis

Rubella in early pregnancy is associated with

a. limb reduction deformities
b. increased miscarriage rate
c. neonatal cataract
d. intrauterine growth retardation
e. cleft palate

A raised serum α-fetoprotein level in pregnancy is associated with

a. exomphalos
b. hydrocephaly
c. threatened miscarriage
d. Down's syndrome
e. multiple pregnancy

Chapter 7. Abnormal pregnancy

With regard to maternal diabetes mellitus in pregnancy:

a. vaginal delivery is contraindicated
b. there is an increased incidence of shoulder dystocia
c. the pregnancy should not proceed beyond 38 weeks of gestation
d. there is an associated increase in cardiac abnormalities in the fetus
e. there is an increase in unexplained fetal death at term, even in well-controlled patients

Chapter 5. Antenatal care

External cephalic version

a. T
b. T
c. F
d. T
e. F

Chapter 6. Fetal progress

Amniocentesis

a. T
b. F
c. T
d. T
e. T

Rubella in early pregnancy is associated with

a. T
b. T
c. T
d. T
e. F

A raised serum α-fetoprotein level in pregnancy is associated with

a. T
b. F
c. T
d. F
e. T

Chapter 7. Abnormal pregnancy

With regard to maternal diabetes mellitus in pregnancy:

a. F
b. T
c. F
d. T
e. T

Eclampsia is characteristically associated with

a. maternal cerebral haemorrhage
b. maternal renal cortical necrosis
c. magnesium sulphate therapy
d. maternal EEG changes in the long term
e. an increasing mortality with increasing age

Silent miscarriage (missed abortion) is associated with

a. dilated cervix
b. uterine size smaller than gestational age
c. bleeding
d. raised temperature
e. viral infections

Hyperemesis gravidarum is associated with

a. hydatidiform mole
b. acute pyelonephritis
c. ectopic pregnancy
d. multiple pregnancy
e. maternal anxiety

Oligohydramnios is characteristically associated with

a. diabetes mellitus
b. anencephaly
c. multiple pregnancy
d. intrauterine growth retardation
e. fetal polycystic kidneys

A glucose tolerance test should be performed in pregnancy in women who have

a. a mother who has diabetes mellitus
b. a history of unexplained stillbirth
c. persistent glycosuria with blood sugar levels < 6.0 mmol/l
d. previous midtrimester abortion
e. a random blood sugar level >7.0 mmol/l

Complications of fibroids during pregnancy include

a. placenta praevia
b. placental abruption
c. malpresentations
d. pain
e. postpartum haemorrhage

Eclampsia is characteristically associated with

a. T
b. T
c. T
d. F
e. T

Silent miscarriage (missed abortion) is associated with

a. F
b. T
c. F
d. F
e. T

Hyperemesis gravidarum is associated with

a. T
b. T
c. F
d. T
e. T

Oligohydramnios is characteristically associated with

a. F
b. T
c. F
d. T
e. F

A glucose tolerance test should be performed in pregnancy in women who have

a. F
b. T
c. F
d. F
e. T

Complications of fibroids during pregnancy include

a. F
b. F
c. T
d. T
e. T

The following have a recognized association in pregnancy:

a. toxoplasmosis : choroidoretinitis in the infant
b. rubella : fetal cardiac abnormalities
c. HIV : transmission to the fetus
d. vulval herpes : absolute indication for caesarean section
e. bacterial vaginosis : midtrimester abortion

Placental abruption is associated characteristically with

a. oliguria
b. postpartum haemorrhage
c. disseminated intravascular coagulation
d. abdominal tenderness
e. proteinuria

Multiple pregnancy

a. is more common amongst Afro-Caribbeans than Caucasians
b. is associated with a decrease in incidence with increasing maternal age
c. occurs in 20% of clomiphene-induced pregnancies
d. is more commonly dizygotic
e. is associated with megaloblastic anaemia

Hypertensive disease of pregnancy is associated with

a. reduced creatinine clearance rate
b. a raised serum urate level
c. a raised platelet count
d. increasing proteinuria
e. a raised sodium level

Chapter 8. Normal labour

Labour is characteristically associated with

a. progressive cervical dilatation
b. descent of the presenting part
c. contractions at least every 15 min
d. ruptured membranes
e. the presenting part being at or below the ischial spines

Chapter 9. Problems in labour

Cephalopelvic disproportion

a. can be reliably diagnosed by pelvimetry
b. having occurred in the first pregnancy, will always recur
c. is associated with deflexion of the fetal head
d. can only be resolved by caesarean section
e. is always present in a mother under 1.5 m

The following have a recognized association in pregnancy:

a. T
b. T
c. T
d. F
e. T

Placental abruption is associated characteristically with

a. T
b. T
c. T
d. T
e. T

Multiple pregnancy

a. T
b. F
c. F
d. T
e. T

Hypertensive disease of pregnancy is associated with

a. T
b. T
c. F
d. T
e. F

Chapter 8. Normal labour

Labour is characteristically associated with

a. T
b. T
c. T
d. F
e. F

Chapter 9. Problems in labour

Cephalopelvic disproportion

a. F
b. F
c. T
d. F
e. F

Prolapse of the umbilical cord is more likely to occur with

a. polyhydramnios
b. twin pregnancy
c. breech presentation
d. placenta praevia
e. preterm labour

Fetal hypoxia in labour is associated with

a. baseline variability in excess of 10 beats/min
b. a fetal blood pH of 7.35 or more
c. late (type 2) decelerations
d. a baseline tachycardia above 180 beats/min
e. a baseline bradycardia below 100 beats/min

Preterm labour is associated with

a. multiple pregnancy
b. chorioamnionitis
c. maternal diabetes mellitus
d. bicornuate uterus
e. hydrocephalus

Chapter 10. The puerperium

The following statements about the puerperium are correct:

a. it is the period following completion of the third stage until the return of the normal non-pregnant state 3 months later
b. lochia contains blood, decidua, trophoblastic tissue and leucocytes
c. prolactin is essential for milk synthesis
d. colostrum contains large amounts of immunoglobulins
e. involution involves anabolic changes in uterine musculature

Disseminated intravascular coagulation is associated with

a. deep-vein thrombosis
b. familial thrombophilia
c. amniotic fluid embolism
d. iron deficiency anaemia
e. placental abruption

Prolapse of the umbilical cord is more likely to occur with

a. T
b. T
c. T
d. F
e. T

Fetal hypoxia in labour is associated with

a. F
b. F
c. T
d. T
e. T

Preterm labour is associated with

a. T
b. T
c. F
d. T
e. F

Chapter 10. The puerperium

The following statements about the puerperium are correct:

a. F

b. T
c. T
d. T
e. F

Disseminated intravascular coagulation is associated with

a. F
b. F
c. T
d. F
e. T

Chapter 11. The baby

The following neonatal conditions are correctly paired:

a. imperforate anus : polyhydramnios
b. renal agenesis : oligohydramnios
c. hypernatraemia : convulsions
d. hyperbilirubinaemia : brain damage
e. hydrocephaly : raised maternal α-fetoprotein level

Chapter 12. Statistics on childbirth

Perinatal mortality

a. is most commonly associated with low birth weight
b. includes terminations of pregnancy
c. is expressed per thousand live births
d. includes stillbirths from 24 weeks of gestation
e. is excluded from infant death rates

Cervical – Gonorrhea
– Chlamydia

Vaginal – candida
BV
T vaginalis.

Genitalia – Herpes
– Genital warts.

Chapter 14. Miscarriage

First trimester miscarriage is characteristically associated with

a. systemic lupus erythematosis
b. viral infections
c. iron deficiency anaemia
d. toxoplasmosis
e. bacterial vaginosis

Chapter 15. Termination of pregnancy

The following statements about first trimester terminations are correct:

a. following termination of a pregnancy, the Chief Medical Officer has to be informed
b. there is a significant increased risk of subsequent incompetence of the cervix
c. in a rhesus-negative woman, anti-D immunoglobulin should be given after the procedure
d. there is an increased rate of failure of sterilization if carried out with occlusive clips at the same time
e. *chlamydia* can be isolated in at least 40% of women undergoing the procedure

Chapter 16. Infections

The following are associated:

a. *Gardnerella vaginalis* : an offensive discharge
b. *Trichomonas vaginalis* : minimal symptoms in the male partner
c. *Condylomata accuminata* : regression in pregnancy
d. HIV : retrovirus
e. Candidiasis : the presence of an intrauterine contraceptive device

Chapter 11. The baby

The following neonatal conditions are correctly paired:

a. F
b. T
c. T
d. T
e. F

Chapter 12. Statistics on childbirth

Perinatal mortality

a. T
b. F
c. F
d. T
e. T

Chapter 14. Miscarriage

First trimester miscarriage is characteristically associated with

a. T
b. T
c. F
d. F
e. F

Chapter 15. Termination of pregnancy

The following statements about first trimester terminations are correct:

a. T
b. F
c. T
d. T
e. F

Chapter 16. Infections

The following are associated:

a. T
b. T
c. F
d. T
e. F

Recognized causes of pruritus vulvae include

a. hyperbilirubinaemia
b. lichen sclerosis
c. diabetes mellitus
d. Bartholin's cyst
e. posterior vaginal wall prolapse

Chapter 17. Menstrual disorders

Secondary amenorrhoea

a. is a consequence of prolonged use of the combined oral contraceptive
b. is associated with a body mass index below 19
c. is associated with elevated serum FSH levels in over 60% of cases
d. is associated with Turner's syndrome
e. is a recognized feature of hyperprolactinaemia

Among those diagnosed with menorraghia

F a. haemoglobin estimation is an accurate diagnostic tool
T b. cyclical norethisterone therapy is effective
T c. tranexamic acid reduces loss by up to 50%
F d. the levonorgestrel-containing intrauterine system reduces loss by up to 75% within 3 months of fitting
e. there is a strong association with subserous fibroids

(handwritten note: during first few months ↑ in menstrual loss (spotting) but this is levened eventually settle)

Chapter 18. Benign lesions

Pelvic endometriosis is recognized as a cause of

a. painful defaecation
b. midcycle pain
c. anovulation
d. intermenstrual bleeding
e. fixed retroversion of the uterus

Polycystic ovarian disease is characteristically associated with

a. raised levels of serum FSH
b. raised levels of serum oestradiol
c. hirsutism
d. recurrent miscarriage
e. endometrial hyperplasia

Recognized causes of pruritus vulvae include

a. T
b. T
c. T
d. F
e. F

Chapter 17. Menstrual disorders

Secondary amenorrhoea

a. F
b. T
c. F
d. F
e. T

Among those diagnosed with menorraghia

a. F
b. F
c. T
d. T
e. F

Chapter 18. Benign lesions

Pelvic endometriosis is recognized as a cause of

a. T
b. T
c. F
d. F
e. T

Polycystic ovarian disease is characteristically associated with

a. F
b. T
c. T
d. T
e. T

Chapter 19. Premalignant lesions

CIN III is characterized by

a. a cytological smear containing dyskaryotic cells
b. a persistent vaginal discharge
c. postcoital bleeding
d. invasion through the basement membrane
e. a strong association with herpes simplex virus

Chapter 20. Malignant lesions

Carcinoma of the cervix

a. is commoner amongst nulliparous women
b. is typically adenomatous
c. is the commonest malignancy in women
d. originates from the transformation zone
e. is commoner amongst women who have had multiple partners

Endometrial carcinoma is more common when

a. there is a history of polycystic ovarian disease
b. associated with diabetes mellitus
c. the patient has a late menopause
d. a postmenopausal patient is treated with tamoxifen for over 10 years
e. a pyometra is present

Chapter 22. Premenstrual syndrome

Premenstrual syndrome

a. is characterized by a variety of symptoms that start at any time after the cessation of menses
b. has a strong relationship with a schizoid personality
c. is more often seen in unmarried women
d. is best treated by the combined contraceptive pill
e. is associated with the luteal phase of the cycle

Chapter 23. The menopause

The menopause

a. can only be diagnosed retrospectively
b. occurs at the mean age of 46 years
c. is associated with a rise in serum cholesterol levels
d. occurs earlier amongst women who smoke
e. is associated with a decline in the rate of myocardial infarction

Chapter 19. Premalignant lesions

CIN III is characterized by

a. T
b. F
c. F
d. F
e. F

Chapter 20. Malignant lesions

Carcinoma of the cervix

a. F
b. F
c. F
d. T
e. T

Endometrial carcinoma is more common when

a. T
b. T
c. T
d. T
e. T

Chapter 22. Premenstrual syndrome

Premenstrual syndrome

a. F
b. F
c. F
d. F
e. T

Chapter 23. The menopause

The menopause

a. T
b. F
c. T
d. T
e. F

Chapter 24. Urogynaecology

Sensory urgency in women

a. is associated with urethral sphincter weakness
b. is improved by retropubic sling procedures
c. is improved by hormone replacement therapy in postmenopausal women
d. is improved by bladder training
e. only affects postmenopausal women

Chapter 25. Prolapse

Cystocele

a. is more common after the menopause
b. is associated with large babies
c. leads to detrusor instability
d. is commonly associated with flatal incontinence
e. dyspareunia

Chapter 27. Paediatric gynaecology

These congenital abnormalities are correctly associated:

a. cryptomenorrhoea : occluding membrane of the vagina
b. bicornuate uterus : an increase of miscarriage
c. vaginal septum : uterine abnormalities
d. Unicornuate uterus : duplex kidney
e. septate uterus : unstable lie in late pregnancy

Vaginal discharge in prepubertal girls is characteristically associated with

a. threadworm infestation
b. sexual assault
c. warts
d. foreign objects in the vagina
e. antibiotic therapy

Chapter 28. Dysmenorrhoea

Secondary dysmenorrhoea is characteristically associated with

a. large loop excision of the transformation zone
b. congenital uterine anomalies
c. adenomyosis
d. the presence of an intrauterine contraceptive device
e. transcervical resection of the endometrium

Chapter 24. Urogynaecology

Sensory urgency in women

a. F
b. F
d. T
d. T
e. F

Chapter 25. Prolapse

Cystocele

a. T
b. T
c. F
d. F
e. F

Chapter 27. Paediatric

These congenital abnormalities are correctly associated:

a. T
b. T
c. T
d. F
e. T

Vaginal discharge in prepubertal girls is characteristically associated with

a. T
b. T
c. F
d. T
e. F

Chapter 28. Dysmenorrhoea

Secondary dysmenorrhoea is characteristically associated with

a. F
b. F
c. T
d. F
e. F

Chapter 29. Fertility

The following are associated with clomiphene citrate treatment:

a. hot flushes
b. midcycle pain
c. multiple pregnancy rate of 20%
d. hirsutism
e. ovarian cysts

Oligozoospermia has a recognized association with

a. sulphasalazine therapy
b. the use of anabolic steroids
c. raised serum FSH levels
d. Klinefelter's syndrome
e. undescended testicles

Chapter 30. Family planning

Regarding intrauterine contraceptive devices:

a. there is an increase in the incidence of endometriosis
b. there is an increase in menstrual loss
c. the optimum time of fitting is immediately before menses
d. the most likely time of expulsion is during the first 3 months after fitting
e. their efficacy is greater with increasing age of the woman

The combined oral contraceptive is associated with

a. a decrease in the incidence of ovarian carcinoma
b. an improvement in primary dysmenorrhoea
c. a decrease in the incidence of arterial disease
d. an increase in the size of pre-existing fibroids
e. an increased pregnancy rate in a woman taking sodium valproate

Chapter 29. Fertility

The following are associated with clomiphene citrate treatment:

a. T
b. T
c. F
d. F
e. T

Oligozoospermia has a recognized association with

a. T
b. T
c. T
d. F
e. T

Chapter 30. Family planning

Regarding intrauterine contraceptive devices:

a. F
b. T
c. F
d. T
e. T

The combined oral contraceptive is associated with

a. T
b. T
c. F
d. F
e. F

Index